THE ART AND SCIENCE OF MEDICAL RADIOGRAPHY

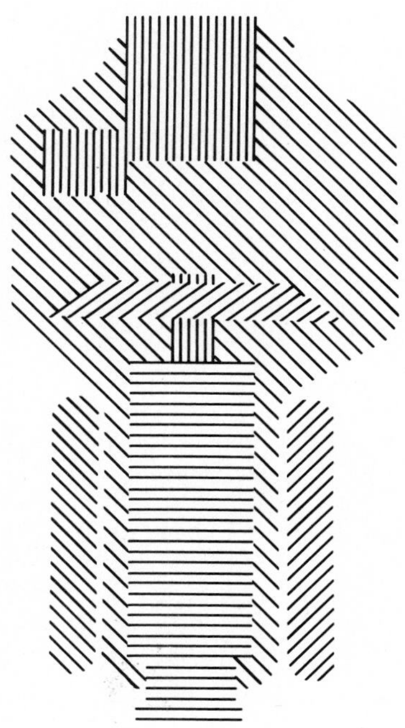

THE ART AND SCIENCE OF MEDICAL RADIOGRAPHY

SEVENTH EDITION

JACK C. MALOTT, AS, RT(R), FASRT, FAHRA
Director, Radiologic Administration
University of Cincinnati Hospital
Professor, Department of Radiology
University of Cincinnati
College of Medicine

JOSEPH FODOR, III, MS, RT(R), FASRT
Vice President for Operations
University of Cincinnati Medical Associates

With 123 illustrations

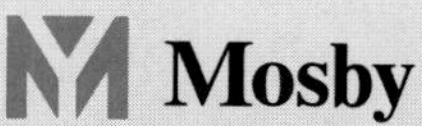

Mosby
St. Louis Baltimore Boston Chicago London Philadelphia Sydney Toronto

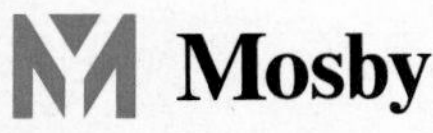

Dedicated to Publishing Excellence

Publisher: David T. Culverwell
Editorial Project Supervisor: Cecilia F. Reilly
Project Manager: Allan S. Kleinberg
Designer: Gail Morey Hudson
Illustrations by: Jack C. Malott and Arnold L. Gomez

SEVENTH EDITION

Printed in the United States of America

Mosby–Year Book, Inc.
11830 Westline Industrial Drive
St. Louis, Missouri 63146

Library of Congress Cataloging-in-Publication Data

Malott, Jack C.
The art and science of medical radiography / Jack C. Malott, Joseph Fodor III.—7th ed.
p. cm.
Fodor's name appears first on the 6th edition.
Includes index.
ISBN 0-8016-6321-0
1. Radiography, Medical—Outlines, syllabi, etc. I. Fodor, Joseph. II. Title.
[DNLM: 1. Technology, Radiologic. WN 160 M257a]
RC78.F563 1993
616.07'572—dc20
DNLM/DLC 92-49306
for Library of Congress CIP

95 CL/WA 9 8 7 6 5 4 3 2

We dedicate this book lovingly
to our wives and children

Karen and **Christopher Malott**
Phyllis, Andrew, and **Casey Fodor**

Contents

Introduction

The Art and Science of Medical Radiography has long been recognized as a pioneering fundamental text for the beginning student. The author of the first five editions, James A. Morgan, RT, is due our gratitude for setting the standard by which subsequent editions must be judged.

The seventh edition is written for the student radiographer and the practicing technologist. The book provides a firm foundation in radiation physics and technique, enabling the student to understand the principles necessary for the practice of radiologic technology. The text includes over 100 illustrations, objectives preceding each chapter, review questions following each chapter, and a glossary of important terms. The format of the book also reinforces important terms through the use of a highlight column throughout the book. The seventh edition of *The Art and Science of Medical Radiography* should prove to be a standard in textbooks for radiographic physics and technique.

The authors express appreciation to General Electric, Fuji, X-Rite, RMI, and Eastman Kodak for their contributions. The photographs in this book are not intended as endorsements of any products or techniques named, known, or described. They are merely used to illustrate current applications.

THE ART AND SCIENCE OF MEDICAL RADIOGRAPHY

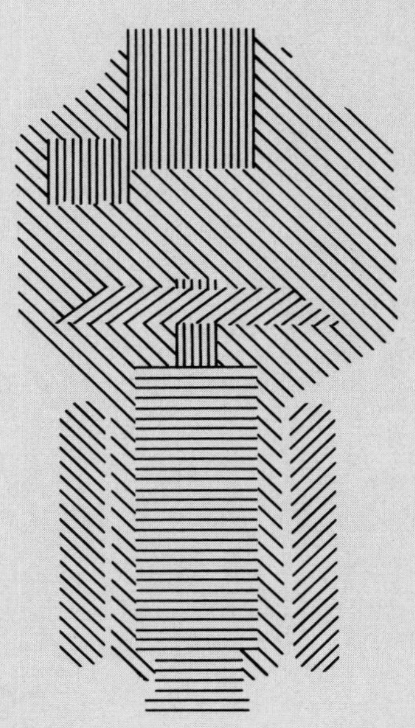

1
Basic Physics

OBJECTIVES

After completing Chapter 1, you should be able to:

1. Define the following terms:
   atom
   atomic number
   atomic weight
   electron
   energy
   inertia
   ionization
   isotope
   kinetic energy
   magnet
   matter
   molecule
   neutron
   nucleus
   potential energy
   proton
   work
2. Discuss electromagnetism and static and current electricity.
3. Define the following terms related to electricity:
   ampere
   resistance
   volt
   watt

A basic knowledge of physics is necessary to understand many of the concepts in this book. These discussions are brief and provide only a basis for the discussion of other concepts in the text. For a more in-depth understanding, you should consult a basic physics text.

Matter

Even a basic understanding of physics is built on some explanation of other physical facts. *Matter* is anything that has mass and occupies space. All matter possesses the property of inertia. *Inertia* is the resistance a body offers to any change in position. Some outside force is necessary to start a body in motion, change its direction, or stop its motion. The law of conservation of matter states that matter can be neither created nor destroyed. Matter can be converted into energy, as is the case in nuclear reactors and nuclear weapons. Matter can take one of three forms—solid, liquid, or gas—and it can be changed from one form to another. The distinction between the three forms of matter is based on the relative distance between molecules in the structure. If matter is a solid, the molecules are closely spaced. In the gaseous state, molecules are farther apart. In the liquid state, molecule spacing is between the extremes of solids and gasses.

Matter *is anything that has mass and occupies space.*

Inertia *is the resistance a body offers to any change in position.*

The law of conservation of matter states that matter can be neither created nor destroyed.

Work is overcoming resistance and involves the physical quantities of force and distance. The definition of work is the force applied multiplied by the distance through which the force acts.

Work *is overcoming resistance and involves the physical quantities of force and distance.*

Energy is the capacity for performing work. Energy indicates how much work a body can do. The two types of energy are potential and kinetic. *Potential energy* is the energy inherent in a body. For example, an object held in the air has the potential to fall. *Kinetic energy* is the result of a body being in motion. For example, an object exhibits kinetic energy when it falls to the floor. Energy conforms to the law of conservation of energy, which states that energy can be neither created nor destroyed. However, energy can be transformed from one form to another. Later we will discuss the conversion of the kinetic energy of electrons to x-rays and heat.

Energy *is the capacity for performing work.*

Potential energy *is the energy inherent in a body.*

Kinetic energy *is the result of a body being in motion.*

Structure of Matter

If a substance was subdivided until it could be subdivided no further, a molecule of the substance would be isolated. A *molecule* is the smallest part of a substance that

A **molecule** *is the smallest part of a substance that retains all the characteristics of the original substance.*

retains all the characteristics of the original substance. A molecule may be a simple molecule, in which case it is an element, or it may be a compound molecule. All atoms of the simple molecule are the same. Pure copper, for example, is all copper; it cannot contain any other combination of elements. Even a microscopic particle of copper is all copper. A compound molecule contains unlike atoms; none have the same properties as the compound molecule. Water is a compound composed of two atoms of hydrogen and one atom of oxygen, H_2O. Breaking down a molecule of water yields two atoms of hydrogen and one of oxygen. Neither hydrogen nor oxygen has the properties of water.

The Atom

The **atom** *is the smallest divided part of matter that can enter into combinations or chemical reactions with other atoms.*

In defining the molecule, the term "atom" was used. Following the molecular stage in the breakdown of matter, molecules are composed of even smaller particles, which are called atoms. The *atom* is the smallest divided part of matter that can enter into combinations or chemical reactions with other atoms. Approximately 90 different types of atoms, or elements, occur naturally, and about 20 do not occur naturally. Everything that exists consists of one or some combination of these atoms.

The atom consists of a central body called the **nucleus.** *The nucleus contains* **protons,** *which have a positive electric charge, and* **neutrons,** *which have no charge.*

Electrons *have a negative electric charge and normally do not leave their orbits or shells.*

According to the theory of atomic structure, as proposed by Niels Bohr, the atom consists of a central body called the *nucleus.* The nucleus contains *protons,* which have a positive electric charge, and *neutrons,* which have no charge. Revolving around the nucleus, in well-defined orbits or shells, are the electrons. *Electrons* have a negative electric charge and normally do not leave their orbits or shells. The proton, neutron, and electron are the fundamental building blocks of all matter. The Bohr atom is illustrated in Figure 1-1.

The electron orbits or electron shells are labeled with identifying letters. Beginning with the innermost shell, closest to the nucleus, they are the K, L, M, N, O, P, and Q shells, as illustrated in Figure 1-2. The shells may contain a maximum of 2, 8, 18, 32, 50, 72, and 98 electrons, respectively. The maximum number of electrons in an orbit is calculated by the equation $2n^2$, where n equals the number of the electron shell (K is shell no. 1, L is shell no. 2, etc.). The number of positive charges in the nucleus determines the total number of shells or orbits and the number of electrons per shell.

The proximity of an electron to the nucleus determines the energy level of an electron shell. The proximity

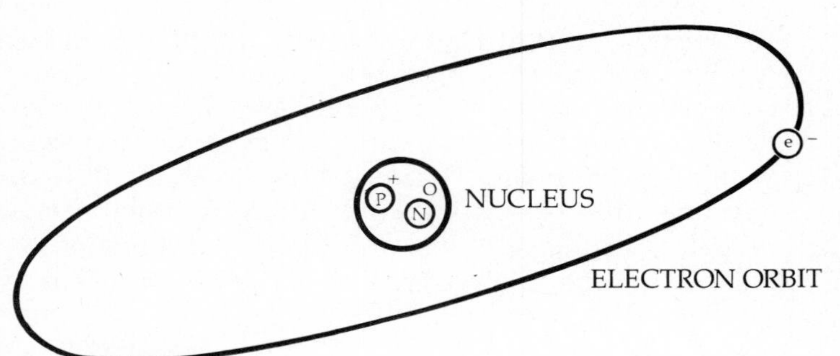

Figure 1-1
The Bohr atom has negatively charged electrons orbiting the positively charged nucleus. The nucleus is composed of positively charged protons and neutral neutrons.

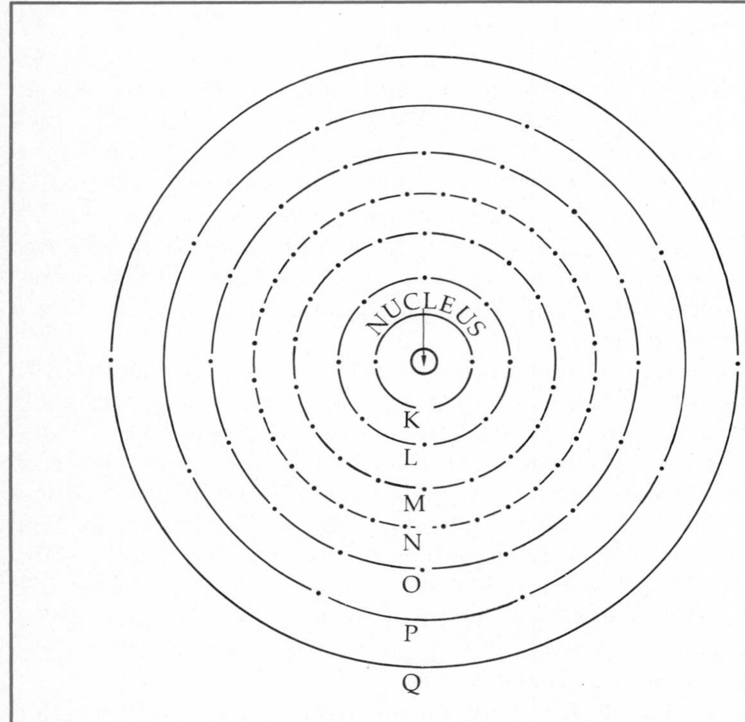

Figure 1-2
The electron shells of an atom are labeled K through Q beginning with the innermost shell.

is an indication of the attractive force with which an electron is bound to the nucleus. It also determines the force required to displace an electron from its shell. Electrons in the K orbit are strongly bound to the nucleus. A great deal of energy is necessary to displace a K-shell electron from its orbit. An electron in the P or Q orbit is loosely bound to the nucleus, and less energy is required to displace it from orbit.

*The **atomic number** is the number of protons or positive charges in the nucleus of the atom.*

Differences in the elements arise from the number and arrangements of electrons, protons, and neutrons. The *atomic number* is the number of protons or positive charges in the nucleus of the atom. Atomic number identifies a substance chemically.

*The **atomic weight** defines the weight of an atom as compared to the weight of the carbon atom.*

Almost all of an atom's weight is in the nucleus in the form of protons and neutrons. Both the proton and the neutron are approximately 1840 times as heavy as the electron. The *atomic weight* defines the weight of an atom as compared to the weight of the carbon atom. The carbon atom has an atomic weight of 12.

Isotopes

***Isotopes** are atoms of an element that have the same atomic number but more or fewer neutrons.*

Isotopes are atoms of an element that have the same atomic number but more or fewer neutrons. The two types of isotopes are stable and unstable. In a stable isotope, the number of protons and neutrons have a stable relationship with each other. In an unstable isotope, an unstable relationship exists between the number of protons and neutrons. Unstable isotopes are radioactive; they decay and emit radiation to reach a stable state. Radioactive isotopes have imaging and therapeutic uses in medicine today.

Ionization

The addition or removal of an electron does not change the identity of an atom.

*The addition or subtraction of an electron is **ionization.***

A neutral atom has an equal number of protons and electrons. The addition or removal of an electron does not change the identity of an atom. The atom retains its identity since the number of protons in the nucleus remains the same. Because of unequal distribution of positive and negative charges, however, the atom is unstable. An atom with a missing electron is positively charged. An atom with an additional electron is negatively charged. The addition or subtraction of an electron is *ionization.* These charged atoms are ions. Ionization occurs in one of two ways: by bombarding matter with x-radiation or by bombarding matter with electrons. The process of ionization is important to the field of radiology and will be discussed later.

Magnetism

An understanding of electricity and the operation of some basic electric components in an x-ray generating system is not possible without a basic understanding of magnetism. A *magnet* is a substance that has the power to attract ferromagnetic substances. Ferromagnetism is a property of a few elements, including iron, nickel, and cobalt, where strong magnetic alignment of the atoms exists. These materials are attracted to a magnet. Two types of magnets exist: natural and artificial. The earth itself, with its magnetic field aligned along a north-to-south axis, is the prime example of a natural magnet. A horseshoe magnet and an electromagnet are examples of artificial magnets.

A **magnet** *is a substance that has the power to attract ferromagnetic substances.*

A magnetic line of force is a line force that flows from the north to the south pole of a magnet, as illustrated in Figure 1-3. The area in space around a magnet where these

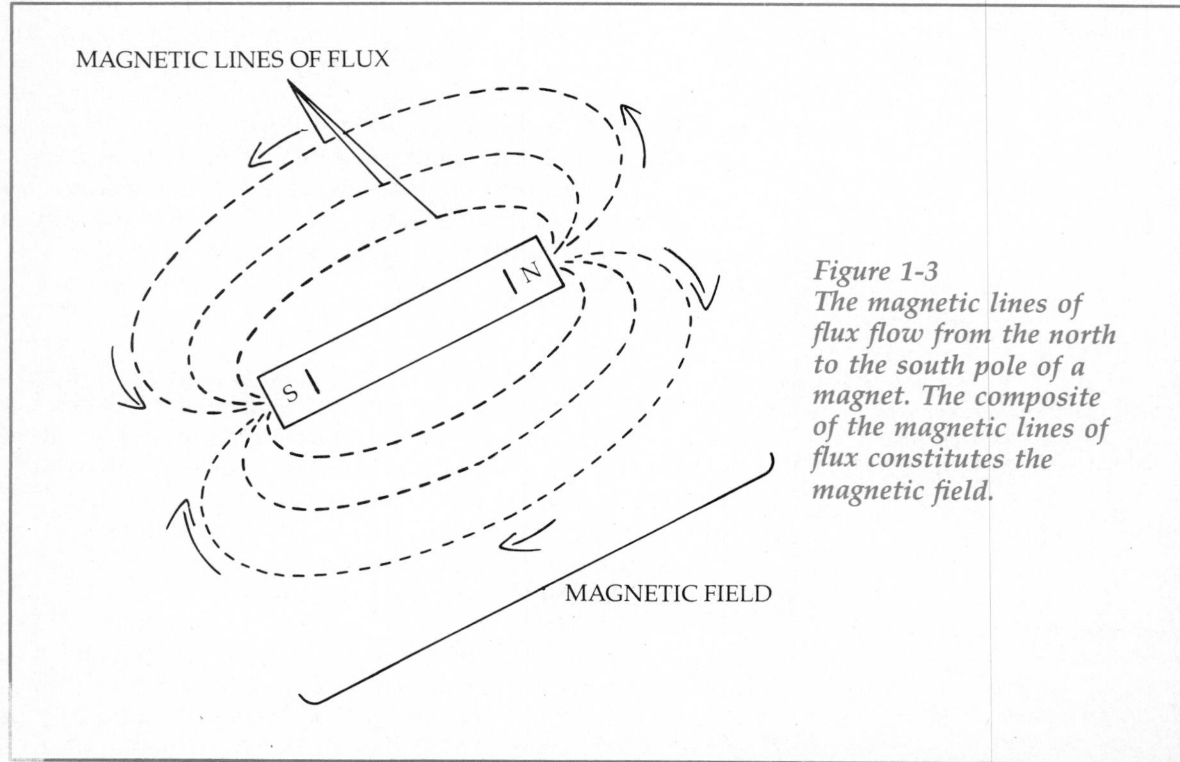

Figure 1-3
The magnetic lines of flux flow from the north to the south pole of a magnet. The composite of the magnetic lines of flux constitutes the magnetic field.

Magnetic flux *is the entire composite of the magnetic lines of force around the magnet.*

magnetic lines of force function is the magnetic field. *Magnetic flux* is the entire composite of the magnetic lines of force around the magnet.

All magnets exhibit certain characteristics according to the laws of magnetism, which include the following:

1. All magnets have a north and south pole at the opposite ends of the magnetic substance.
2. Like magnetic poles repel each other, and unlike magnetic poles attract each other.
3. The force between two poles of a magnet is directly proportional to the strength of the two poles and inversely proportional to the distance between them.
4. Breaking a magnet into pieces will result in each piece of the magnet behaving as a freestanding magnet with a north and south pole.

Electromagnetism

Magnetism and electricity are two separate but closely related phenomena since an electric current will always produce a magnetic field. Passing an electric current through a length of wire sets up a magnetic field around the wire at a right angle. Reversing the polarity of the current flow in the wire reverses the direction of the magnetic field. Changing the polarity of the current creates a moving magnetic field.

In 1831 Faraday discovered that creating a moving magnetic field with a coil of wire creates an electric current in a surrounding coil of wire. This occurs even though no connection exists between the two coils. Therefore, a conductor that forms part of a closed circuit and cuts across magnetic lines of force will have voltage and current induced in it. All transformers function on this principle of mutual inductance. The two coils of wire in a transformer are positioned so the magnetic field from one coil cuts the turns of wire in the second coil. Changing the magnetic field of the first coil induces a voltage in the second coil. The function of transformers will be discussed in more detail in Chapter 4.

Static and Current Electricity

Static electricity *is a quantity of electricity in which the electric charge is at rest.*

The two kinds of electricity are static and current. *Static electricity* is a quantity of electricity in which the electric charge is at rest. The only difference between static and current electricity is the absence of the flow of electrons. *Current electricity* is the flow of electrons along a conductor. Electron flow is always from a point of high potential to a point of low potential.

Current electricity *is the flow of electrons along a conductor.*

Two types of current electricity exist: direct and alternating. Direct current, such as delivered from a battery, rises to a maximum value and always flows in the same direction, as illustrated in Figure 1-4. The uniformity and consistency of flow in direct current are not useful for the operation of transformers. The second type of electric current, alternating current, is the type used to power most household appliances. Alternating current is a movement of electrons in which polarity changes from positive to negative and back to positive at regular intervals. Each change in polarity is a pulse, with two pulses constituting a cycle. The number of cycles per second dictates the frequency of the current.

Direct current *rises to a maximum value and always flows in the same direction.*

Alternating current *is a movement of electrons in which polarity changes from positive to negative and back to positive at regular intervals.*

Figure 1-5 is a graphic representation of alternating current. Voltage starts at zero (A) and builds up to a maximum positive value (MP). The voltage then declines to zero (B) and flows to a maximum negative value (MN) and finally returns to zero (C). The time from point A to point

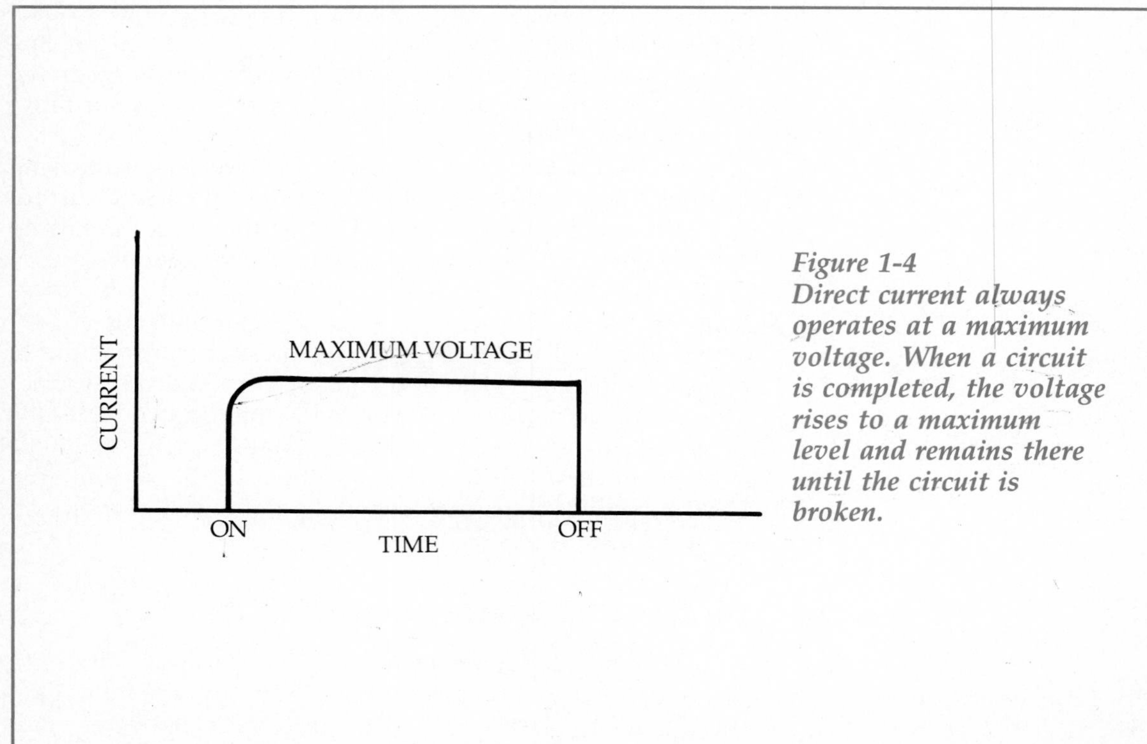

Figure 1-4
Direct current always operates at a maximum voltage. When a circuit is completed, the voltage rises to a maximum level and remains there until the circuit is broken.

B, or point B to point C, is one pulse. The time from point A to point C is one cycle. The maximum positive and the maximum negative value are equivalent. Assuming 60 cycle current, the time of one pulse is 1/120 of a second, and a cycle is 1/60 of a second. Sixty cycle current is the most common frequency in the United States. Fifty cycle current is the most common in Europe and Asia.

When discussing electricity, several terms require definition. Some of these terms have particular importance to the technologist.

The **ampere** *(A) is a quantitative term of current.*

The *ampere* (A) is a quantitative term of current. The ampere indicates the number of electrons passing a given point in a circuit in a period of 1 second. The ampere is a purely quantitative term that provides no information concerning the amount of force causing the electrons to move. The milliampere (mA) is 1/1000 of an ampere and is often used in the selection of x-ray technique.

The **milliampere** *(mA) is 1/1000 of an ampere and is often used in the selection of x-ray technique.*

The **volt** *(V) is the electric pressure or force that causes the electrons to move.*

The *volt* (V) is the electric pressure or force that causes the electrons to move. As voltage increases, the potential energy of the electrons increases. The volt is the potential difference carrying a current of 1 ampere and dissipating

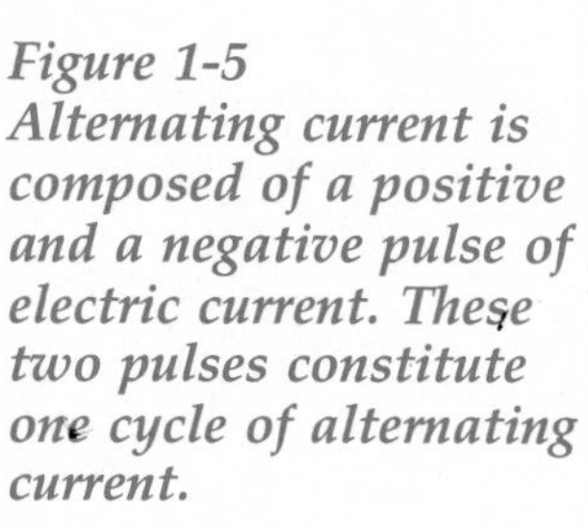

Figure 1-5
Alternating current is composed of a positive and a negative pulse of electric current. These two pulses constitute one cycle of alternating current.

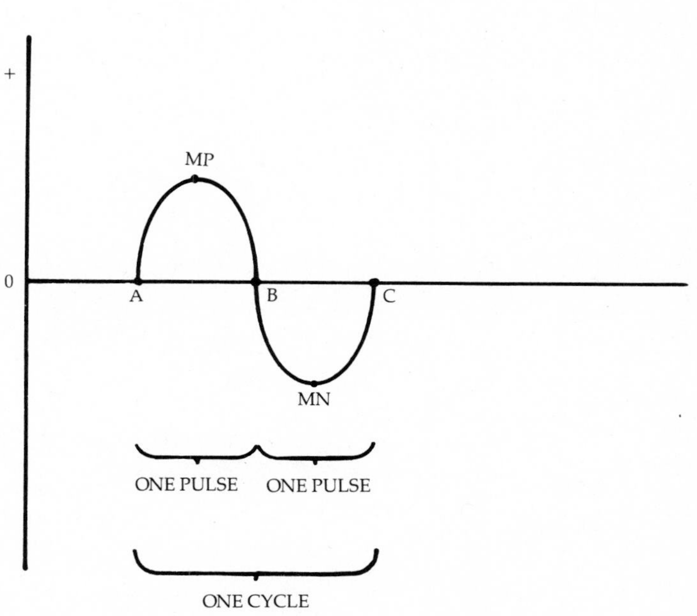

thermal energy at the rate of 1 watt. The kilovolt (kV) is 1000 volts and is often used in the selection of x-ray technique. The maximum voltage or peak voltage applied across an x-ray tube is termed the kilovoltage peak (kVp). Kilovoltage peak is often used in the selection of x-ray technique.

The *watt* (W) is a unit of power and defines the power required to cause 1 ampere of current to flow. The watt is the product of current multiplied by voltage. The kilowatt (kW) is 1000 watts and is frequently used to quantify the maximum output of x-ray generators.

Resistance is the hindrance to the flow of electricity encountered in all electric circuits. The unit of measurement for resistance is the ohm (Ω). The ohm is the amount of resistance that permits 1 ampere of current to flow under the pressure of 1 volt in a circuit. Ohm's law states that resistance (R) is directly proportional to voltage (V) and inversely proportional to current (I):

$$R = \frac{V}{I}$$

The **kilovolt** *(kV) is 1000 volts and is often used in the selection of x-ray technique.*

The **watt** *(W) is a unit of power and defines the power required to cause 1 ampere of current to flow.*

Resistance *is the hindrance to the flow of electricity encountered in all electric circuits.*

Ohm's law *states that resistance (R) is directly proportional to voltage (V) and inversely proportional to current (I):*

$$R = \frac{V}{I}$$

Chapter 1—Review Questions

1. The smallest part of a substance that retains all the characteristics of the original substance is:
   a. a compound
   b. matter
   c. an atom
   d. a molecule
   e. none of the above
2. Atoms of an element that have the same atomic number but more or fewer neutrons are:
   a. matter
   b. molecules
   c. isotopes
   d. ions
   e. none of the above
3. The quantitative term of current is the:
   a. ampere
   b. volt
   c. polarity
   d. ohm
   e. resistance
4. The unit of power is the:
   a. ohm
   b. watt
   c. volt
   d. kilovolt peak
   e. none of the above
5. According to Ohm's law:
   a. Resistance is inversely proportional to voltage and current.
   b. Resistance is inversely proportional to voltage and directly proportional to current.
   c. Resistance is directly proportional to current and voltage.
   d. Resistance is directly proportional to voltage and inversely proportional to current.
   e. two of the above
6. One cycle of alternating current is:
   a. comprised of a change in polarity
   b. defined by the frequency
   c. equal to two pulses
   d. the hindrance to the flow of electricity
   e. two of the above

7. A quantitative term of current often used in the selection of x-ray technique is the:
   a. kilovolt
   b. ampere
   c. volt
   d. watt
   e. none of the above
8. A line of force that flows from the north to the south pole of a magnet is:
   a. magnetic flux
   b. a magnetic line of force
   c. magnetism
   d. ferromagnetic
   e. none of the above
9. The atomic number:
   a. defines the weight of an atom
   b. identifies a substance chemically
   c. is the number of neutrons in the nucleus
   d. two of the above
   e. all of the above
10. The resistance a body offers to any change in position is:
    a. mass
    b. inertia
    c. work
    d. ohms
    e. energy
11. Which of the following is the best example of kinetic energy?
    a. a bowling ball suspended above the ground
    b. a magnetic field
    c. an ionized atom
    d. an automobile traveling 10 miles per hour
    e. a potential difference of 24 volts
12. Which of the following is true of energy?
    a. It involves the physical quantities of force and distance.
    b. It is the capacity for performing work.
    c. It can be neither created nor destroyed.
    d. two of the above
    e. none of the above

13. A bowling ball at rest on the ground has:
    a. kinetic energy
    b. potential energy
    c. no energy
14. The electron orbits are labeled K, L, M, N, O, P, and Q and respectively contain a maximum of how many electrons?
    a. 2, 4, 8, 18, 32, 32, 32
    b. 2, 8, 18, 32, 50, 72, 98
    c. 2, 8, 16, 32, 32, 32, 32
    d. none of the above
15. An electron in which of the following shells has the greatest kinetic energy and would be the most difficult to displace?
    a. Q
    b. K
    c. all the electrons are equally difficult to displace
    d. electrons cannot be displaced from their orbits
    e. none of the above

2

X-Radiation

OBJECTIVES

After completing Chapter 2, you should be able to:

1. Define the following terms:
   attenuation
   bremsstrahlung radiation
   characteristic radiation
   classical scattering
   Compton effect
   cumulative maximum permissible dose
   differential absorption
   electromagnetic radiation
   electromagnetic spectrum
   maximum permissible dose
   pair production
   photodisintegration
   photoelectric effect
2. Discuss the production of radiation.
3. Discuss the five basic ways that x-rays interact with matter and their importance in diagnostic radiology.
4. Define and interrelate the following units of radiation measurement:
   becquerel
   coulomb per kilogram
   curie
   Gray
   rad
   rem
   roentgen
   sievert
5. Discuss the principles of radiation protection for occupational exposure.

Properties of X-Radiation

X-radiation is a form of electromagnetic radiation that has the power to penetrate and ionize matter. Ionization is the removal of an orbital electron from an atom of material; this is the phenomenon that makes x-radiation useful for medical applications. Ionization is also responsible for the harmful effects on living tissue. When recording a radiographic image, it is the ionization of atoms in the intensifying screens or film that results in the production of the latent image in the film emulsion. X-rays can also ionize air. This results in production of an electric charge, which is the basis for many radiation detection devices. These properties of x-rays will be discussed in detail throughout the book.

X-radiation *is a form of electromagnetic radiation that has the power to penetrate and ionize matter.*

The Electromagnetic Spectrum

Electromagnetic radiation is the movement of electric and magnetic fields through space at the speed of light. Common examples of electromagnetic radiation include radio waves, microwaves, infrared radiation, visible light, ultraviolet light, x-rays, and gamma rays. These forms of electromagnetic radiation constitute the electromagnetic spectrum. The *electromagnetic spectrum* is a ranking of these radiations in order of wavelength, frequency, and energy.

Electromagnetic radiation *is the movement of electric and magnetic fields through space at the speed of light.*

The **electromagnetic spectrum** *is a ranking of these radiations in order of wavelength, frequency, and energy.*

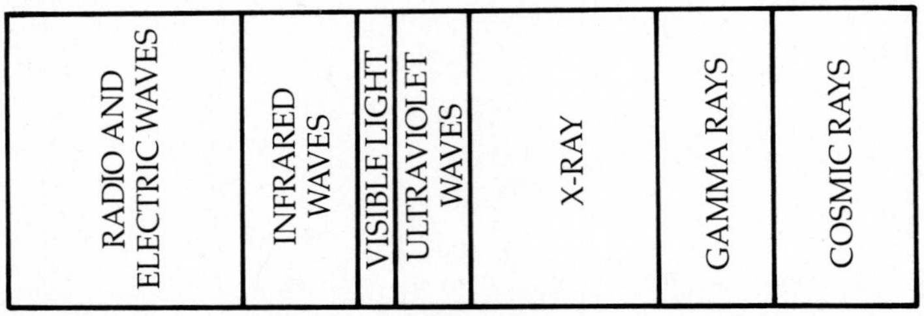

Figure 2-1
The electromagnetic spectrum is a ranking of electromagnetic radiation based on wavelength and energy.

Figure 2-1 is an illustration of the electromagnetic spectrum. The usual illustration of the electromagnetic spectrum would appear to indicate a sharp line of demarcation between forms of radiant energy. Actually, some overlapping occurs between the shortest wavelength of one type and the longest wavelength of the immediately adjacent portion of the spectrum. For example, grenz rays are the area of overlap of ultraviolet radiation and x-rays.

Wavelength *defines the penetrating power of any form of radiant energy and is the distance between two successive crests or troughs in the waveform.*

The unit of measurement for wavelength (λ) is the angstrom. One angstrom unit is equal to 10^{-10} meters. *Wavelength* defines the penetrating power of any form of radiant energy and is the distance between two successive crests or troughs in the waveform. Wavelength and penetrating power or energy are inversely proportional. As wavelength decreases or shortens, the penetrating power of the radiation increases. Wavelength and frequency (ν) are also inversely proportional. As wavelength decreases or shortens, frequency increases. This is true because all forms of electromagnetic radiation travel at the speed of light in a vacuum.

Production of X-Radiation

Less than 1 percent of the kinetic energy results in the production of x-rays.

The production of x-rays occurs when fast-moving electrons are suddenly decelerated by interaction with matter. During the interaction, the kinetic energy of the high-speed electrons is converted into x-radiation and heat. The production of x-rays is an inefficient process since more than 99 percent of the kinetic energy of the electrons produces heat. *Less than 1 percent of the kinetic energy results in the production of x-rays.* Also, the energy of the resultant x-radiation is directly proportional to the kinetic energy of the incident electrons. As the kinetic energy of the fast-moving incident electron increases, a corresponding increase occurs in the energy of the x-rays produced. The production of x-rays takes place through one of two electron interactions with matter. These interactions produce bremsstrahlung radiation or characteristic radiation.

Bremsstrahlung Radiation

Bremsstrahlung radiation *occurs when a high-speed electron passes near the nucleus of an atom.*

Bremsstrahlung radiation occurs when a high-speed electron passes near the nucleus of an atom. The positive charge of the nucleus deflects the electron from its original path of travel. The deflection results in a reduction of the kinetic energy of the electron. Since energy can be neither created nor destroyed, the lost kinetic energy results in the production of either heat or x-radiation, as illustrated in Figure 2-2. The

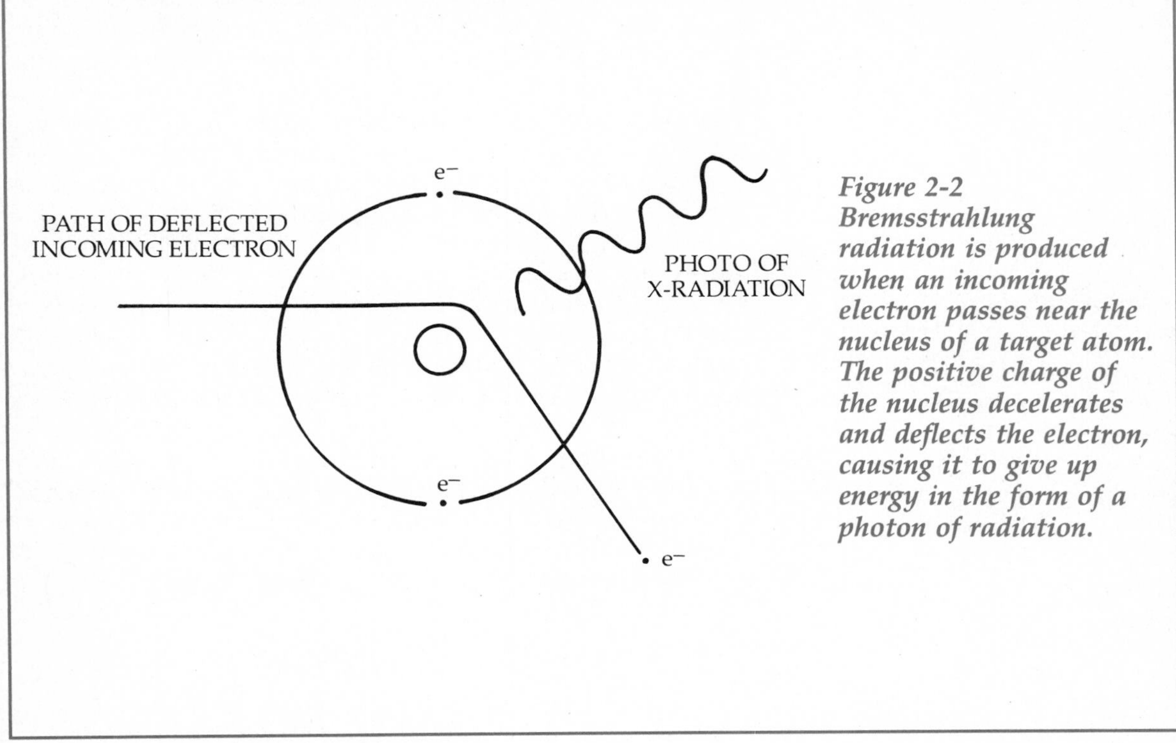

Figure 2-2
Bremsstrahlung radiation is produced when an incoming electron passes near the nucleus of a target atom. The positive charge of the nucleus decelerates and deflects the electron, causing it to give up energy in the form of a photon of radiation.

energy of the x-radiation produced by this interaction depends on three factors: (1) the energy of the incident electron, (2) the charge of the nucleus, and (3) the proximity of the incident electron to the nucleus. Occasionally, an incident electron will collide with the nucleus of an atom. The electron then gives up all its kinetic energy as a single photon of x-radiation. Bremsstrahlung radiation is also referred to as general or braking radiation ("bremsstrahlung" is the German word for braking).

Characteristic Radiation

The production of *characteristic radiation* occurs when an incident electron ejects an orbital electron from an inner shell of an atom in the bombarded material. The ejection of the inner-shell orbital electron creates a temporary "hole," and the atom becomes unstable. An outer-shell electron then moves in to fill the void in the inner shell to stabilize the atom. The binding energy of outer-shell electrons differs from the binding-energy level of the inner-shell elec-

Characteristic radiation *occurs when an incident electron ejects an orbital electron from an inner shell of an atom in the bombarded material.*

Figure 2-3
Characteristic radiation is produced when an incoming electron interacts with an inner-shell electron, ejecting it from its orbit. In an attempt to stabilize the atom, an electron from an outer shell moves in to fill the void. The difference in energy between the two shells is given up as a photon of radiation. The energy of the photon is characteristic of the target atom.

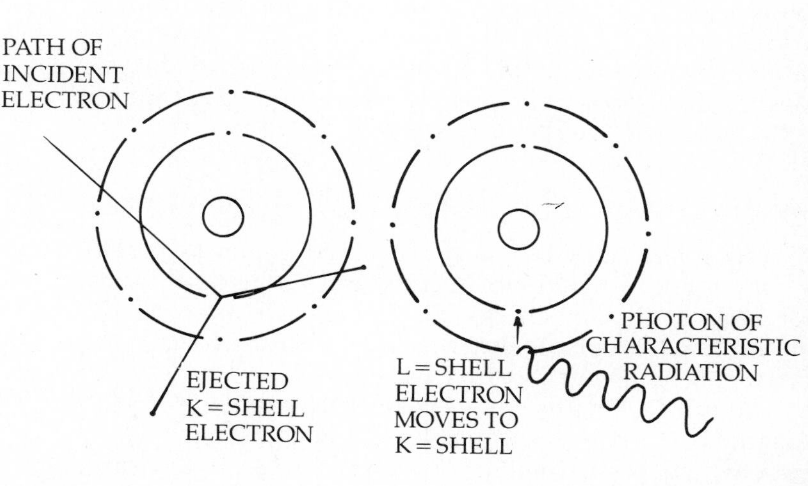

trons. The difference between the binding energies results in the production of x-radiation. (See Figure 2-3.)

Normally this interaction occurs with the ejection of a K-shell electron from the atom and a replacement electron from the L shell. The energy of the x-radiation produced will always be the same for given shells of a given element. For example, the difference in energy of the K and L shell of the tungsten atom is approximately 59 kiloelectron volts (keV). The x-radiation produced following the ejection of a K-shell electron can only have an energy of approximately 59 keV. Subsequently, an M-shell electron will fill the "hole" left in the L shell, the N shell will move into the M, and so forth until the atom is stable. Each of these interactions will produce a photon. The energy of these photons will be characteristic of the difference in the binding energy of the shells. The incident electron and the ejected electron involved in the original interaction both leave the atom. They equally share the kinetic energy of the incident photon minus the energy expended to overcome the binding energy of the ejected electron.

Propagation of X-Radiation

As x-radiation travels and interacts with matter, both the wave theory and the quantum or particle theory can describe its properties. First, x-radiation travels much as sound does in a waveform. Some of its properties can be best explained by using the waveform model. When x-radiation reacts with matter, however, it behaves as discrete packets of energy or photons. The particle theory can best explain most of x-radiation's behavior.

Interactions of X-Radiation and Matter

All interactions between x-rays and matter take place at the atomic level.

All interactions between x-rays and matter take place at the atomic level; x-rays interact with individual atoms, not molecules. Low-energy x-rays tend to interact with whole atoms, moderate-energy x-rays with the orbital electrons, and high-energy x-rays with nuclei.

A group of atoms will stop the same number of x-rays regardless of their physical state. Oxygen as a gas and oxygen bound to hydrogen (as water) will stop the same number of photons atom for atom. The important factor is the atomic makeup of a substance, not the molecular structure. X-rays interact with matter in five basic ways:

1. Coherent or classical scattering
2. Compton effect
3. Photoelectric effect
4. Pair production
5. Photodisintegration

Classical Scattering

During **classical scattering,** *a low-energy photon interacts with a target atom.*

Classical scattering is also referred to as unmodified, coherent, and Rayleigh or Thompson scattering. During *classical scattering,* a low-energy photon interacts with a target atom. The photon transfers its energy and excites the atom, causing it to vibrate. The excited atom immediately returns to a nonexcited state by giving off the absorbed energy as a photon. This photon has the exact same wavelength and energy as the incident photon but differs in direction. This is the only interaction between x-rays and matter that does not cause ionization. The only effect of classical scattering is to change the direction of the incident photon. The percentage of photons undergoing classical scattering is less than 5 percent, and this interaction occurs throughout the diagnostic range of energies. Most classically scattered radiation is in a forward direction and contributes slightly to fog on radiographic film. (See Figure 2-4.)

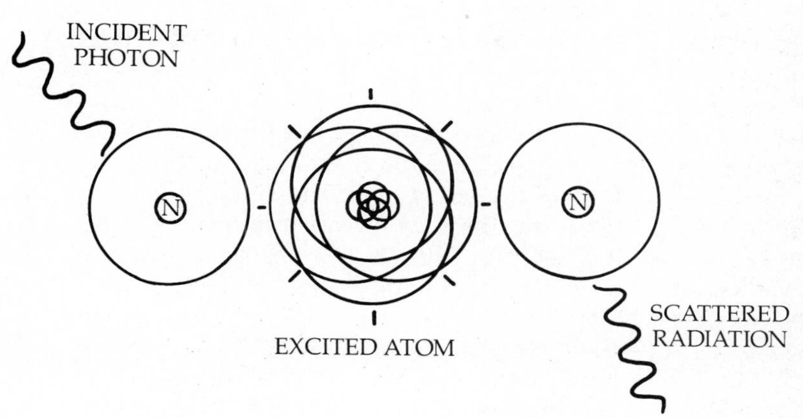

Figure 2-4
In classical scattering, an incident photon interacts with an entire atom. All the photon's energy is momentarily transferred to the atom. This energy is given up by the atom as a photon of the same energy in an altered direction.

Compton Effect

In the **Compton effect (scattering),** *the incident photon interacts with an outer-shell electron, ejecting it from its orbit and ionizing the atom.*

The Compton effect, also called Compton scattering, is a basic interaction that occurs with moderate-energy photons throughout the diagnostic energy range. Almost all the scatter radiation encountered in diagnostic radiology comes from Compton scattering. In the *Compton effect (scattering),* the incident photon interacts with an outer-shell electron, ejecting it from its orbit and ionizing the atom. Compton interactions occur with electrons whose binding energies are much less than the energy of the incident photon. With the photon energies used in diagnostic radiology, these interactions occur with outer-shell electrons of atoms with high atomic numbers or with electrons of atoms with low atomic numbers, such as those found in soft tissues, whose binding energies are low.

The ejected electron is a secondary, recoil, or Compton electron. The photon continues in an altered direction with decreased energy. The energy of the Compton-scattered photon is equal to the difference between the incident photon and the energy used to break the binding energy of the electron and any kinetic energy imparted to the electron. The scattered photon retains most of its energy. Both the scattered photon and the secondary electron may have enough energy to undergo more ionizing interactions before losing all their energy.

Two factors determine the amount of energy the photon retains: (1) its initial energy and (2) the angle of deflection or change in photon direction.

Two factors determine the amount of energy the photon retains: (1) its initial energy and (2) the angle of deflection or change in photon direction. The more forward the direction of the scattered photon, the more energy the photon will retain. Conversely, the greater the angle of deflection, the more energy the photon will lose in the interaction. Also, the lower the energy and the greater the photon's angle of deflection, the greater the amount of energy transferred to the electron. Ultimately, absorption of the scattered photon will occur photoelectrically. The secondary electron will drop into an atomic shell hole previously created by an ionizing event. (See Figure 2-5.)

Some photons scatter approximately 180 degrees or in the opposite direction of the incident photon. This scatter is backscatter radiation. Lead foil is placed in the back of

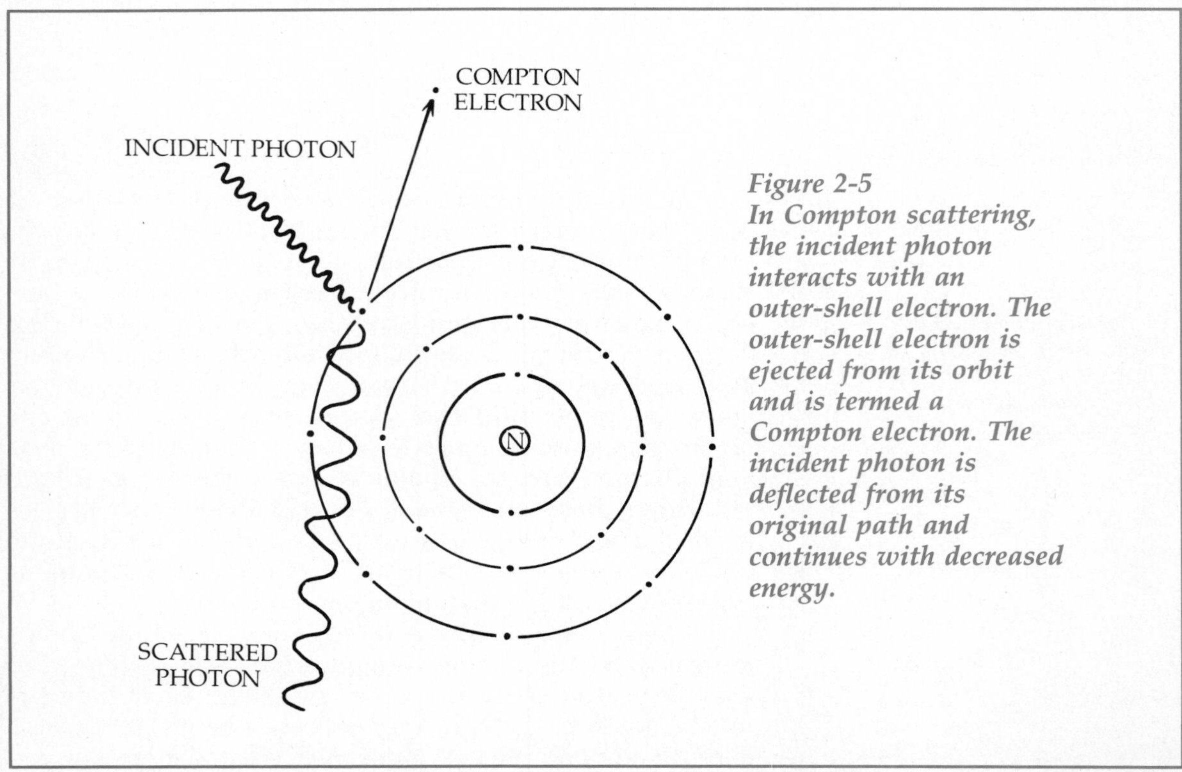

Figure 2-5
In Compton scattering, the incident photon interacts with an outer-shell electron. The outer-shell electron is ejected from its orbit and is termed a Compton electron. The incident photon is deflected from its original path and continues with decreased energy.

x-ray cassettes to prevent backscatter from fogging the film.

The probability of a Compton interaction is a complex function of the energy of the incident photon and depends on the total number of electrons in the absorber. This in turn depends on the density and the number of electrons per gram. As the energy of the photon increases, the probability of a Compton interaction decreases. This occurs because a high-energy photon is more likely to pass through the body than a low-energy photon.

The Compton-scattered x-ray contributes to film fog.

Compton scattering occurs throughout the diagnostic range and is therefore of considerable importance. The Compton-scattered x-ray contributes to film fog, however, resulting in an inferior radiograph.

The Compton-scattered x-rays are a serious radiation exposure hazard.

The Compton-scattered x-rays are also a serious radiation exposure hazard, particularly in fluoroscopy. Even when a photon scatters as much as 90 degrees, it still retains most of its initial energy. This means the scatter radiation arising in the patient is almost as energetic as the primary beam. This radiation exposure occurs to radiologic personnel and is responsible for most of their dose. These scatter radiation levels even necessitate shielding of the x-ray rooms.

Photoelectric Effect

The **photoelectric effect** *is a photoabsorption interaction.*

The *photoelectric effect* is a photoabsorption interaction. An incident photon, with slightly more energy than the binding energy of a K-shell electron, encounters a K-shell electron ejecting it from orbit. The photon disappears as it gives all its energy to the electron. The atom completely absorbs the photon. Most of the energy is used to overcome the binding energy of the electron. The rest of the energy gives the ejected electron kinetic energy. This free electron flies off as a photoelectron, a negatively charged ion. Since charged particles have little penetrating power, absorption of the photoelectron takes place almost immediately. Also, the atom minus one electron becomes a positive ion. An electron from another shell, usually from the L shell and occasionally from the M shell, fills the void in the K shell. As the electron drops into the K shell, it gives up the excess energy as a photon. The amount of energy is characteristic for each element. The radiation produced in the interaction by the movement of the electrons within the atom is characteristic radiation, as discussed earlier. (See Figure 2-6.)

Characteristic radiation is usually termed *secondary radiation* rather than *scatter radiation*. The distinction hardly

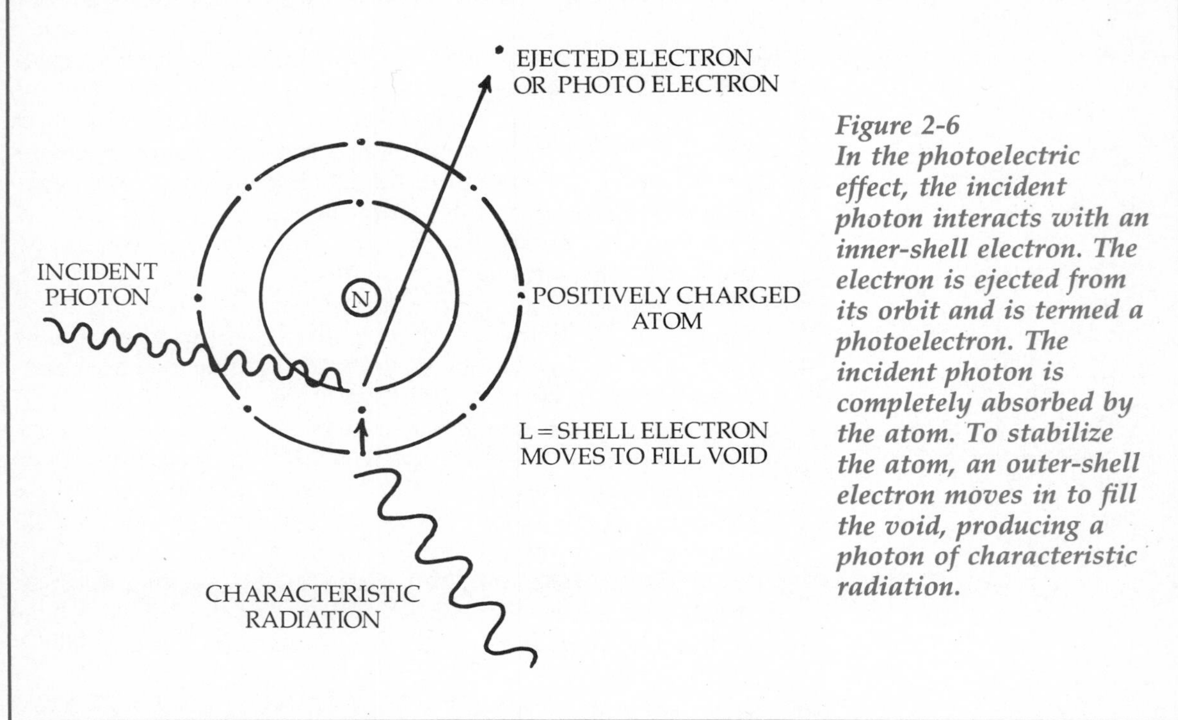

Figure 2-6
In the photoelectric effect, the incident photon interacts with an inner-shell electron. The electron is ejected from its orbit and is termed a photoelectron. The incident photon is completely absorbed by the atom. To stabilize the atom, an outer-shell electron moves in to fill the void, producing a photon of characteristic radiation.

seems necessary since the result is the same for both: a photon deflected from its original path. The photoelectric effect always yields three end products:

1. Characteristic radiation (a photon)
2. A negative ion (a photoelectron)
3. A positive ion (an electron-deficient atom)

Three simple rules govern the probability of a photoelectric interaction:

1. The incident photon must have enough energy to overcome the binding energy of the electron. However, the probability is inversely proportional to the third power of photon energy. In other words, as photon energy increases, the number of photoelectric interactions decreases.
2. A photoelectric interaction is most likely to occur when the photon energy and the K-shell binding energy are nearly the same.
3. The tighter an electron is bound in its orbit, the more likely it is to undergo a photoelectric interaction. The probability is directly proportional to the third power of the atomic number. As the atomic

number increases, the number of photoelectric interactions also increases.

Photoelectric interactions will most likely occur with low-energy photons and elements of high atomic number.

Therefore, photoelectric interactions will most likely occur with low-energy photons and elements of high atomic number, provided the photon has sufficient energy to overcome the forces binding the electrons in their shells.

The photoelectric effect has two impacts in the field of diagnostic radiology, one positive and one negative. First, it produces images of excellent quality because the photoelectric effect (1) does not produce energetic scatter radiation and (2) enhances the natural soft tissue contrast. Contrast is greatest when subject contrast is high. Thus, the photoelectric effect enhances the differences in tissues composed of different elements, such as soft tissue and bone. On the negative side, the photoelectric effect increases patient dose. Patients receive more radiation dose from this interaction than any other. The patient absorbs all of the photon energy in this interaction. As kilovoltage peak (kVp) increases, the likelihood of a photoelectric interaction declines. High-kVp techniques lower the number of photoelectric interactions and patient dose, although film quality suffers.

Pair Production

In **pair production** *a high-energy photon interacts with the nucleus of an atom.*

In *pair production* a high-energy photon interacts with the nucleus of an atom. The photon disappears, and its energy undergoes conversion into matter in the form of two particles: an electron and a positron. A positron is a particle with the same mass as an electron having a positive charge. The mass of one electron is equal to 0.51 million electron volts (MeV); therefore, the mass of two particles would total 1.02 MeV. The incident photon energy must be at least 1.02 MeV for pair production to occur. Photon energy in excess of 1.02 MeV is given up as kinetic energy to the two particles. Pair production is of no consequence in diagnostic radiology. (See Figure 2-7.)

Photodisintegration

In **photodisintegration,** *a high-energy photon interacts with the nucleus of an atom.*

In *photodisintegration,* a high-energy photon interacts with the nucleus of an atom, ejecting part of the nucleus. The ejected part may be a neutron, a proton, an alpha particle, or a cluster of particles. For this interaction to occur, a photon must have extremely high energy in the range of 7 to 15 MeV. This high energy is necessary to break the binding energy of the particles in the nucleus. Again, since the photon energy required exceeds the energies used in diagnostic radiology, this interaction is of no consequence to this field. (See Figure 2-8.)

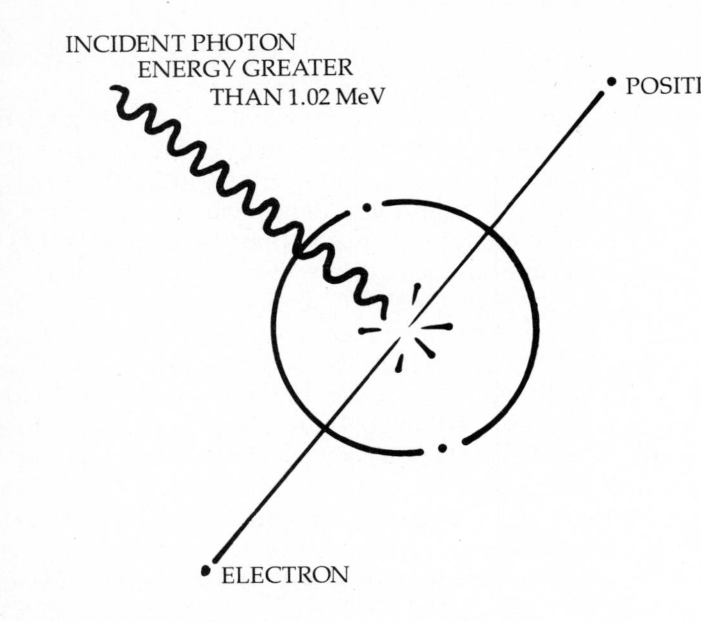

Figure 2-7
In pair production, a high-energy photon (greater than 1.02 MeV) interacts with the nucleus of an atom. The photon energy is transformed into matter in the form of a positron and an electron.

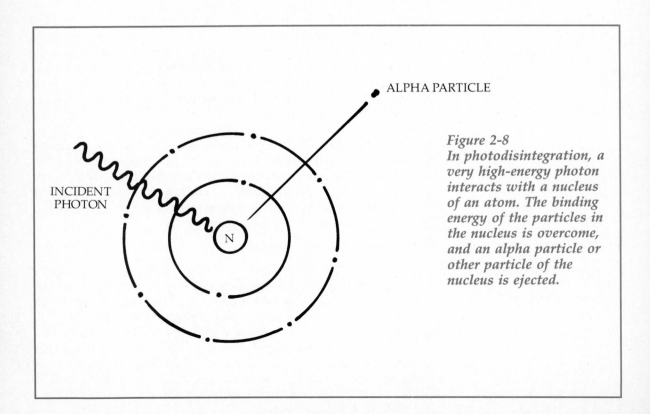

ALPHA PARTICLE

INCIDENT PHOTON

N

Figure 2-8
In photodisintegration, a very high-energy photon interacts with a nucleus of an atom. The binding energy of the particles in the nucleus is overcome, and an alpha particle or other particle of the nucleus is ejected.

Technique Considerations

Of the five ways that x-rays can interact with matter, only two are important in diagnostic radiology: the Compton effect and the photoelectric effect. Compton-scattered x-rays provide no useful information on the resultant radiograph: their only contribution is in the form of film fog. The application of special equipment and techniques reduces the number of scattered x-rays reaching the film.

Photons undergoing a photoelectric interaction provide diagnostic information in a negative sense. Since these photons are absorbed, they help image structures that are radiopaque. The photoelectric effect is responsible for the light or low-density areas on the film, such as those corresponding to bone. As one lowers kVp, the number of photoelectric interactions increases.

X-rays that do not interact with the tissue or pass through the body are responsible for the black or high-density areas on the film, such as those corresponding to air. Gray or medium-density areas correspond to tissue where some photoelectric interactions have taken place, and some x-rays pass through without interaction.

Differential absorption *is the difference between those photons absorbed photoelectrically and those not absorbed at all.*

By comparing these situations, one can define differential absorption. *Differential absorption* is the difference between those photons absorbed photoelectrically and those not absorbed at all. Kilovoltage peak controls differential absorption. As one lowers kVp, more photoelectric interactions occur, producing the maximum differential. Therefore, differential absorption increases as one lowers kVp. Conversely, as kVp increases, more photons pass through the body and fewer photoelectric interactions are taking place. As kVp increases, differential absorption decreases. To image small differences in subject contrast, as in mammography, one must use low-kVp techniques to maximize differential absorption. This is why one must apply optimum kVp ranges when examining different parts of the anatomy.

Contrast Media

Contrast material has a high atomic number—barium, 56; iodine, 53—compared to that of bone at 13.8. Therefore, a significantly higher number of photoelectric interactions will occur due to the higher atomic number of the contrast agent. Air, when used as a contrast agent, produces the opposite effect. It decreases the number of photoelectric interactions taking place, allowing more photons to pass through without interaction.

Attenuation

The interaction of x-rays by absorption and scatter is attenuation. *Attenuation* is the total reduction in the number of x-rays remaining in the x-ray beam following penetration through a given thickness of matter. X-rays undergo exponential attenuation. Attenuation of a certain percentage of photons occurs in each incremental thickness of an absorber. For example, if a given tissue sample attenuates 50 percent of the x-ray beam per centimeter of tissue traversed and is 5 cm thick, the following would take place:

> With 1000 photons in the incident x-ray, it begins to traverse the tissue sample. Attenuation of 50 percent of the photons occurs in the first centimeter of tissue, leaving 500. In the next centimeter of tissue, attenuation of 50 percent of the remaining 500 photons occurs, leaving 250. This continues through each centimeter of tissue until only 32 photons remain.

The total effect of the above attenuation was that only 3 percent of the incident photons were transmitted through the tissue sample.

Attenuation *is the total reduction in the number of x-rays remaining in the x-ray beam following penetration through a given thickness of matter.*

Units of Radiation Measurement

Four units of measurement exist for radiation. Each unit of measurement has specific units, but all are interrelated. Each unit of measurement also has a metric (International System, or SI) equivalent.

The *roentgen* (R) is the unit of radiation exposure or intensity. The R is that amount of radiation that will create 2.08×10^9 ion pairs in a cubic centimeter of air. The R quantifies radiation output or exposure.

The **roentgen** *(R) is the unit of radiation exposure or intensity.*

The *rad* is the unit of *r*adiation *a*bsorbed *d*ose. The rad is that amount of radiation that deposits 100 ergs/gram (g), where the erg is a unit of energy and the gram is a unit of mass. The rad can be quantified for any type of radiation striking any target material. The rad describes the dose received by human beings or animals.

The **rad** *is the unit of radiation absorbed dose.*

The *rem* is the *r*adiation *e*quivalent *m*an and quantifies radiation dose for human beings. The rem takes into account the biological effectiveness of different types of radiation. The rem finds its major application in recording doses from radiation monitoring devices.

The **rem** *is the radiation equivalent man and quantifies radiation dose for human beings.*

In diagnostic radiology the R, the rad, and the rem are all equivalent; 1 R equals 1 rad equals 1 rem. This is true since the linear energy transfer (LET), or the rate of energy deposited in tissue, and the relative biological effectiveness (RBE), or the ability of radiation to produce a biological effect, are one.

The **curie** *(Ci) is the unit of radioactivity.*

The *curie* (Ci) is the unit of radioactivity and actually quantifies the amount of radioactive material and not the radiation emitted. The Ci is that amount of material in which 3.7×10^{10} atoms disintegrate every second. This unit is of particular importance in nuclear medicine.

The equivalent to the R is the **coulomb per kilogram** *(C/kg).*

The equivalent to the rad is the **Gray** *(Gy).*

The equivalent to the rem is the **sievert** *(Sv).*

The equivalent to the Ci is the **becquerel** *(Bq).*

As previously mentioned, each unit has an SI system equivalent. The equivalent to the R is the *coulomb per kilogram* (C/kg), which is electric charge per unit mass of air. The coulomb is the measure of electric charge, and the kilogram is the unit of mass. One roentgen equals 2.58×10^{-4} C/kg. The equivalent to the rad is the *Gray* (Gy), which equals 1 erg/g. One rad equals 10^{-2} Gy. The equivalent to the rem is the *sievert* (Sv). The sievert shares the same relationship with the Gray that the rem does with the rad; therefore, 1 rem equals 10^{-2} Sv. The equivalent to the Ci is the *becquerel* (Bq). The becquerel quantifies that amount of radioactive material in which one atom disintegrates every second. One Ci equals 3.7×10^{10} Bq. To date, widespread acceptance of these units has not occurred.

It is important to understand the use and interrelationships of the units of radiation measurement. This understanding will be helpful in the evaluation of equipment, estimation of patient dose, and determination of personnel dose.

Radiation Protection

As previously mentioned, photoelectric interactions are the primary contributors to patient radiation dose. In addition, lowering the kVp increases the number of photoelectric interactions and patient dose. Therefore, to help reduce patient dose, one can use high-kVp techniques. This lowers patient dose but may also have a negative impact on film quality. Thus, optimum kVp ranges should be used for all radiographic examinations since they represent the best compromise between patient dose and film quality.

Optimum kVp ranges should be used for all radiographic examinations since they represent the best compromise between patient dose and film quality.

With the use of higher kVp, the number of Compton interactions will increase. This increases the production of scatter radiation, which increases personnel exposure for those in the room during the exposure. This primarily occurs during fluoroscopy or mobile radiography. One must remember that a photon scattered as much as 90 degrees retains most of its energy. This indicates the need for good radiation protection techniques.

Personnel Radiation Protection

Occupational exposure to radiation is relatively low and safe for radiologic technologists, provided appropriate radiation protection measures are taken. It is important for the technologist to have a good understanding of radiation protection principles to minimize his or her occupational exposure. Although in most instances the technologist works in a shielded control area, there are procedures, such as mobile radiography and fluoroscopy, during which the technologist will be exposed to radiation. Failure to observe proper radiation protection techniques can result in increased exposure and potential health effects. In the early history of radiology, before the effects of low-level radiation exposure were known, radiologists had increased incidences of leukemia and shorter life spans when compared with other physicians. Using contemporary radiation protection techniques, radiologists' incidence of leukemia and life span do not significantly differ from those of other physicians.

The Cardinal Rules of Radiation Protection

There are three basic principles for personnel radiation protection. These three basic principles, termed the Cardinal Rules of Radiation Protection, are time, distance, and shielding.

Time refers to the length of time an individual is exposed to ionizing radiation. The length of exposure time has a direct relationship to dose; if exposure time is reduced by 50%, then dose is reduced by 50%. In many instances, the technologist will have minimal control over this factor, since exposure time will be governed by technique requirements or the physician's fluoroscopic technique. While the technologist's presence in the room may be imperative during some fluoroscopic procedures, in others the technologist may be able to move to a shielded area. Care should be taken to confirm the acceptability of your absence with the radiologist. Whenever possible, technologists should attempt to minimize the amount of time they are exposed to radiation.

The length of time of exposure has a direct relationship to dose; if the length of time is reduced by 50%, then dose is reduced by 50%.

Distance can be a very effective method of radiation protection. *As the distance from the source of radiation increases, the dose is reduced according to the inverse square law* (see Chapter 9). Doubling of the distance from the source of radiation exposure will reduce the technologist's exposure four times, to 25%. The technologist must also be aware that the primary source of occupational exposure is scatter radiation from the patient. Therefore, increasing the

As the distance from the source of radiation increases, the dose is reduced according to the inverse square law.

distance from the patient during mobile radiographic or fluoroscopic procedures will result in decreased dose to the technologist. This principle is the reason for the long exposure cords on mobile radiographic equipment.

Shielding can be used to protect a radiologic technologist when exposure to radiation is unavoidable.

Shielding can be used to protect a radiologic technologist when exposure to radiation is unavoidable. Shielding devices are designed to protect the radiosensitive structures including the thyroid, the gonads, and the hemopoietic or blood forming tissues. Shielding devices include lead aprons, lead gloves, thyroid shields, leaded or photogrey glasses, and permanent or moveable partitions.

Lead aprons, gloves, and thyroid shields are typically constructed of lead-impregnated rubber or vinyl. Lead-impregnated rubber and vinyl are fairly fragile and are typically covered with a durable material. These items must not be creased, because cracks may develop that decrease their effectiveness. In 1991, the National Council on Radiation Protection stated that lead aprons shall provide radiation attenuation equal to 0.5 mm of lead (NCRP Report no. 102). Lead gloves shall provide radiation attenuation equal to 0.25 mm of lead.

Glasses with lead-impregnated or photogrey lenses can significantly reduce the dose to the eyes. However, since the technologist is seldom looking at the source of radiation exposure during a procedure, protective side flaps on the glasses are recommended.

Permanent shielded partitions, such as in the control areas, as well as mobile shields, are very effective in reducing exposure. The fixed exposure controls on fixed radiographic units are intended to prevent the technologist from making an exposure in an unshielded area. It should be noted that most shielding devices are designed to protect the technologist from secondary radiation only. Unless a partition is specifically designed as a primary barrier it does not offer adequate protection against primary radiation.

It should also be noted that shielding can, and should, be used to decrease patient exposure. Gonadal shielding or covering the radiosensitive parts of the patient's body that are not in the area of interest are sound patient protection techniques.

Personnel Monitoring

Radiation exposure is monitored for occupationally exposed individuals because of the concern about the latent effects of low level radiation and the unavoidable exposure to personnel.

Radiation exposure is monitored for occupationally exposed individuals because of the concern about the latent effects of low level radiation and the unavoidable exposure to personnel. Devices used for personnel monitoring include pocket ionization chambers, thermoluminescent dosimeters and film badges.

Pocket ionization chambers, also termed small pocket dosimeters, utilize an ionization chamber to measure radiation exposure. As the ionizing radiation interacts with the air in the chamber, ions are created, producing an electrical charge in the chamber. The change in the charge allows quantification of the radiation dose. These devices have the advantage of allowing immediate determination of dose and can be useful in areas of potentially high exposure. Disadvantages include the requirement to read doses daily and rough handling sensitivity from both an accuracy and function standpoint.

Pocket ionization chambers, *also termed small pocket dosimeters, utilize an ionization chamber to measure radiation exposure.*

Thermoluminescent dosimeters use an energy storing crystal, lithium fluoride, to monitor radiation dose. When exposed to radiation, lithium fluoride stores some portion of the energy absorbed from the radiation. When heated, these crystals release the stored energy in the form of light. The amount of light emitted is proportional to the radiation to which the crystal was exposed. Measurement of the light emitted yields a highly accurate determination of dose. These devices have the advantage of increased sensitivity to low doses of radiation and the ability to be utilized for longer periods of time. Unfortunately, they are more expensive to use than film badges. Primary applications for personnel monitoring include extremity monitoring; there are special applications such as monitoring the dose to the eyes.

Thermoluminescent dosimeters *use an energy storing crystal, lithium fluoride, to monitor radiation dose.*

Film badges are the most commonly employed method of personnel monitoring. These devices use a small strip of film in a light tight, waterproof packet. Measuring the photographic effect on the film allows accurate estimation of the dose at a relatively low cost. Special holders are used to hold the film packet. These holders incorporate filters that allow estimation of the radiation energy as well as the dose.

Film badges *are the most commonly employed method of personnel monitoring.*

In an effort to minimize occupational injury as a result of occupational exposure, the *maximum permissible dose (MPD)* has been established for various parts of the body based on radiosensitivity. The *whole body MPD* is 5 rem annually; other MPDS are listed below.

In an effort to minimize occupational injury as a result of occupational exposure, the **maximum permissible dose (MPD)** *has been established for various parts of the body based on radiosensitivity.*

The **whole body MPD** *is 5 rem annually.*

Combined whole body occupational exposure	5 rem in any one year
Lens of the eye	15 rem in any one year

All others (e.g., red bone marrow, breasts, lung, gonads, skin, and extremities)	50 rem in any one year
Human fetus during pregnancy	0.5 rem in gestational period

Since radiation has a cumulative effect, a **cumulative MPD** *has also been established. The* **cumulative MPD** *is based on age and the whole body MPD. The historic method of calculating cumulative MPD is 5(N−18) = MPD_c. The current method of calculating MPD is 1 × Age = MPD_c.*

Since radiation has a cumulative effect, a *cumulative MPD* has also been established. The *cumulative MPD* has historically been based on age and the whole body MPD. The historic cumulative MPD assumed no occupational exposure occurred before the age of 18 and was expressed:

$$5\ (N-18) = MPD_c \quad \text{(where N = age)}$$

Therefore, the cumulative MPD for a 45-year-old technologist is

$$5\ (45-18) = 135 \text{ rem}$$

In 1987, the National Council on Radiation Protection changed the cumulative MPD recommendations to 1 rem times the age in years (NCRP Report No. 91). The new cumulative MPD recommendation is expressed as:

$$1 \times N = MPD_c \quad \text{(where N = age)}$$

Therefore, the cumulative MPD for a 45-year-old technologist using the new recommendations is

$$1 \times 45 = 45 \text{ rem}$$

Obviously, the new recommendations result in a significantly lower cumulative MPD than was recommended for the previous method of calculating the cumulative MPD.

Following the basic principles of radiation protection coupled with careful personnel monitoring can minimize personnel dose. It is the technologist's responsibility to minimize occupational exposure; doing so will result in radiology continuing to be a safe profession.

Chapter 2—Review Questions

1. Which of the following is *not* true concerning x-radiation?
   a. It is a form of electromagnetic radiation.
   b. It does not ionize air.
   c. It can cause harmful biological effects.
   d. It is a type of ionizing radiation.
   e. none of the above
2. The two methods of x-ray production are:
   a. bremsstrahlung and characteristic radiation
   b. electromagnetic and ionizing radiation
   c. propagating and ionizing radiation
   d. x-rays and gamma rays
   e. grenz and deceleration radiation
3. Ionization is:
   a. responsible for the harmful effects on living tissue
   b. capable of producing an electrical charge in air
   c. the removal of an orbital electron from an atom of material
   d. two of the above
   e. all of the above
4. The unit of measurement for wavelength is the:
   a. frequency
   b. pulse
   c. electromagnetic spectrum
   d. angstrom
   e. none of the above
5. Which of the following factors determine the photon energy of bremsstrahlung radiation?
   a. the energy of the incident electron
   b. the proximity of the incident electron to the nucleus of the target atom
   c. the conversion of kinetic energy into x-radiation and heat
   d. the positive charge of the nucleus
   e. a and d
   f. a, b, and d
   g. a, b, and c
   h. none of the above

6. Which of the following factors determine the photon energy of characteristic radiation?
   a. the energy of the incident electron
   b. the proximity of the incident electron to the nucleus of the target atom
   c. the conversion of kinetic energy into x-radiation and heat
   d. the positive charge of the nucleus
   e. a and d
   f. a, b, and d
   g. a, b, and c
   h. none of the above
7. Which of the following is *not* true concerning the production of x-radiation?
   a. As electron energy increases, the energy of the radiation produced increases.
   b. Fast-moving electrons are suddenly decelerated.
   c. Most of the electron's kinetic energy is converted into x-radiation.
   d. It occurs by one of two electron interactions with matter.
   e. none of the above
8. Which of the following statements is true concerning interactions between x-rays and matter?
   a. Interactions take place at the molecular level.
   b. Low-energy x-rays interact with electrons.
   c. The physical state of the matter determines the number of x-rays a group of atoms will stop.
   d. High energy x-rays tend to interact with the entire atom.
   e. none of the above
9. Which of the following statements is true concerning classical scattering?
   a. This interaction with matter does not cause ionization.
   b. The scattered photon travels in the same direction with reduced energy
   c. A low-energy photon interacts with a target atom.
   d. two of the above
   e. all of the above

10. In which of the following interactions is a K-shell electron ejected from its orbit?
    a. Compton effect
    b. photodisintegration
    c. photoelectric effect
    d. unmodified scattering
    e. none of the above

11. The probability of Compton interaction is a complex function of:
    a. the total number of electrons in the absorber
    b. the difference in the energy of the incident photon and the binding energy of the electron
    c. the energy of the incident photon
    d. two of the above
    e. none of the above

12. Compton scattering results in which of the following?
    a. total absorption of the incident photon
    b. film fog
    c. increase in the patient's radiation exposure
    d. enhancement of soft tissue contrast
    e. reduction in personnel radiation exposure

13. Which of the following is *not* an end product of the photoelectric effect?
    a. a photoelectron
    b. a positively charged ion
    c. a photon of characteristic radiation
    d. a negatively charged ion
    e. none of the above

14. Which of the following rules govern the probability of a photoelectric interaction?
    a. The higher the energy of the incident photon, the higher is the probability of a photoelectric interaction.
    b. The lower the atomic number of the absorber, the higher is the probability of photoelectric interaction.
    c. The smaller the difference between the photon energy and the K-shell binding energy, the higher is the probability of a photoelectric interaction.
    d. two of the above
    e. all of the above

15. Which of the following statements is true concerning pair production?
    a. The incident photon energy must be at least 0.51 MeV.
    b. A high-energy photon interacts with the nucleus of an atom.
    c. The photon energy undergoes conversion into matter.
    d. two of the above
    e. all of the above

16. Of the five ways x-rays can interact with matter, which two are the most important in diagnostic radiology?
    a. Compton effect and photoelectric effect
    b. pair production and photoelectric effect
    c. photodisintegration and Compton effect
    d. classical scattering and pair production

17. Differential absorption is:
    a. the difference between those photons absorbed photoelectrically and those not absorbed at all
    b. decreased as kVp is decreased
    c. the reason for optimum kVp ranges
    d. two of the above
    e. all of the above

18. Attenuation is:
    a. the interaction of x-rays by absorption and scatter
    b. the total reduction in the number of x-rays remaining in the x-ray beam following penetration through a given thickness of matter
    c. exponential for x-radiation
    d. two of the above
    e. all of the above

19. A given tissue sample attenuates 50 percent of the x-ray beam per centimeter of tissue traversed. If 4 cm of this tissue is penetrated with an x-ray beam containing 10,000 photons, how many photons will be attenuated?
    a. 1250 photons
    b. 625 photons
    c. 8750 photons
    d. 9375 photons
    e. 313 photons

20. The unit of radiation exposure or intensity is the:
    a. rem
    b. rad
    c. roentgen
    d. curie

21. The amount of radiation that deposits 100 ergs/gram is the:
    a. Gray
    b. becquerel
    c. roentgen
    d. rad

22. What is the unit of radiation measurement that takes into account the biological effectiveness of radiation?
    a. RBE
    b. rad
    c. rem
    d. LET

23. What is the SI system equivalent to the rad?
    a. coulomb per kilogram
    b. Gray
    c. sievert
    d. becquerel

24. What is the unit of radioactivity that actually quantifies the amount of radioactive material and not the amount of radiation emitted?
    a. roentgen
    b. erg
    c. Gray
    d. curie

25. What is the cumulative MPD for a 29-year-old technologist under both the historic and current recommendations?
    a. 55 R (historic), 29 R (current)
    b. 145 R (historic), 29 R (current)
    c. 145 rem (historic), 29 rem (current)
    d. 55 rem (historic), 29 rem (current)

3

The X-Ray Tube

OBJECTIVES

After completing Chapter 3, you should be able to:

1. Define the following terms:
   anode
   cathode
   focusing cup
   glass envelope
   heat unit
   heel effect
   off-focus radiation
   thermionic emission
2. Discuss the concepts and construction of rotating-anode x-ray tubes.
3. Discuss the concepts behind the line-focus principle.
4. Demonstrate the use of x-ray tube rating charts and cooling curves.
5. Briefly discuss the following:
   special application x-ray tubes
   field-emission x-ray tubes
   graphite-backed anode x-ray tubes
   mammography x-ray tubes
   metal-center-section x-ray tubes
6. Discuss use and abuse of x-ray tubes.

The x-ray tube is a special type of diode used to produce x-radiation. The three major parts of the x-ray tube are the cathode, the anode, and the glass envelope.

The Cathode

The *cathode* is the negatively charged electrode in the x-ray tube that serves as the source of electrons. The cathode is composed of a filament and a focusing cup (Figure 3-1). The filament is the actual source of electrons and is a tight coil of tungsten alloy wire. The tungsten alloy is ideal to use for a filament. It has a high melting point, does not vaporize at high temperatures, and can be drawn into a fine wire. When a current is applied to the filament, electrons are liberated about the surface of the filament. The liberated electrons form an electron "cloud" surrounding the filament. This is termed the space charge. Typically, the current applied to the filament is 4 to 6 amperes at 10 to 12 volts. The process by which the electrons are liber-

The **cathode** *is the negatively charged electrode in the x-ray tube that serves as the source of electrons.*

The process by which the electrons are liberated or "boiled off" the filament is **thermionic emission.**

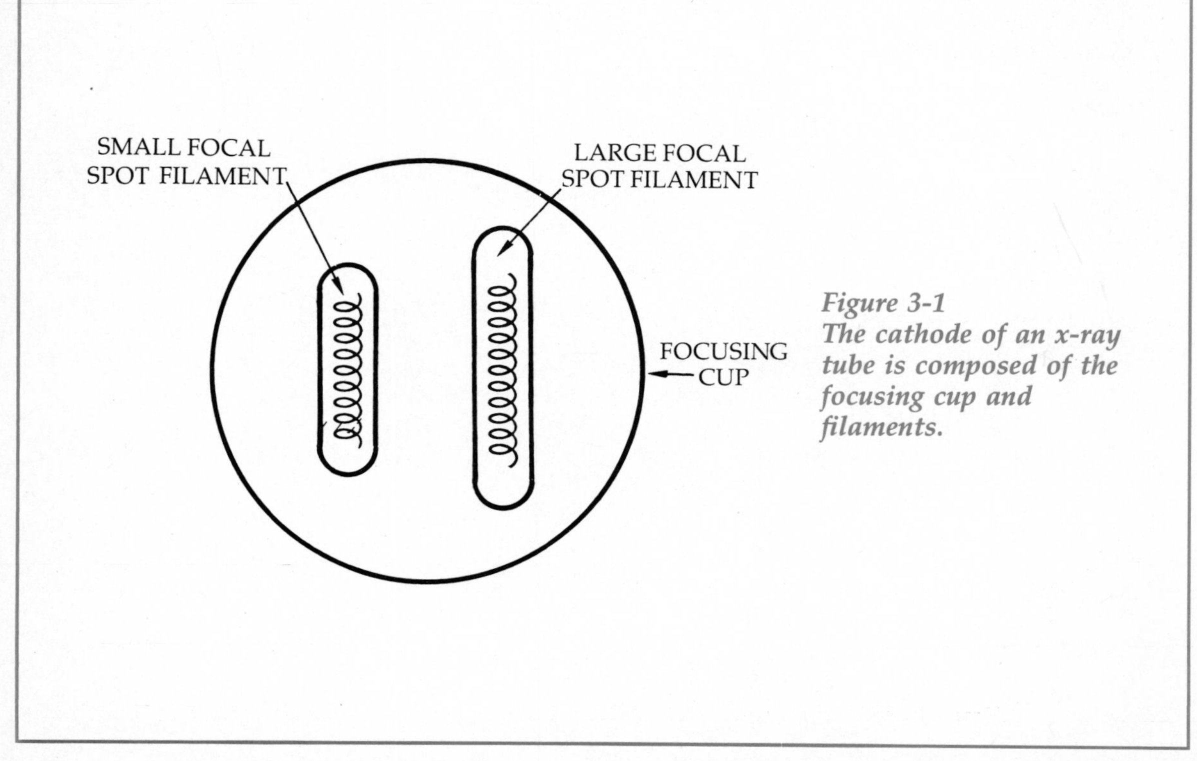

Figure 3-1
The cathode of an x-ray tube is composed of the focusing cup and filaments.

The purpose of the **focusing cup** *is to condense or focus the cloud of electrons.*

ated or "boiled off" the filament is *thermionic emission*.

The purpose of the *focusing cup* is to condense or focus the cloud of electrons. Since all the electrons have a negative charge, they repel one another and spread out or "bloom." The focusing cup houses the filament and is negatively charged. Thus, the electrons are repelled by the negative charge of the focusing cup and compressed together around the filament. This minimizes focal spot bloom and improves resolution.

The Anode

The **anode** *is the positively charged electrode of the x-ray tube.*

The *anode* is the positively charged electrode of the x-ray tube. It serves to decelerate the electrons as well as store and dissipate heat. The target is the area of actual electron deceleration and x-ray production. The target is usually composed of tungsten. Tungsten is used because it has a high atomic number and a high melting point. The tungsten target is imbedded in a heat sink. In the case of

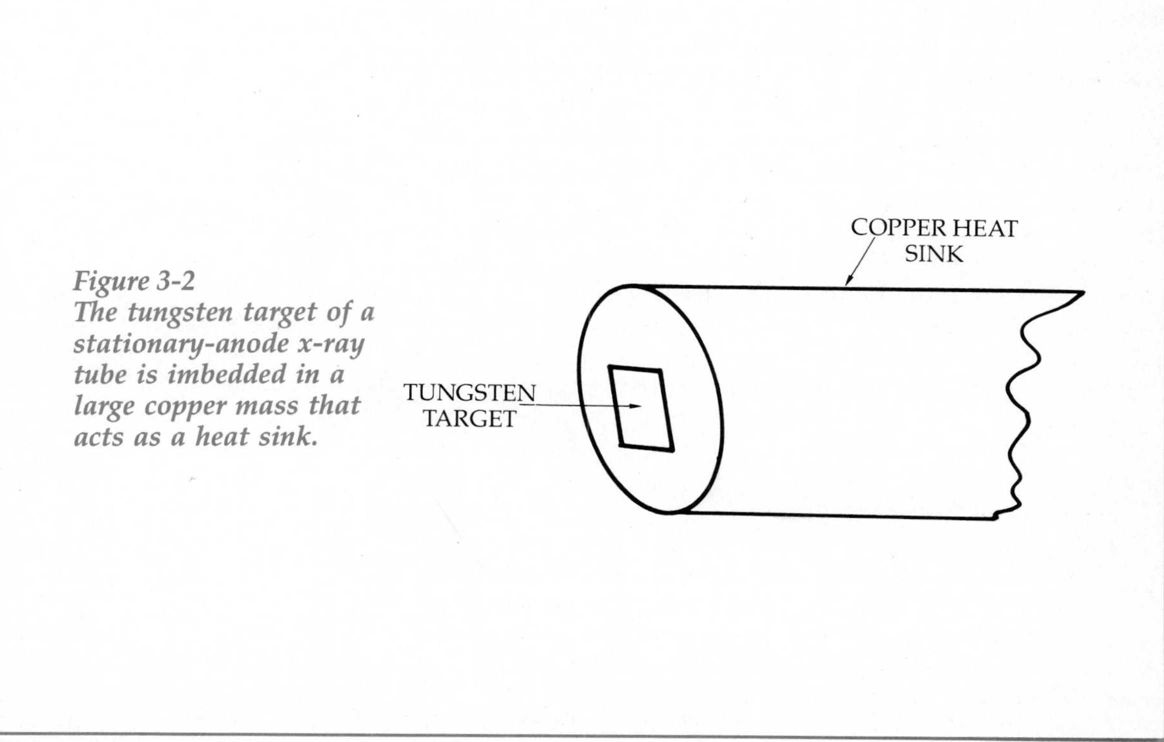

Figure 3-2
The tungsten target of a stationary-anode x-ray tube is imbedded in a large copper mass that acts as a heat sink.

the stationary-anode x-ray tube, the target is imbedded in a large copper mass (Figure 3-2). The copper mass serves to support the target, carry heat away from the target, and store the heat until it can dissipate. The heat-loading capabilities of an x-ray tube are often the limiting factor in maximum exposure.

The Glass Envelope

The *glass envelope* serves two major purposes: it is the structural support for the anode and cathode and contains the vacuum necessary for x-ray production. The glass envelope is constructed of Pyrex glass due to the high temperature encountered with the production of x-rays. A special port or window is located where the radiation exits the glass envelope. The port is thinner than the rest of the envelope to reduce x-ray attenuation.

The **glass envelope** *serves two major purposes: it is the structural support for the anode and cathode and contains the vacuum necessary for x-ray production.*

Rotating-Anode X-Ray Tubes

The anode of the x-ray tube must serve as an effective heat sink, capable of storing and carrying away large amounts of heat. This is necessitated by the inefficiency of x-ray production. Remember: *during production of x-rays, more than 99 percent of the electric energy is given up as heat and less than 1 percent is converted to x-rays.* In the discussion of x-ray tube construction, the target was imbedded in a large copper mass. The copper serves to carry heat away from the target. Unfortunately, for the large exposures required in contemporary radiology, the stationary copper anode is inadequate. This resulted in the development of the rotating-anode x-ray tube (Figure 3-3). The purpose of the rotating anode is to increase the surface area bombarded by electrons, spreading the heat over a larger area. This increases the heat-loading capabilities of the x-ray tube.

The purpose of the rotating anode is to increase the surface areas bombarded by electrons, spreading the heat over a larger area.

Anode construction in the rotating x-ray tube typically includes the following: (1) a tungsten-rhenium focal track; (2) a molybdenum disk to store heat (the molybdenum disk is usually about 4½ inches in diameter); and (3) an induction motor to turn the anode disk (this motor works similar to a transformer). Most rotating-anode x-ray tubes rotate at 3600 rpm. High-speed rotating-anode x-ray tubes rotate at about 10,000 rpm. The rotating anode increases the heat-loading capabilities of x-ray tubes by nearly 200 times.

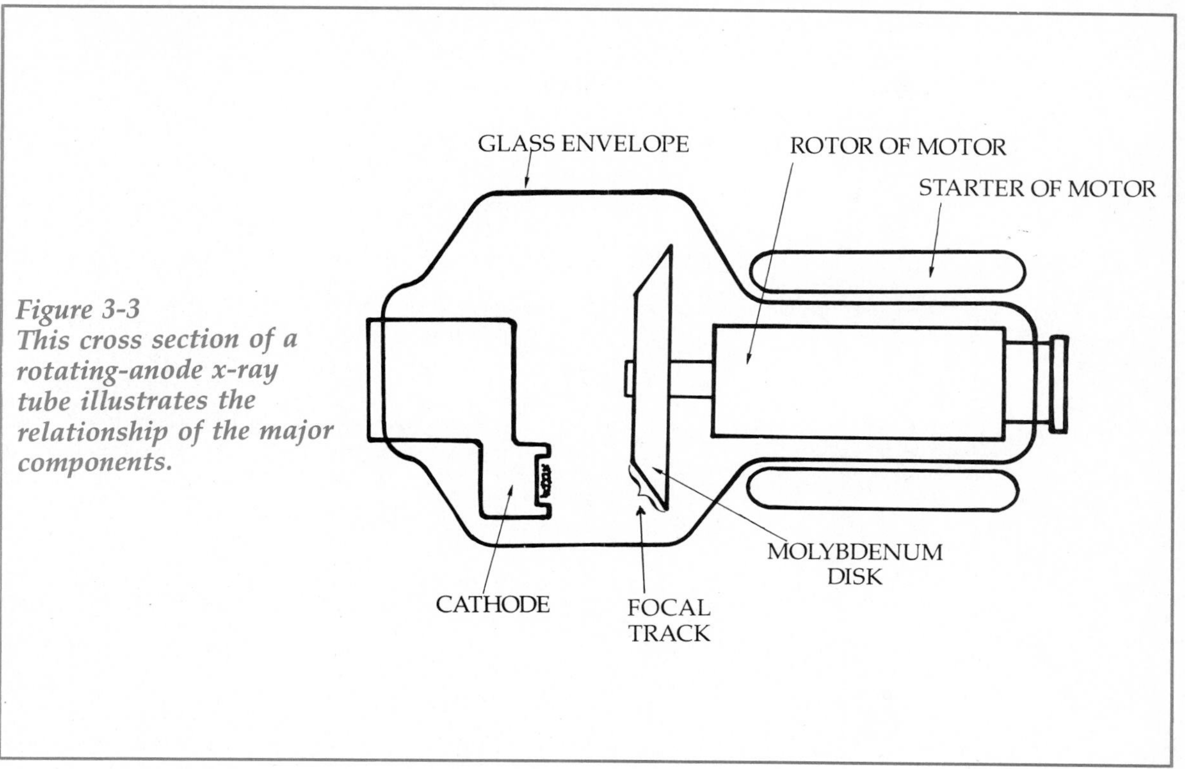

Figure 3-3
This cross section of a rotating-anode x-ray tube illustrates the relationship of the major components.

Line-Focus Principle

The line-focus principle increases the heat-loading capability of the x-ray tube while improving the resolution capabilities.

Another method to increase the heat-loading capabilities of the x-ray tube is the line-focus principle. In diagnostic radiology, the use of small focal spots is advantageous because they improve resolution. As the focal spot decreases in size, however, the area of target that is heated also decreases. This limits the exposure that can be safely made and usually results in limiting the size of the focal spot used. The line-focus principle requires the use of a steep target angle. This allows a large area of the target to be bombarded with electrons, whereas the effective or projected focal spot is much smaller (Figure 3-4). The lower the target angle, the smaller is the effective focal spot. Therefore, the line-focus principle increases the heat-loading capability of the x-ray tube while improving the resolution capabilities. Also, as target angles decrease, x-ray field size can be limited, and the heel effect, which is described later, will become more prominent.

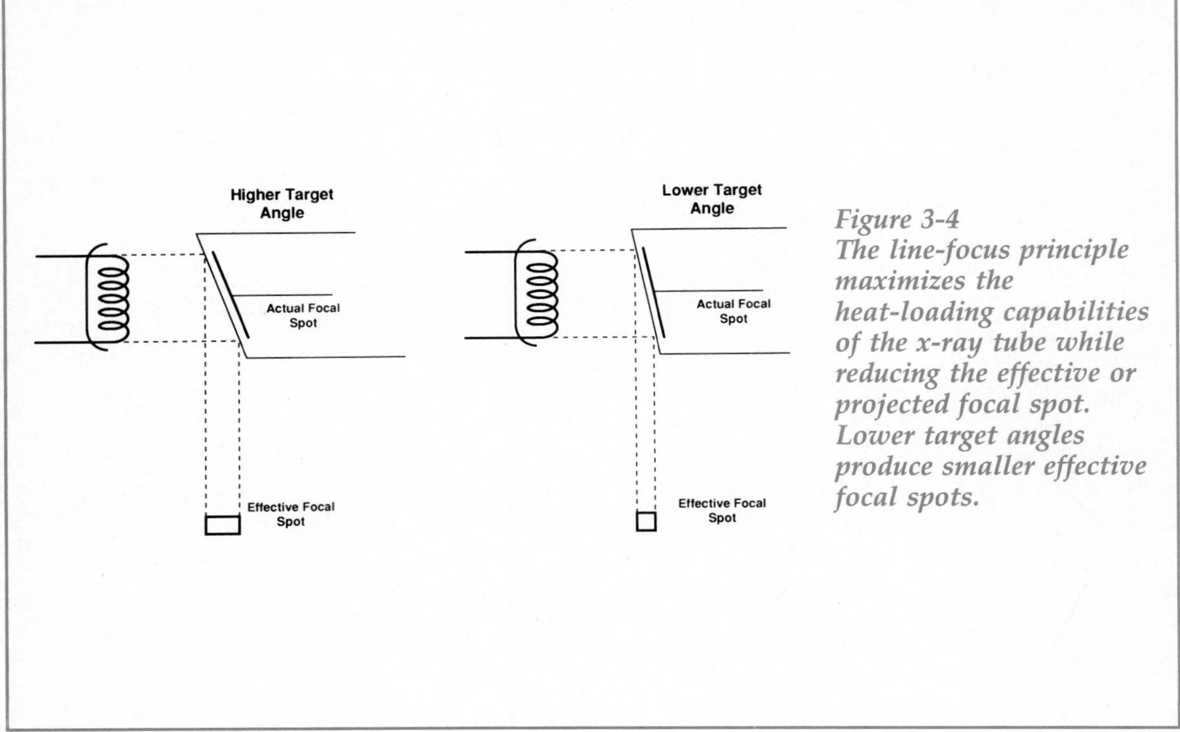

Figure 3-4
The line-focus principle maximizes the heat-loading capabilities of the x-ray tube while reducing the effective or projected focal spot. Lower target angles produce smaller effective focal spots.

X-Ray Tube Rating Charts and Cooling Curves

The amount of heat produced on the target of an x-ray tube is a product of milliamperes (mA), kilovoltage peak (kVp), and time. The unit of measure of this energy is the heat unit (HU). The *heat unit* is defined as the product of mA × kVp × seconds (S) for single-phase equipment and the product of mA × kVp × S × 1.35 for three-phase equipment. To determine the maximum safe exposure for a given x-ray tube, the technologist can consult the tube rating charts provided by the equipment manufacturer. The three most important types of charts are the radiographic rating chart, the anode cooling chart, and the housing cooling chart.

*The **heat unit** is defined as the product of mA × kVp × seconds (S) for single-phase equipment and the product of mA × kVp × S × 1.35 for three-phase equipment.*

The radiographic rating chart shows the maximum safe techniques for a particular tube. This chart has several curves that represent the mA that can be used on the equipment. The horizontal axis represents the time of ex-

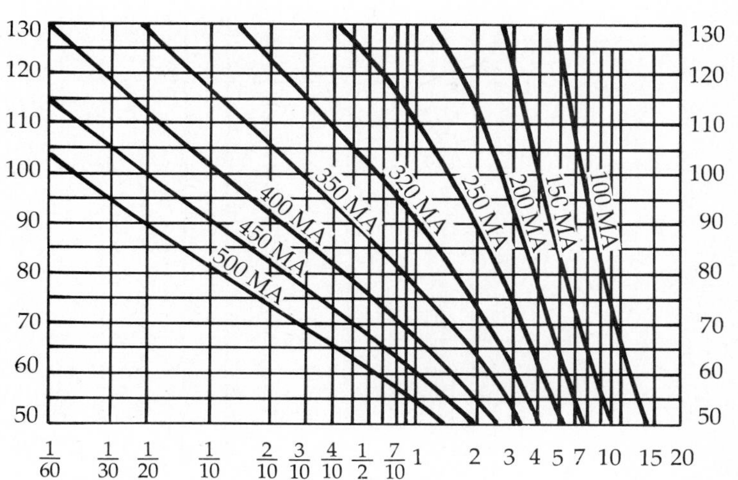

Figure 3-5
Typical radiographic rating chart. Using this chart, an exposure of 80 kVp at 500 mA for 0.1 second is safe since it falls below the 500 mA line. However, an exposure of 0.2 second at 500 mA and 80 kVp is unsafe because it lies above the 500 mA line. (Courtesy of General Electric)

posure, and the vertical axis represents the kVp used (Figure 3-5). Any combination of kVp and time that intersects below the curve for the mA used is within the safe operating range of the tube. If the intersection lies above the curve for the mA used, it exceeds the safe operating limits of the tube.

The technologist must make certain he or she is using the appropriate radiographic rating chart when evaluating the safety of exposures. Several charts often will be provided, with different ones for small focal spot, large focal spot, single-phase operation, three-phase operation, standard-speed anode rotation, and high-speed anode rotation. Using the wrong chart could result in serious damage to the x-ray tube.

The anode cooling chart is used to calculate the amount of time necessary to dissipate the heat stored in the anode. The chart consists of a curve demonstrating the cooling rate, with the vertical axis showing the heat units stored and the horizontal axis showing time (Figure 3-6).

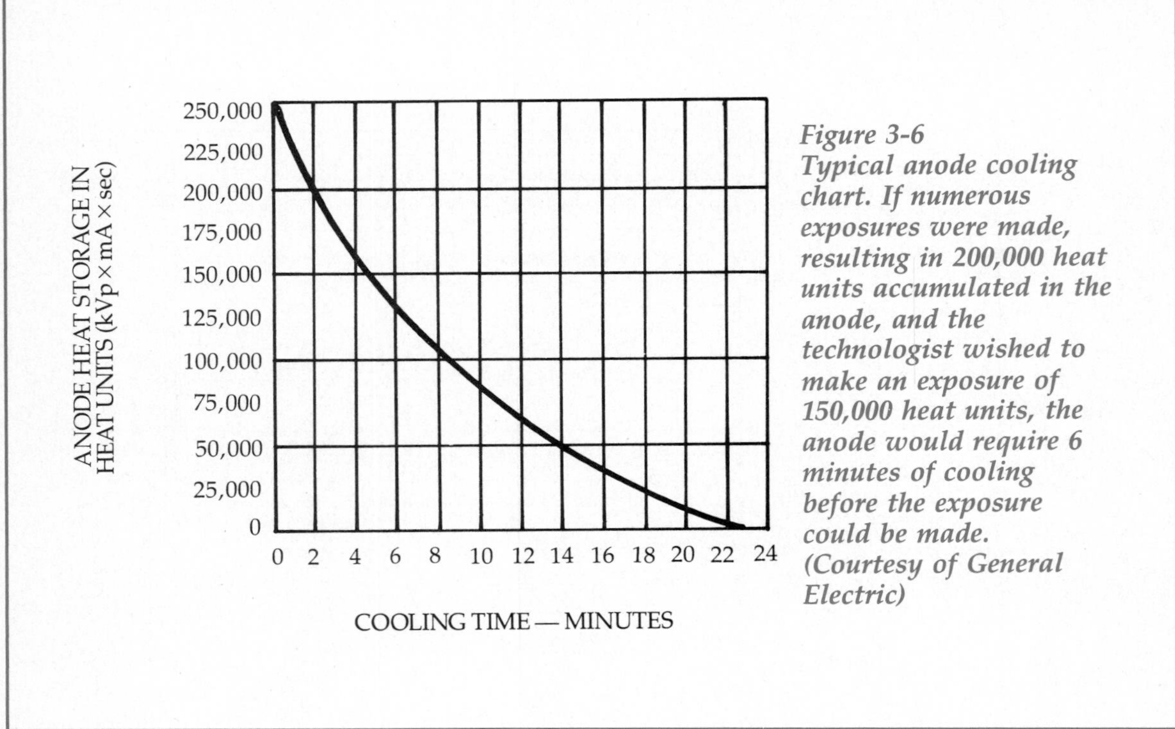

Figure 3-6
Typical anode cooling chart. If numerous exposures were made, resulting in 200,000 heat units accumulated in the anode, and the technologist wished to make an exposure of 150,000 heat units, the anode would require 6 minutes of cooling before the exposure could be made. (Courtesy of General Electric)

The anode cooling chart is used to determine the maximum amount of heat units the anode can tolerate and the amount of time required to dissipate that heat.

The housing cooling chart is used to calculate the amount of time necessary to dissipate the heat stored in the tube housing. X-ray tube housings can characteristically store 1.5 million HU, but they require long amounts of time to dissipate heat. The addition of an oil cooler or muffin fan to the tube housing can dramatically reduce the amount of time necessary for cooling.

Heel Effect

The *heel effect* is the result of decreased x-ray intensity at the anode end of the x-ray tube. This is a consequence of the line-focus principle. In general, those x-rays emitted toward the anode end of the x-ray tube must traverse a greater thickness of target material. Some of those x-rays are absorbed by the target material, resulting in decreased

The **heel effect** *is the result of decreased x-ray intensity at the anode end of the x-ray tube.*

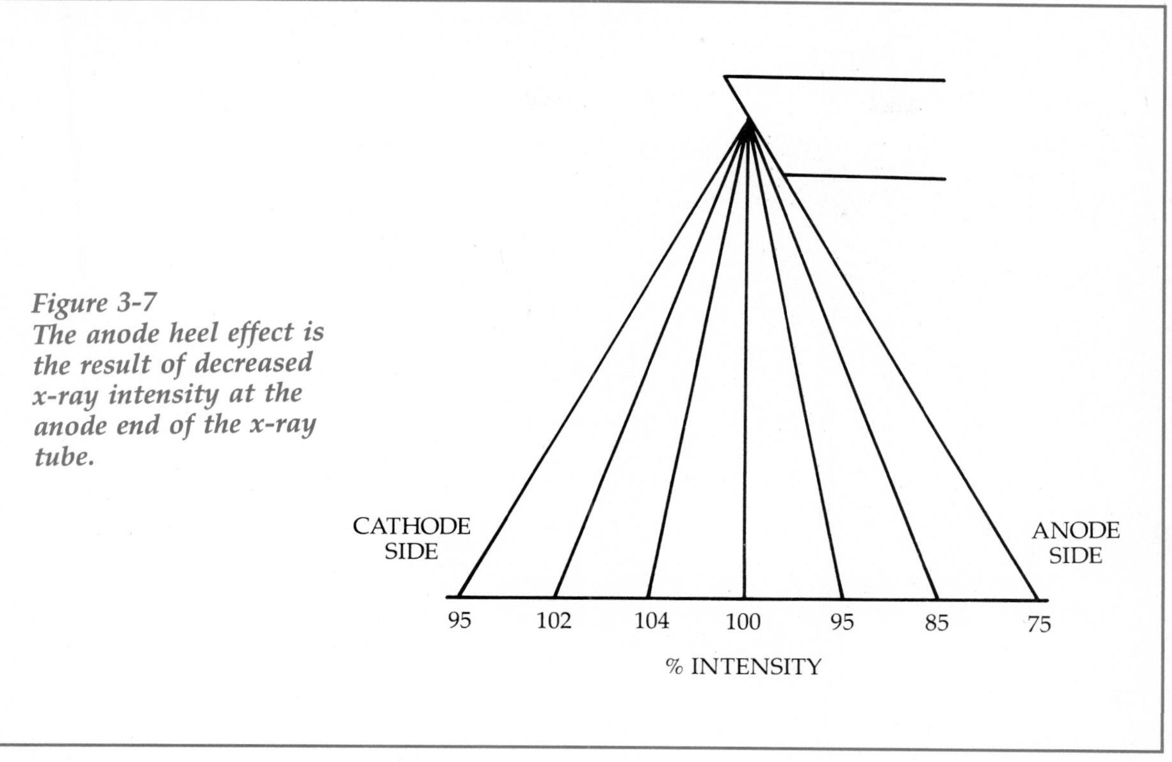

Figure 3-7
The anode heel effect is the result of decreased x-ray intensity at the anode end of the x-ray tube.

intensity at the anode end of the tube (Figure 3-7). This variation in intensity can be significant in some cases. Heel effect is most pronounced with (1) lower target angles, (2) short-source image-receptor distances, and (3) large fields with little or no collimation. (Collimation limits the useful x-ray beam and thereby spares adjacent tissue from needless exposure.)

From a technical standpoint, the heel effect should be considered when performing radiography on body parts that vary significantly in thickness. Common examples include the thoracic spine and the femur. When performing radiography in these areas, the anode should be positioned at the thinner end of the body part. This results in an evening out of the density across the film despite the varying thickness in the parts. Failure to position the patient in this way will result in exaggeration of the density differences, with the inability to produce a diagnostic image of the entire part.

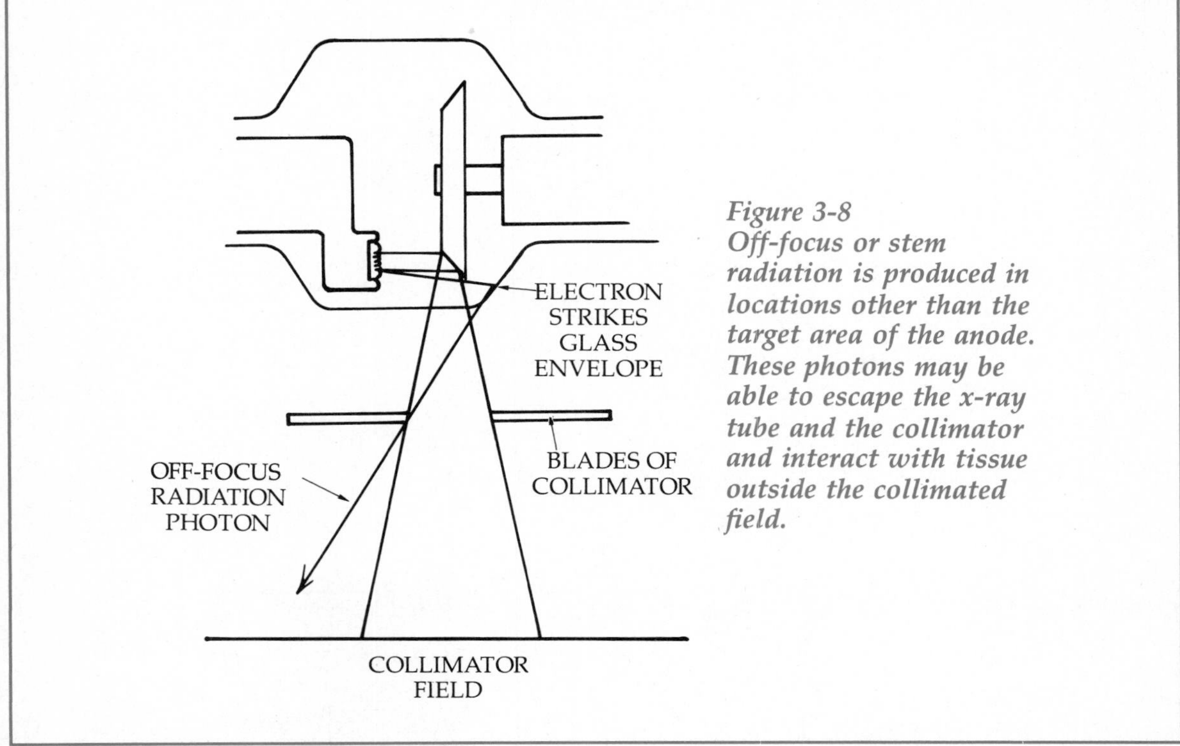

Figure 3-8
Off-focus or stem radiation is produced in locations other than the target area of the anode. These photons may be able to escape the x-ray tube and the collimator and interact with tissue outside the collimated field.

Off-Focus Radiation

Off-focus or *stem radiation* is radiation produced in the x-ray tube when electrons interact with matter other than the target. The most likely sites for the production of off-focus radiation are the nontarget portion of the anode, the glass envelope, and tungsten deposits on the glass envelope. Since off-focus radiation arises from areas other than the focal spot, it detracts from image quality. In addition, off-focus radiation increases patient exposure since these photons do not contribute to the diagnostic image and may interact with tissue outside the collimated field (Figure 3-8). Steps must be taken to control the escape of off-focus radiation from the x-ray tube. Chapter 10 discusses the control of off-focus radiation.

Off-focus *or* **stem radiation** *is radiation produced in the x-ray tube when electrons interact with matter other than the target.*

Special-Application X-Ray Tubes

Several x-ray tubes are specially constructed for specific applications. The best example is probably the mammography x-ray tube. The mammography tube is constructed with a special low-atomic-number target and window. The molybdenum target results in production of the lower-energy photons needed to image the breast. The beryllium window permits the low-energy photons to exit the tube.

Another special x-ray tube used for mammography and magnification radiography is the microfocus x-ray tube. These tubes employ focal spots of 0.1 mm or less. The small focal spot enhances the resolution on the resultant radiograph.

Metal center-section x-ray tubes have a metal section in the glass envelope. The metal section is grounded and protects against arcing and subsequent damage to the tube. The tubes are typically used for angiography, where numerous high-milliampere exposures result in excessive evaporation and deposits of tungsten on the inside of the tube surface.

In computed tomography (CT), x-ray tubes often have a graphite backing on the anode. The graphite serves as a heat sink, transmitting and storing heat from the face of the anode. This greatly increases the heat-loading capabilities of the x-ray tube and increases tube life. This is an important advance in the construction of CT tubes.

X-ray tubes for cineradiography are triodes and contain a grid between the cathode and anode. The grid can be negatively charged, which prevents electrons from the cathode crossing the tube and striking the anode. The grid provides a method of starting and stopping the exposure very quickly. This allows the synchronization of the exposures to the cinecamera. This will be discussed later in Chapter 5.

The field-emission or cold-cathode tube is another special application x-ray tube. In the field-emission tube, the cathode is not heated, and thermionic emission does not occur. The cathode is a series of fine needle points that surround the anode (Figure 3-9). When high-voltage current is applied to the tube, electrons are pulled from the needle points and strike the anode. Field-emission tubes are often found in the capacitor-discharge type of mobile units.

Use and Abuse of X-Ray Tubes

The technologist can do several things to extend the life of the x-ray tube. Conversely, improper use of the x-ray tube will shorten its life. An x-ray tube costs thousands of dollars and the technologist is responsible for using it properly and preventing unnecessary damage.

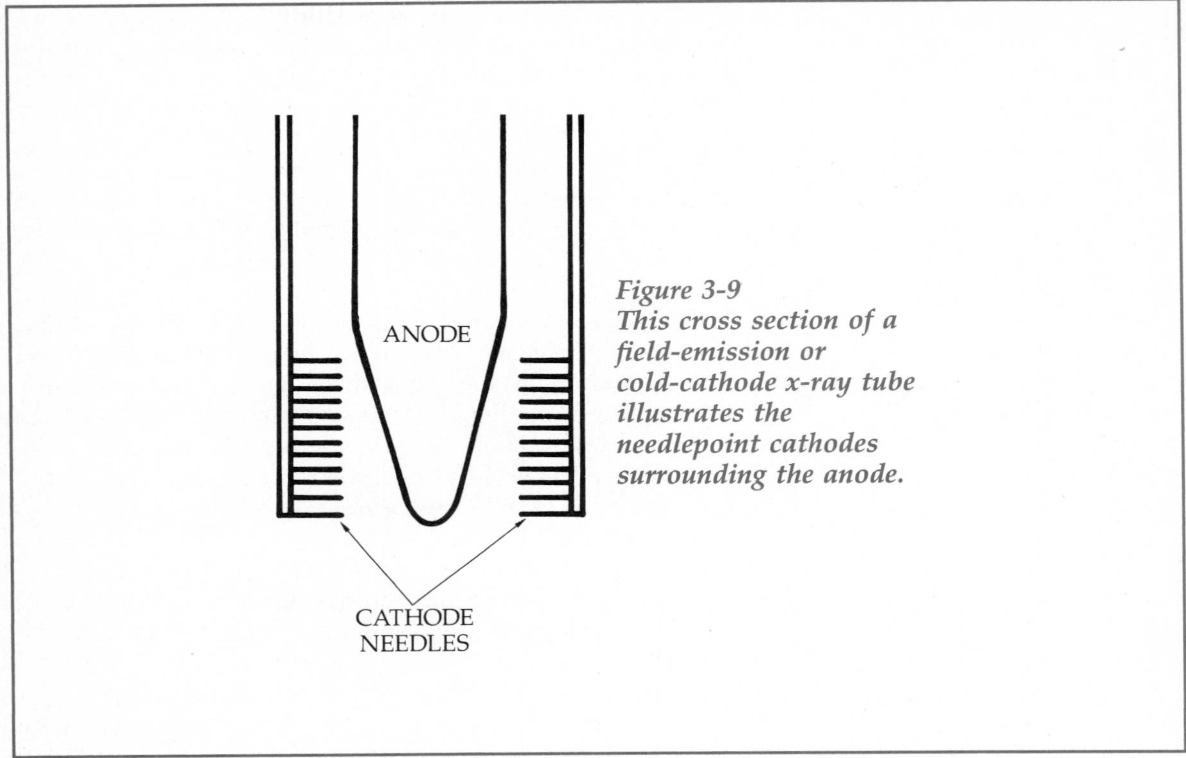

Figure 3-9
This cross section of a field-emission or cold-cathode x-ray tube illustrates the needlepoint cathodes surrounding the anode.

Before using radiographic equipment, the technologist should first preheat the x-ray tube. A large, instantaneous exposure produces great heat on the surface of the rotating anode. The heated surface of the anode expands, causing thermal stress, which may fracture the anode. If the x-ray tube has not been used for 30 minutes or more, it has probably cooled to near room temperature. A great difference between the surface temperature and that of the rest of the anode increases the probability of a fracture occurring. Preheating the x-ray tube significantly reduces the possibility of fracturing the anode.

The technique required to preheat the x-ray tube is quite simple. Select a low-milliampere (50 to 200 mA), large focal spot, moderate kVp (65 to 75), and a long time (4 to 6 seconds). Make two to three exposures at this setting, allowing several seconds between exposures for heat dissipation into the anode. Preheating should be repeated any time the x-ray tube has stood idle for 30 minutes or more. It is important to preheat all the x-ray tubes on units with multiple tubes, such as fluoroscopy or angiography units.

The proper technique is to give all instructions to the patient, then engage both rotor and exposure switches.

When performing an examination that will produce great heat, it is best to perform the view requiring the largest exposure first.

Another important consideration for the technologist is rotor preparation time or "hurting time." When the rotor and exposure are activated simultaneously, a delay occurs while the x-ray tube's rotor reaches its appropriate speed. Once the rotor has reached its appropriate operating speed, the exposure is made. However, few technologists engage both the rotor and the exposure switch simultaneously. The more common practice is to engage the rotor, allowing it to reach speed, while giving the patient breathing instructions. Several seconds elapse before the technologist depresses the exposure button. Although this is a typical practice, it is not a good one. During the time the rotor switch is engaged, two phenomena occur: the rotor accelerates to its proper speed, and the filament of the cathode heats white hot. The cathode of the x-ray tube has a finite life span. The longer the filament is heated per exposure, the fewer the number of exposures before the tube fails.

A more proper technique is to give all instructions to the patient, then engage both rotor and exposure switches. As soon as the exposure terminates, the switches should be released. Since most equipment's rotor preparation time is 1 second or less, this should not pose a serious problem for most examinations. An uncooperative or pediatric patient may require advanced preparation of the rotor.

The technologist should also consider the sequence of exposures for a particular examination. When considering heat-dissipation principles, one follows a logical sequence of exposures. An anode dissipates heat faster when it is hotter. When performing an examination that will produce great heat, it is best to perform the view requiring the largest exposure first. During a lumbar spine examination, one should perform the lateral views, then the oblique views, and finally the anteroposterior (AP) views. This produces the greatest amount of target heating early, and cooling would be more rapid during the entire series.

More serious abuses of the x-ray tube result in serious damage or immediate failure. One of the most common serious abuses is exceeding the heat-sink rate. This problem occurs when exposures are made in rapid sequence and the anode cannot dissipate the heat as fast as it is generated. No single exposure exceeds the capabilities of the tube, but the rapid sequence does not allow cooling time. This is a common problem in angiographic runs. Exceeding the heat-sink rate can cause thermal stress and cracking of the anode. During extreme cases, the molybdenum stem can soften and bend, resulting in destruction of the x-ray tube. The technologist should calculate the total number of heat units and check the anode rating charts before initiating a series of large exposures.

It may be difficult to calculate the heat in the anode at any given time because of the anode's continuous cooling. Several vendors manufacture heat calculators that keep track of the percentage of heat load. Most heat calculators also prevent exposures above a preset percentage. Early heat calculators used a fiberoptic system to measure the infrared emissions of the anode. More contemporary units use a microprocessor that continuously calculates heating and cooling in the anode. They constantly display the percentage of heat contained in the anode. Although these devices are almost foolproof, they can be defeated. Interrupting the power to the unit erases the memory and resets the unit to zero, regardless of the actual heat load of the anode.

One final consideration when using the x-ray tube is gyroscopic effect. A high-speed x-ray tube behaves similar to a toy gyroscope and resists any change in direction. If the anode is rotating at high speed and the direction of the tube is changed quickly, there is resistance to direction change. The resistance may be great enough to break the glass envelope. For this reason, most modern x-ray tubes use a dynabrake, which is a device that slows the rotating anode immediately after exposure. This reduces gyroscopic effect and possible damage to the tube. However, the technologist should avoid rapidly changing direction on a rotating-anode x-ray tube.

Chapter 3—Review Questions

1. The cathode:
   a. is the positively charged electrode in the x-ray tube
   b. serves as the source of electrons
   c. is composed of a filament and a focusing cup
   d. two of the above
   e. all of the above
2. Which of the following properties of tungsten make it ideal for the construction of the filament?
   a. It has a high melting point.
   b. It can be drawn into a fine wire.
   c. It has a low atomic number.
   d. two of the above
   e. all of the above
3. The boiling off of electrons is termed:
   a. space-charge effect
   b. the electron cloud
   c. thermionic emission
   d. field emission
   e. electron boiling
4. Which of the following statements about the focusing cup is true?
   a. The focusing cup houses the filament.
   b. The focusing cup is positively charged.
   c. The focusing cup contributes to focal spot bloom.
   d. two of the above
   e. all of the above
5. The anode:
   a. serves to decelerate the electrons
   b. is the positively charged electrode of the x-ray tube
   c. serves to store and dissipate heat
   d. two of the above
   e. all of the above
6. Which of the following structures provides support for the anode and the cathode and contains the vacuum necessary for x-ray production?
   a. the glass envelope
   b. the tube housing
   c. the focusing cup
   d. the diode
   e. none of the above

7. What is the primary purpose of the rotating anode in an x-ray tube?
   a. to take advantage of the line-focus principle
   b. to increase the heat-loading capabilities of the x-ray tube
   c. to increase the mass of the heat sink
   d. two of the above
   e. all of the above

8. Which of the following statements about the line-focus principle is true?
   a. The lower the target angle, the smaller the effective focal spot becomes.
   b. As the target angle is decreased, the x-ray field size is increased.
   c. As the target angle is decreased, the heel effect becomes less pronounced.
   d. As the target angle is increased, the heat-loading capabilities are decreased.
   e. none of the above

9. Which of the following is the correct formula for heat units for three-phase equipment?
   a. $HU = kVp^2 \times mA \times S \times 1.35$
   b. $HU = kVp \times mA \times S$
   c. $HU = kVp \times mA \times S \times 1.35$
   d. $HU = mA \times S \times 1.35$
   e. none of the above

10. Which of the following modifications of the typical x-ray tube increases the heat-loading capabilities?
    a. the use of a molybdenum target
    b. the use of a metal-center section
    c. the use of a cold cathode
    d. the use of graphite backing on the anode
    e. all of the above

11. Which of the following statements is true about the heel effect?
    a. It is the result of decreased x-ray intensity at the cathode end of the x-ray tube.
    b. It is a consequence of the line-focus principle.
    c. It is most pronounced with short source image receptor distance (SID) and large fields.
    d. two of the above
    e. all of the above

12. Radiation produced in the x-ray tube when electrons interact with matter other than the target is termed:
    a. characteristic radiation
    b. off-focus radiation
    c. stem radiation
    d. two of the above
    e. all of the above

13. Which of the following materials is used in the construction of mammography tubes?
    a. molybdenum target
    b. beryllium window
    c. tungsten filament
    d. two of the above
    e. all of the above

14. Which of the following are characteristics of an exposure used to warm up an x-ray tube?
    a. small focal spot
    b. short exposure time
    c. high kVp
    d. high mA
    e. two of the above
    f. all of the above
    g. none of the above

15. What is the proper sequence for making a radiographic exposure?
    a. Activate the rotor, give breathing instructions, and then make the exposure.
    b. Give breathing instructions, activate the rotor, wait several seconds, then make the exposure.
    c. Activate the rotor and exposure buttons, then give breathing instructions quickly.
    d. Give breathing instructions, then activate the rotor and exposure buttons simultaneously.

4

The X-Ray Generating System

OBJECTIVES

After completing Chapter 4, you should be able to:

1. Define the following terms:
   line voltage compensator
   rectification
   transformer
2. Discuss the three types of transformers used in an x-ray generating system.
3. Discuss the primary controls of the x-ray circuit.
4. Discuss rectification and single-phase versus three-phase power.

The x-ray generating system is a complex electronic device; an extensive discussion of its elements is beyond the scope of this text. This chapter presents the major components of the x-ray generating system to familiarize the technologist with their function.

The x-ray generating system can be divided into two major sections: the high-voltage side and the low-voltage side. The high-voltage side components include the milliampere meter, the high-voltage transformer, and the x-ray tube. The low-voltage side components include the line voltage compensator, autotransformer, kilovoltage selector, and timer.

Transformers

The purpose of a *transformer* is to change voltage from one level to another. A transformer consists of two coils of wire, insulated from one another and wrapped around a single iron core. These coils are the primary and secondary coils. Depending on the design, transformers can increase or decrease voltage. A transformer that increases voltage is a *step-up transformer*, and a transformer that decreases voltage is a *step-down transformer*.

The purpose of a **transformer** *is to change voltage from one level to another.*

A transformer that increases voltage is a **step-up transformer,** *and a transformer that decreases voltage is a* **step-down transformer.**

To function, transformers take advantage of the principle that when an electric current passes through a wire or coil, a magnetic field arises around the wire or coil. Conversely, if a wire or coil passes through a magnetic field, an electric current is induced. In the transformer, a moving magnetic field is created as alternating current is applied to the primary coil. As the magnetic field created by the primary coil expands and contracts about the secondary coil, an electric current is induced. *The change in voltage between the primary and secondary coils of a transformer is directly proportional to the ratio of turns of wire in each coil.* One hundred turns of wire in the primary coil and 100 turns of wire in the secondary coil would result in no change in voltage induced in the secondary coil. However, 100 turns in the primary coil and 5000 turns in the secondary coil would result in an output voltage 50 times greater than the input. This is stated as:

The change in voltage between the primary and secondary coils of a transformer is directly proportional to the ratio of turns of wire in each coil.

$$\frac{\text{Secondary voltage}}{\text{Primary voltage}} = \frac{\text{Primary turns}}{\text{Secondary turns}}$$

If the input voltage is 240 volts in a transformer with 100 turns in the primary coil and the desired output is 150,000 volts, how many turns are necessary in the secondary coil?

$$\frac{150{,}000 \text{ volts}}{240 \text{ volts}} = \frac{x}{100 \text{ turns}}$$
$$240x = 150{,}000 \times 100$$
$$x = 62{,}500 \text{ turns}$$

To determine the "turns ratio" of this transformer, divide the number of turns of wire in the primary side of the transformer by the number of turns in the secondary side. The turns ratio of this transformer is 625:1.

As stated earlier, energy can be neither created nor destroyed. The total energy applied to a transformer is the product of the voltage and the amperage. Therefore, for any change in voltage, there must be a corresponding change in amperage. If voltage increases, amperage proportionally decreases. Conversely, if voltage decreases, amperage proportionally increases. This is stated as:

$$\frac{\text{Secondary amperage}}{\text{Primary amperage}} = \frac{\text{Primary voltage}}{\text{Secondary voltage}}$$

If a transformer has a secondary amperage of 500 mA with a secondary voltage of 150,000 volts and a primary voltage of 240 volts, what is the primary amperage?

$$\frac{500 \text{ mA}}{x} = \frac{240 \text{ volts}}{150{,}000 \text{ volts}}$$
$$240 \text{ volts} \times x = 500 \text{ mA} \times 150{,}000 \text{ volts}$$
$$240x = 75{,}000{,}000$$
$$x = 312{,}500 \text{ mA or } 312.5 \text{ amperes}$$

The milliamperage can also be calculated using the number of turns in the coils of the transformer or the turns ratio.

Types of Transformers

The purpose of the step-up (high-voltage) transformer is to supply the x-ray tube with the voltage necessary to operate.

The primary purpose of the step-down (filament) transformer is to supply the filament of the x-ray tube with the low voltage it needs to operate.

An x-ray generating system has three types of transformers: (1) the step-up transformer, (2) the step-down transformer, and (3) the autotransformer. The purpose of the step-up (high-voltage) transformer is to supply the x-ray tube with the voltage necessary to operate. The operating voltage is in the range of 25,000 to 150,000 volts (Figure 4-1). The primary purpose of the step-down (filament) transformer is to supply the filament of the x-ray tube with the low voltage it needs to operate. The filament operates at 6 to 10 volts (Figure 4-2). The *autotransformer* is somewhat different in design and more complicated in operation than the step-up and step-down transformers. The

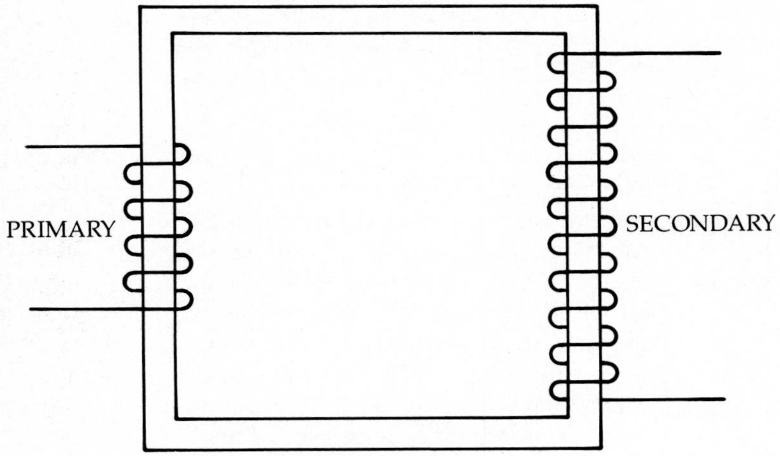

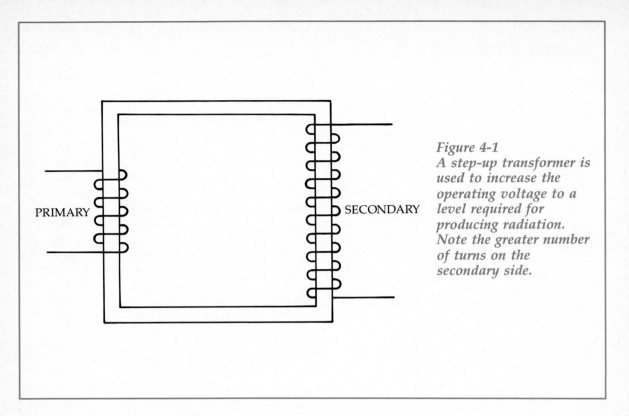

PRIMARY

SECONDARY

Figure 4-1
A step-up transformer is used to increase the operating voltage to a level required for producing radiation. Note the greater number of turns on the secondary side.

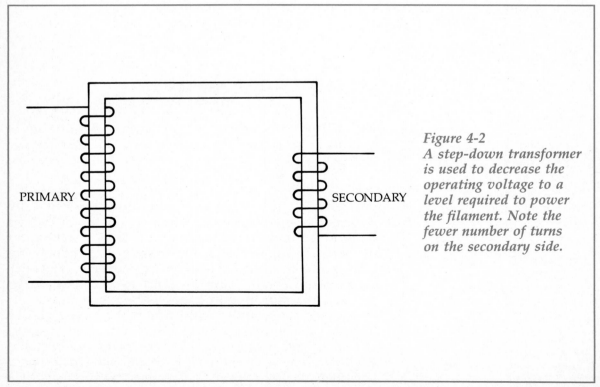

PRIMARY

SECONDARY

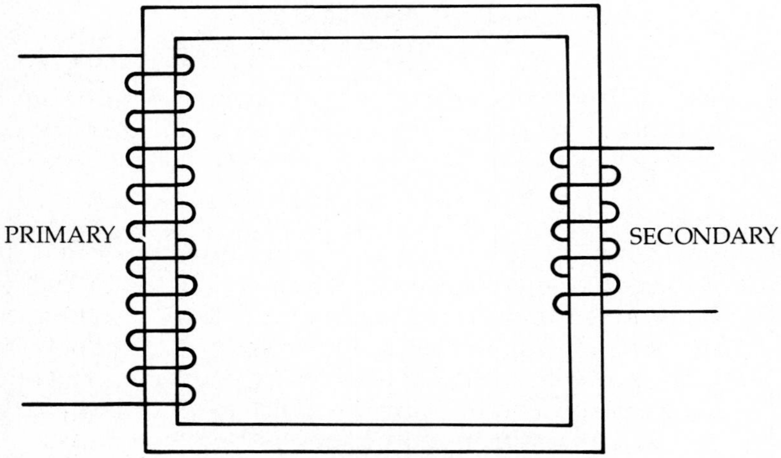

Figure 4-2
A step-down transformer is used to decrease the operating voltage to a level required to power the filament. Note the fewer number of turns on the secondary side.

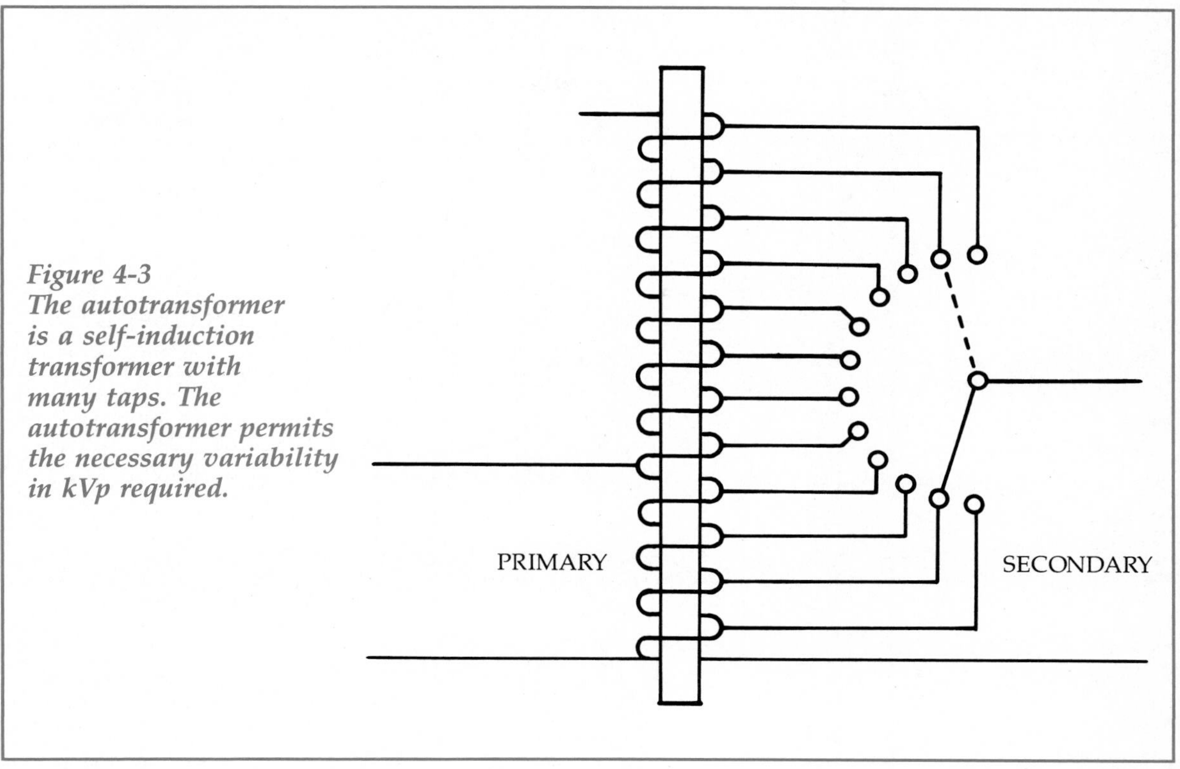

Figure 4-3
The autotransformer is a self-induction transformer with many taps. The autotransformer permits the necessary variability in kVp required.

The purpose of the autotransformer is to allow selection of the voltage applied across the x-ray tube.

purpose of the autotransformer is to allow selection of the voltage applied across the x-ray tube. This is essential to medical radiography and the use of optimum kilovoltage peak (kVp) techniques.

The autotransformer is a single coil of wire and functions through self-induction. The autotransformer also has many taps, which permit changes in the volts/turn ratio and the output voltage. The output voltage of the autotransformer is the input voltage for the high-tension transformer. This permits the variability of kVp necessary for the operation of the x-ray tube (Figure 4-3).

Line Voltage Compensation

The *line voltage compensator* is a device that senses changes in the incoming voltage. This device also allows for either automatic or manual adjustment for the changes. The line voltage compensator is usually on the primary side of the autotransformer. It consists of a number of taps, which permit selection of the appropriate number of windings for the incoming voltage. The line voltage compensator is an important device, since a change of only a few volts in the incoming voltage will change the voltage to the x-ray tube by a few thousand volts. This may result in poor-quality radiographs. The line voltage compensator requires monitoring if it is not automatic.

Primary Controls of the X-Ray Circuit

Despite the differences in radiographic equipment, all radiographic generators have certain controls in common. The technologist must understand these essential controls to control the x-ray beam properly. They include the on/off switch, the filament control or milliampere selector, the milliampere meter, the kilovoltage selector, and the timer. A diagram of an oversimplified x-ray circuit is illustrated in Figure 4-4.

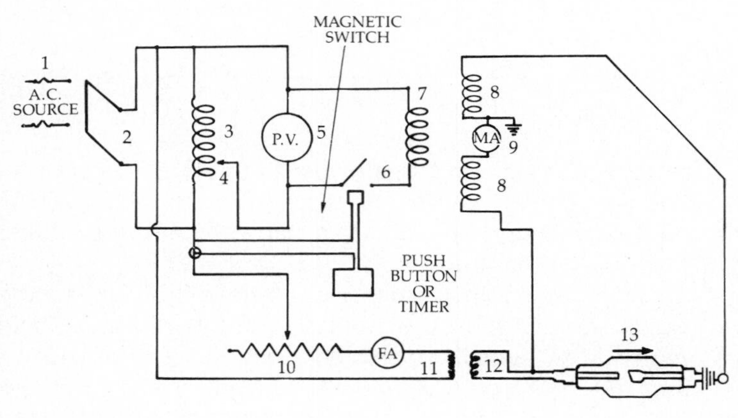

Figure 4-4
Diagram of an oversimplified x-ray circuit helps to demonstrate the relationship of the primary controls.

1. FUSES
2. LINE SWITCH
3. AUTOTRANSFORMER
4. X-RAY VOLTAGE
5. PRIMARY VOLTMETER
6. X-RAY SWITCH
7. X-RAY TRANSFORMER, PRIMARY
8. X-RAY TRANSFORMER, SECONDARY
9. GROUNDED mA METER
10. X-RAY FILAMENT CONTROL
11. FILAMENT TRANSFORMER, PRIMARY
12. FILAMENT TRANSFORMER, SECONDARY
13. X-RAY TUBE

The On/Off Switch

The purpose of the on/off switch is to complete a connection of the generating system to an incoming power supply. Radiographic generators typically require only a few seconds to warm up. Therefore, the radiographic generator should be turned off when not in use. In addition to the on/off switch, the technologist should also be familiar with the location of the main power disconnect switch. In an emergency, the main power disconnect switch will turn off the power to all components of the radiographic unit.

Filament Control or Milliampere Selector

The filament control or milliampere selector controls the tube current. The tube current determines the number of electrons flowing across the x-ray tube. As the filament current increases, filament temperature also increases. As a result, more electrons are "boiled off" from the filament wire.

The milliampere selector functions by changing the resistance in the filament circuit and in turn changing the filament current. Most generators offer a wide variety of milliampere selections, ranging from 50 to 3000 mA. In many generators, selection of milliamperage controls filament or focal spot selection, reducing the possibility of tube failure. Typically, the maximum milliamperage for use with a small focal spot is 100 to 200 mA.

Milliampere Meter

The milliampere meter indicates the actual milliamperage or current passing through the x-ray tube during an exposure. The milliampere meter functions in the high-voltage side of the circuit and displays only during the actual exposure. This meter can detect problems with milliampere calibration. When making an exposure, the technologist should glance at the mA meter. This may provide valuable information relating to equipment calibration.

Kilovoltage Selector

As stated earlier, the autotransformer permits selection of kilovoltage. The kilovoltage selector allows the technologist to control the kilovoltage by selecting the appropriate taps on the autotransformer.

Timer

The timer functions in the low-voltage side of the x-ray circuit and controls the duration of the exposure. Typically, exposure times vary from 1/120 of a second to 6 seconds. The three types of timers used on radiographic units are (1) the mechanical timer, (2) the synchronous timer, and (3) the electronic timer. The mechanical timer resembles a spring-driven kitchen timer. The synchronous timer takes advantage of the alternating current used in the x-ray machine. A small motor that turns one revolution per second powers the synchronous timer. Electronic timers are probably the most frequently used timers in medical radiography equipment. They have these advantages:

1. They produce more accurate and reproducible exposures.
2. They are capable of shorter exposure times.
3. They are typically less prone to failure, thus requiring less service.

Time is one of the two primary factors used to control the quantity of x-rays produced. Together, milliamperage multiplied by exposure time produce *mAs,* the quantity factor for radiation in radiography. Many generators have an mAs meter that displays the selected mAs.

Rectification

The x-ray tube can only safely function when the anode has a positive charge with respect to the cathode. Alternating current changes polarity or direction of flow with each cycle. Therefore, a method to prevent the flow of electrons from the anode to the cathode is necessary. This process is termed *rectification.*

The two types of rectification are half wave and full wave. *Half-wave rectification* takes place in one of two ways. The first type is self-rectification. In *self-rectification,* electrons will only pass across the x-ray tube when the anode is positively charged and the cathode is negatively charged. This occurs because electrons are not available at the anode since the anode temperature is below that necessary for electron emission. If the anode is sufficiently heated, electrons can flow from the anode to the cathode, resulting in cathode damage. Therefore, only dental units and small-output mobile units use this type of rectification.

Rectification *prevents the flow of electrons from the anode to the cathode.*

Half-wave rectification can also be accomplished with a valve tube or rectifier. The *valve tube* or *rectifier* is a diode that only permits the flow of electrons in one direction. Its use suppresses the negative portion of the waveform. Half-wave rectification is inefficient because it uses only one half of the available energy of the alternating current. However, this type of equipment is usually lightweight and inexpensive.

The **valve tube** *or* **rectifier** *is a diode that only permits the flow of electrons in one direction.*

In ***full-wave rectification,*** *the waveform to the x-ray tube is modified to create two positive pulses for each cycle of the alternating current.*

The second type, *full-wave rectification,* requires the use of valve tubes or rectifiers. In full-wave rectification, the waveform to the x-ray tube is modified to create two positive pulses for each cycle of the alternating current. This allows the use of all the energy in each cycle. Full-wave rectification is more efficient than half-wave rectification because it produces two pulses of radiation per cycle rather than one. If a system is using single-phase power, it requires four rectifiers working in two pairs. Each pair permits the positive or negative half-cycle to pass from cathode to anode, respectively, as illustrated in Figure 4-5. Three-phase power requires 6 or 12 rectifiers for full-wave rectification.

Figure 4-5
Diagram of a full-wave rectified x-ray circuit.

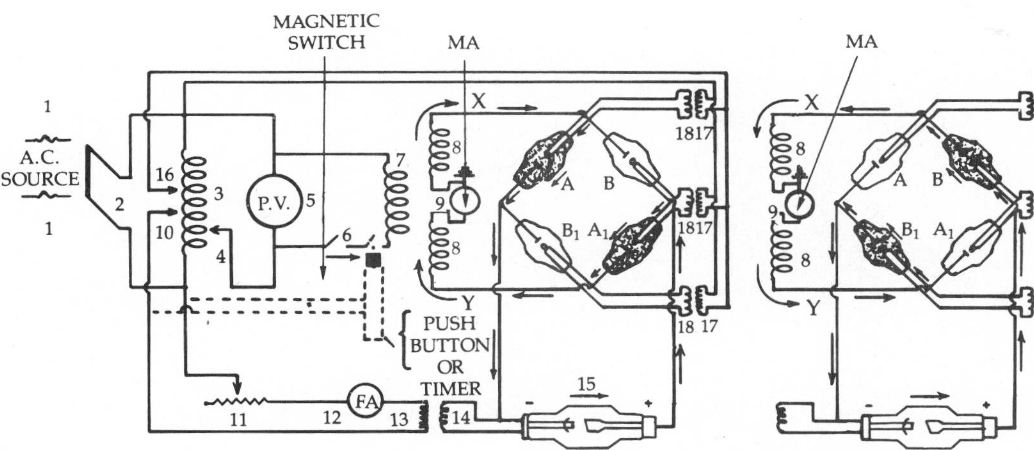

1. FUSES
2. LINE SWITCH
3. AUTO TRANSFORMER
4. X-RAY VOLTAGE CONTROL
5. PRIMARY VOLTMETER
6. X-RAY SWITCH
7. X-RAY TRANSFORMER PRIMARY
8. X-RAY TRANSFORMER, SECONDARY
9. GROUNDED MA-METER (AC)
10. X-RAY FILAMENT VOLTAGE ADJUSTER
11. X-RAY FILAMENT CONTROL
12. FILAMENT AMMETER
13. X-RAY FILAMENT TRANSFORMER, PRIMARY
14. X-RAY FILAMENT TRANSFORMER, SECONDARY
15. X-RAY TUBE
16. VALVE TUBE FILAMENT ADJUSTER
17. VALVE TUBE FILAMENT TRANSFORMER, PRIMARY
18. VALVE TUBE FILAMENT TRANSFORMER, SECONDARY

A-A_1 B-B_1 — VALVE TUBES

Single-Phase versus Three-Phase Power

To this point, our discussion has centered around single-phase power. *Single-phase power* has a frequency of 60 cycles per second, and each cycle consists of a positive and negative pulse. Full-wave rectification inverts the negative peak of an alternating current, resulting in two positive pulses. The production of x-rays using single-phase power is inefficient. This is because of the relatively short time that high voltage passes across the tube and the relatively long period that low voltage passes across the tube, as demonstrated in Figure 4-6.

Single-phase power *has a frequency of 60 cycles per second, and each cycle consists of a positive and negative pulse.*

One method of increasing the efficiency of x-ray production is the use of three-phase power. *Three-phase power* consists of three single-phase waveforms that are 120 degrees out of phase from one another, as demonstrated in Figure 4-7. Three-phase power is full-wave rectified, producing a six-pulse waveform similar to Figure 4-8. When the waveform passes across the x-ray tube, it uses only the high-voltage component. This increases the efficiency of

Three-phase power *consists of three single-phase waveforms that are 120 degrees out of phase from one another.*

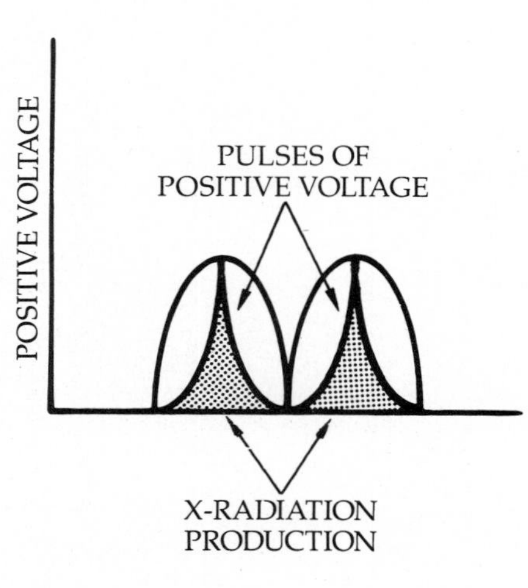

Figure 4-6
Diagram demonstrating the inefficiency of single-phase waveforms. The amount of radiation produced is significantly less than that of the electric energy applied across the x-ray tube.

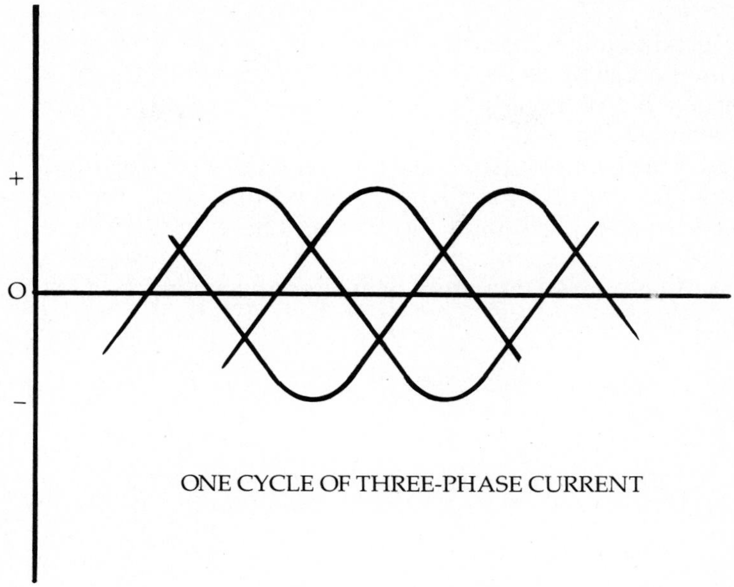

+

O

−

ONE CYCLE OF THREE-PHASE CURRENT

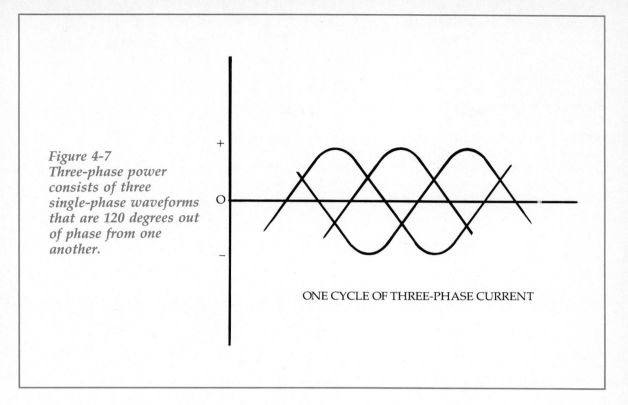

Figure 4-7
Three-phase power consists of three single-phase waveforms that are 120 degrees out of phase from one another.

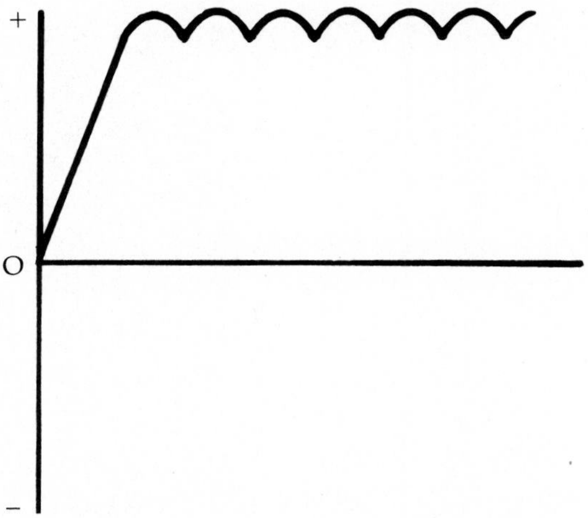

+

O

−

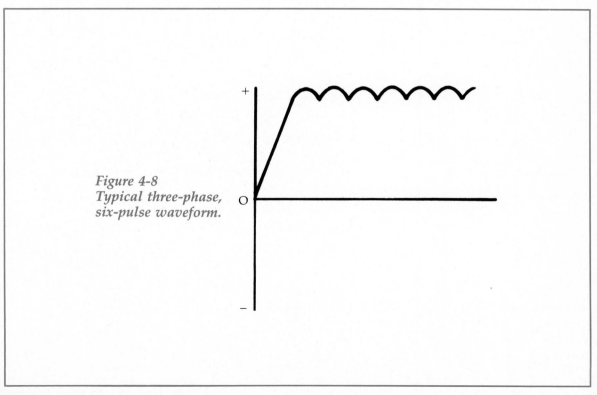

Figure 4-8
Typical three-phase, six-pulse waveform.

x-ray production, since the ratio of high voltage/low voltage time increases to the high side. This results in the production of a greater number of photons at all energy levels. The average energy of the resultant beam is slightly higher. The three-phase generator decreases patient dose slightly and permits a reduction in exposure. Also, the increased efficiency permits the use of higher milliampere stations and extremely short exposure times. A primary use of three-phase generators is in special procedures such as angiography.

Chapter 4—Review Questions

1. Which of the following statements about transformers is true?
   a. Transformers function to change voltage from one level to another.
   b. A moving magnetic field is created as alternating current is applied to a primary coil.
   c. The total energy applied to a transformer is the product of the voltage and the amperage.
   d. If the voltage is increased, the amperage is proportionally decreased.
   e. two of the above
   f. all of the above
2. A transformer has a secondary amperage of 300 mA with a secondary voltage of 100,000 volts and a primary voltage of 220 volts. What is the primary amperage?
   a. 136,363.63 amperes
   b. 136.36 mA
   c. 0.136 amperes
   d. 13.63 amperes
   e. 136.36 amperes
3. What type of transformer is used to supply the filament of the x-ray tube?
   a. step-up transformer
   b. step-down transformer
   c. autotransformer
4. What type of transformer is constructed of a single coil of wire and functions through self-induction?
   a. step-up transformer
   b. step-down transformer
   c. autotransformer
5. What device in the x-ray circuit senses changes in the incoming voltage and allows for adjustment of the incoming voltage?
   a. autotransformer
   b. step-up transformer
   c. line voltage compensator
   d. rectifier
   e. none of the above

6. Which device controls the number of electrons flowing across the x-ray tube?
   a. filament control
   b. rectifier
   c. mA meter
   d. line voltage compensator
   e. none of the above
7. What device permits the selection of kV?
   a. step-up transformer
   b. line voltage compensator
   c. autotransformer
   d. rectifier
   e. none of the above
8. What device in the x-ray circuit only permits the flow of electrons in one direction?
   a. autotransformer
   b. mA meter
   c. filament control
   d. rectifier
   e. none of the above
9. What is the primary difference between the self-rectified and full-wave rectified waveforms?
   a. the absence of negative pulses of electricity
   b. the number of positive pulses for each cycle of alternating current
   c. the maximum positive potential of the waveform
   d. two of the above
   e. none of the above
10. How far out of phase are the three single-phase waveforms that comprise three-phase power?
    a. 90 degrees
    b. 120 degrees
    c. 180 degrees
    d. 240 degrees
    e. none of the above

5

Dynamic Imaging

OBJECTIVES

After completing Chapter 5, you should be able to:

1. Define the following terms:
   accelerating anode
   brightness gain
   cinefluorography
   electrostatic focusing lenses
   fluoroscopy
   flux gain
   image intensifier
   input phosphor
   minification gain
   output phosphor
   photocathode
   photopic vision
   scotopic vision
   vignetting
2. Identify the various components of the image intensifier.
3. Describe the relationships and purposes of the various components of cine systems, spot-film cameras, and television systems.
4. Discuss the interrelationships of the imaging subsystems.

Conventional Fluoroscopy

The image produced by x-rays as they pass through an object is not visible until the energy of the x-ray photons is converted by some type of image-recording system. The first images of the human body were demonstrated on fluorescent screens, and fluoroscopy remains an important diagnostic technique today. *Fluoroscopy* is a dynamic imaging technique, or one where motion is evident. This is particularly useful in diagnosis because the motion of various organs and body parts may give important information concerning disease or injury.

Fluoroscopy *is a dynamic imaging technique, or one where motion is evident.*

The simplest type of equipment used to perform fluoroscopy is the fluoroscope. The fluoroscope consists of two major components, an x-ray tube and a fluorescent screen. Normally, the x-ray tube and the fluorescent screen are mounted on a C-arm in order to maintain their alignment (Figure 5-1). The operator positions the patient between the x-ray tube and the screen and moves the C-arm over the parts of the patient to be visualized. Fluoroscopy performed using the simple fluoroscope is often referred to as *conventional fluoroscopy.* The x-ray tube used for conven-

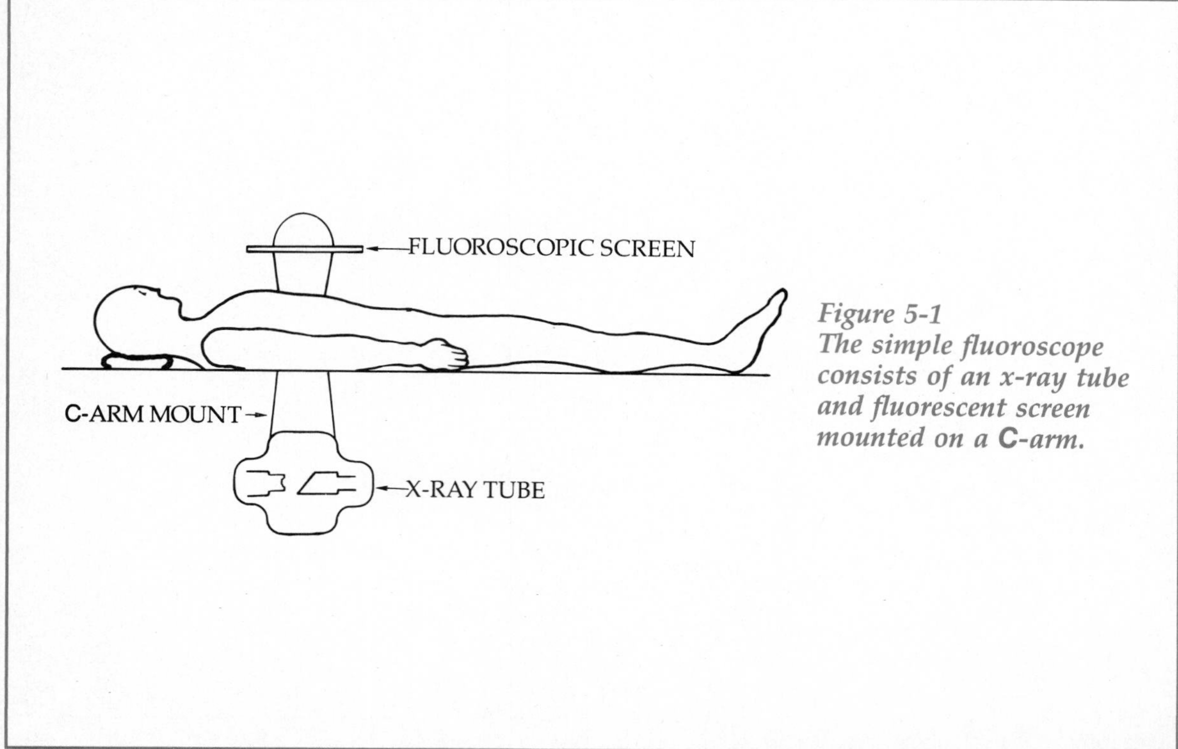

Figure 5-1
The simple fluoroscope consists of an x-ray tube and fluorescent screen mounted on a C-arm.

tional fluoroscopy is identical to the ones used for radiography. However, the tube operates at lower milliampere settings, typically ranging from 3 to 5 mA. The fluorescent screen is usually composed of zinc cadmium sulfide and emits light in the yellow-green spectrum. Since a large amount of radiation will pass through the screen, a sheet of lead glass is placed on top of the screen for radiation protection purposes.

Although the simple fluoroscope was used for many years in radiology and may still be used in some areas, it has several limitations. The light output of the fluorescent screen is very low, and the observer must view the image in complete darkness. Radiologists using conventional fluoroscopy must dark-adapt their eyes for 20 to 30 minutes. Dark adaptation is a physiologic phenomena of the eye in which the eye becomes more sensitive to light after a period in low-level light. This type of vision at a low-light level, *scotopic vision,* is a function of the rods in the retina of the eye. Vision at higher-light levels, *photopic vision,* is a function of the cones in the retina of the eye. Radiologists often wore red goggles between fluoroscopic cases because the red light did not reduce their level of dark adaptation. This permitted them to leave the darkened room and pursue other activities between cases. Unfortunately, the dark-adapted eye is less able to discern detail. Scotopic vision is approximately 10 times less acute than is photopic vision. Therefore, the radiologist's ability to interpret fine detail was reduced by the function of the eye in low-light levels.

The type of vision at a low-light level, **scotopic vision,** *is a function of the rods in the retina of the eye. Vision at higher-light levels,* **photopic vision,** *is a function of the cones in the retina of the eye.*

Scotopic vision is approximately 10 times less acute than is photopic vision.

Image-Intensified Fluoroscopy

In the early 1950s, the development of the image intensifier or image amplifier revolutionized fluoroscopy. The image intensifier allowed the viewer to see the image with photopic vision. This increased visual acuity and eliminated the need for dark adaptation. In addition, image intensification produced an image bright enough to allow the use of cine systems, spot-film cameras, and television for image recording.

The *image intensifier* is an electronic device that receives the x-ray image, converts it to a light image, and then substantially increases the light intensity of the image. The image-intensifier tube is an evacuated glass envelope with five major components: (1) the input phosphor, (2) the photocathode, (3) the accelerating anode, (4) the electrostatic focusing lenses, and (5) the output phosphor, as illustrated in Figure 5-2.

The **image intensifier** *is an electronic device that receives the x-ray image, converts it to a light image, and then substantially increases the light intensity of the image.*

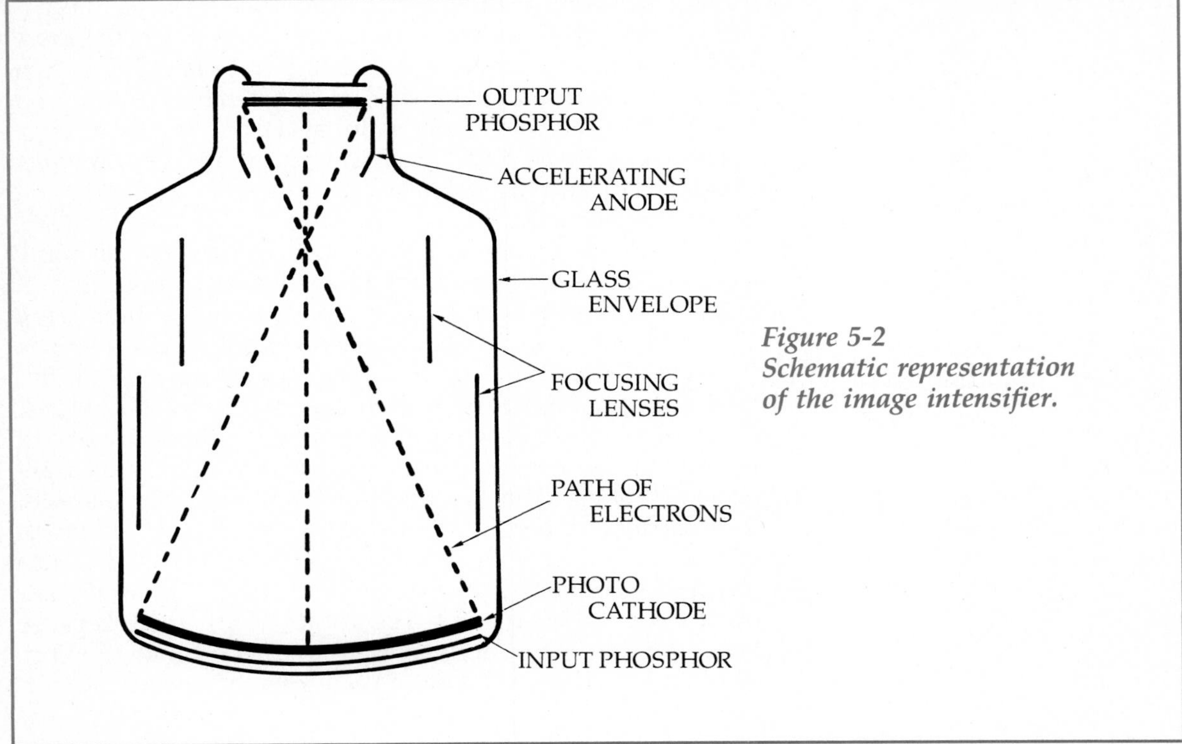

Figure 5-2
Schematic representation of the image intensifier.

The *input phosphor* of an image intensifier is a fluorescent screen composed of zinc cadmium sulfide in first-generation intensifiers or cesium iodide in second-generation intensifiers. The input phosphor is located on the inside surface of the intensifier, where it receives the incoming x-ray photons and converts them into a light image. The input phosphor of the image intensifier is round, and its diameter is the value used to describe the size of the intensifier. Common input phosphor sizes include 14, 12, 10, 9, 7, and 5 inches.

The ***input phosphor*** *converts incoming x-ray photons into a light image.*

The *photocathode* is placed on top of the input phosphor, and the two layers are in intimate contact, separated only by a very thin transparent layer. The transparent layer serves only to prevent the photocathode and input phosphor from chemically reacting with each other. The photocathode is usually composed of compounds of cesium and antimony, which convert the light, produced by the input phosphor, to electrons. This process of converting light to electrons is *photoemission,* and the photocathode is referred to as the *photoemissive layer.* The pattern of electrons produced by the photocathode corresponds to the

The ***photocathode*** *converts the light produced by the input phosphor into electrons.*

The process of converting light to electrons is ***photoemission,*** *and the photocathode is referred to as the* ***photoemissive layer.***

light image produced by the input phosphor. Areas of bright light will produce more electrons, and areas of less light will produce fewer electrons. The major function of the photocathode is to convert the light image of the input phosphor to a corresponding electrostatic image. Also, the photocathode serves as the cathode of the image intensifier and is at ground potential.

The **accelerating anode** *functions to draw the electrons from the photocathode and accelerate them.*

The *accelerating anode* is located at the opposite end of the image intensifier. Its function is to draw the electrons away from the photocathode and accelerate them, with tremendous velocity, toward the output screen. The accelerating anode has a positive charge of 25,000 volts.

The **electrostatic focusing lenses** *focus and invert the electron beam.*

The *electrostatic focusing lenses* are a series of metal rings, usually plated around the interior sides of the intensifier. The lenses have a positive charge, each successive lens being of a higher voltage (e.g., +300, +2000, and +5000 volts) than the previous. As the electrons generated by the photocathode travel toward the output phosphor, the electrostatic focusing lenses focus and invert the electron beam. The focusing lenses influence the electrons but do not capture them due to their high level of acceleration and kinetic energy. For proper focusing, each electron must travel exactly the same distance before striking the output phosphor. To achieve this, the input phosphor and photocathode are curved so that every point on the photocathode is approximately equidistant from the output phosphor.

The **output phosphor** *converts the accelerated electron into a light image of greater brightness.*

The *output phosphor* is a thin layer of very small particles of zinc cadmium sulfide. The accelerated electrons strike the output phosphor with great energy, resulting in more light photons being generated than were originally present on the input phosphor. The thin layer and small particulate size of the output phosphor help to maintain the detail present in the original image on the input phosphor. Output phosphor size is usually 1 inch.

Flux gain *is the increase in brightness as a result of the acceleration of the electron.*

Minification gain *is the increase in brightness as a result of minifying the image.*

The gain in brightness produced by the image intensifier is a product of two separate phenomena. First, the acceleration of the electrons from the input phosphor to the output phosphor results in approximately a 50-fold increase in light output and is termed *flux gain.* Second, the reduction in size of the image from the input phosphor to the output phosphor results in more light photons in a smaller area. This results in increased brightness and is termed *minification gain.* Minification gain is determined by the square of the diameter of the input phosphor divided by the square of the diameter of the output phosphor. An image intensifier with a 9-inch input phosphor and a

1-inch output phosphor would produce a minification gain of 81 times the intensity of the input phosphor. The product of flux gain and minification gain is termed the *brightness gain* of the intensifier. The brightness gain of contemporary image intensifiers ranges from 1000 to 5000; however, it decreases with use and age.

Brightness gain *is the product of flux gain and minification gain.*

The image intensifier is contained in a lead-lined metal cover that is open at the input and output ends. The intensifier is mounted on a fluoroscope where the fluorescent screen would be for conventional fluoroscopy. The output phosphor is coupled to one of two viewing devices. The first and simplest viewing device, termed *mirror optics,* is a series of lenses and mirrors that magnify and reflect the image to a viewer. Mirror optics are still widely used, but they are limited by the loss of some of the image brightness, and only one viewer at a time can see the image. The other viewing option involves the use of a television system to view the image on the output phosphor. Television systems are discussed later in this chapter.

The brightness of the image on an image intensifier can be increased by increasing the fluoroscopic milliamperage (mA) or kilovoltage potential (kVp). As patient size or body part density increases, the brightness may decline due to a reduction of x-ray photons reaching the input phosphor. It is necessary to increase the number or energy of the incident x-ray photons to maintain the appropriate brightness of the image. On earlier fluoroscopic equipment, fluoroscopic mA and kVp controls can be adjusted by the operator to maintain an optimum image. On newer equipment, a photoelectric cell is often positioned to measure the brightness of the output phosphor. The photoelectric cell is attached to a circuit that adjusts the fluoroscopic kVp or mA to maintain a preset level of brightness at the output phosphor. Some fluoroscopic units are capable of adjusting both mA and kVp to maintain brightness. This may be advantageous because increasing the kVp alone may increase output phosphor brightness, but this may also result in quantum mottle, which is a grainy image from too few photons interacting with the input phosphor. The automatic adjustment of technical factors to maintain the brightness of the fluoroscopic image is called automatic brightness control (ABC) or automatic brightness stabilization (ABS).

The automatic adjustment of technical factors to maintain the brightness of the fluoroscopic image is called **automatic brightness control (ABC) or automatic brightness stabilization (ABS).**

The image quality of an image intensifier is somewhat difficult to compare to conventional fluoroscopy. The most significant factor in image quality of the image intensifier is that the *brightness level of the image increases.* Image bright-

The most significant factor in image quality of the image intensifier is that the **brightness level of the image increases.**

ness increases enough that the radiologist can use photopic vision and see detail not previously visible. In addition, the image intensifier increases contrast, which also aids in the perception of detail. However, the image intensifier does not resolve as much detail as a conventional fluoroscopic screen. The apparently improved image is simply a result of the radiologist's use of photopic vision.

Vignetting *is a fall off of brightness at the periphery of the field of an image intensifier.*

The image intensifier also distorts the image slightly by enlarging the image at the periphery of the field. The resolution at the periphery of the field is also slightly less than at the center of the field. Intensifiers also produce a "fall off" in brightness at the periphery of the field, which is termed *vignetting.* All three of these phenomena may not be particularly objectionable during routine fluoroscopy, but they do result in a reduction of image quality as the structures observed leave the center of the field.

Image intensifiers with smaller input phosphors have superior images; however, many applications require larger image intensifiers. In an effort to resolve the need for high-quality images and larger fields of view, dual- or triple-field intensifiers were developed. These multiple-field intensifiers are large-input phosphor devices that are electronically focused to view a smaller field size. Triple-field intensifiers may have 14-, 7- and 5-inch fields, whereas dual fields often have 9- and 6-inch fields. The dual-field or triple-field intensifier may seem to be the perfect solution to the field size problem; however, they have two drawbacks. First, multiple-field intensifiers are more expensive than a single-field intensifier. Second, when the intensifier focuses to a smaller field size, the minification gain is reduced. Thus, the x-ray machine automatically increases the exposure factors to compensate for the loss of brightness.

Cine Systems

Cinefluorography *is recording the fluoroscopic image with a motion picture or cine camera.*

The first widely accepted method to record the dynamic image produced by the image intensifier was cinefluorography. *Cinefluorography* is recording the fluoroscopic image with a motion picture or cine camera. The motion picture camera used is a commercial variety, and cinefluorography cameras are available in either 16 mm or 35 mm. Although 16 mm cameras are still in use, most cine systems today are for cardiac angiography and use 35 mm cameras, which are better suited to cardiac studies.

In a typical cine system, the image from the image intensifier enters an image distribution box, where the image can be diverted by mirrors to one or more recording systems. When using a cine camera, the distribution box diverts part of the image to the cine camera via a semitransparent mirror. The image enters the camera through a lens and passes through the rectangular aperture of the camera. The aperture is simply an opening allowing the light to pass through to the film. Since the film cannot be exposed while it is transported, the light coming through the aperture is blocked while the film is moving and allowed to pass through while the film is still. This is accomplished by the shutter, which is a rotating half-disk, as illustrated in Figure 5-3. The rotation of the shutter is synchronized with the motion of the pull-down arm. The pull-down arm engages the drive holes in the film and advances the film one frame, positioning it to receive the next exposure. The film is held in position against the aperture by a pressure plate. This ensures that the film stays in the focal plane of the lenses. A schematic of the cine camera is illustrated in Figure 5-4.

An electric synchronous motor drives the cine camera, and the number of frames per second that are re-

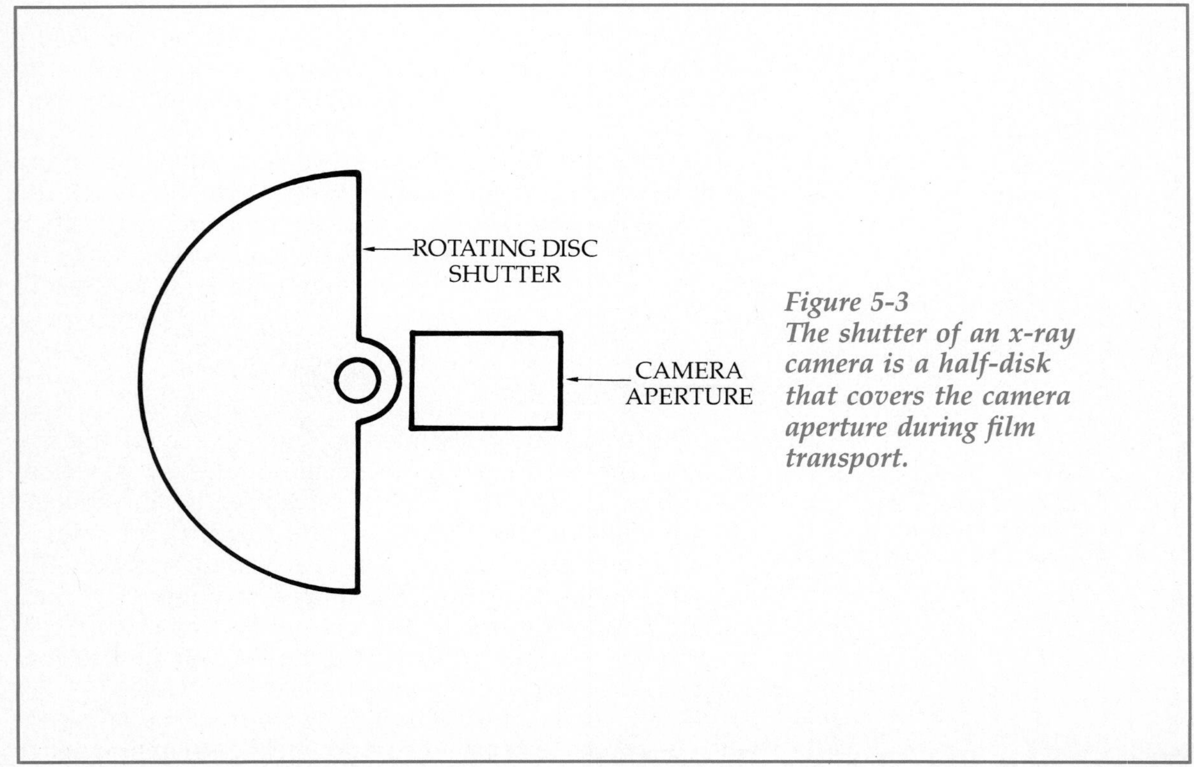

Figure 5-3
The shutter of an x-ray camera is a half-disk that covers the camera aperture during film transport.

corded is normally divisible by 60. The most common frame rates include 7.5, 15, 30, and 60 frames per second. As stated earlier, the shutter is closed during the transport of the film. It takes approximately the same amount of time to transport the film as it does to expose it.

When performing cinefluorography at 60 frames per second, the maximum exposure time of the film is 1/120 of a second. Since the shutter of the camera is closed approximately 50 percent of the time during a cine run, it makes little sense to expose the patient continuously to radiation. It would reduce the heat units on the x-ray tube and substantially reduce the patient exposure if the x-ray exposure was pulsed and synchronized to the open phases of the shutter. The pulsing of the x-ray tube is accomplished with a thyratron or grid-controlled x-ray tube, which allows the instantaneous on/off control of the x-ray exposure.

Cine requires considerably more milliamperage than conventional fluoroscopy. This is largely due to the short time available to allow the light entering the camera to produce an image on the film. The greater amount of radiation results in fairly high exposure to the patient. This is one of

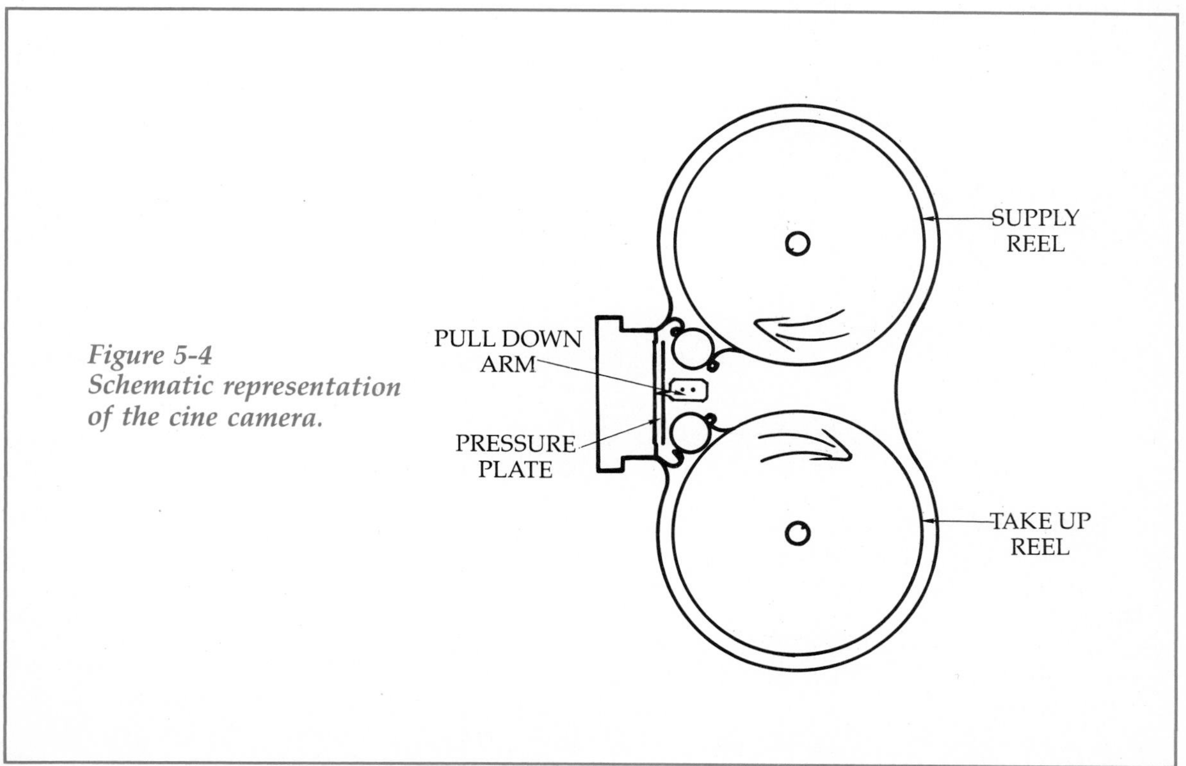

Figure 5-4
Schematic representation of the cine camera.

the major disadvantages to cinefluorography. Patient exposure depends on many factors, including frame rate, image intensifier field size, and the type of film used. Other disadvantages of cinefluorography include (1) stress on the x-ray tube, (2) the cost of the equipment, and (3) the need for special processing and special viewing projectors. The major advantages of cinefluorography, when compared to other dynamic imaging techniques, are (1) excellent detail resolution, (2) the ability to stop motion, and (3) the ability to examine individual high-resolution still frames.

Spot-Film Cameras

The spot-film camera is very similar in function to a cine camera. The spot-film camera, however, uses larger film and usually is not capable of more than 12 frames a second. Spot-film cameras use 90 mm to 105 mm roll film or 100 mm sheets of cut film. The larger film format allows viewing of the images without the use of projection or magnification devices. Since the image is recorded from the image intensifier, less radiation exposure is required when compared to conventional spot films; however, the exposure is higher than that required for fluoroscopy.

The major advantages of spot-film cameras include (1) lower patient exposure, (2) less wear and tear on the x-ray tube, (3) multiple films per second capability, (4) elimination of the need to change cassettes, (5) reduced examination time for many procedures, and (6) reduced film cost. The major disadvantages of spot-film cameras include (1) lesser resolution (compared to conventional spot films), (2) limited field size (controlled by the size of the image intensifier), (3) the cost and maintenance of the equipment, and (4) the problem of processing roll or cut film in automatic processors.

Television Systems and Videotape Recording

As stated earlier, one of the two options for viewing the output of the image intensifier is a television system. With a television monitoring system, the output phosphor of the image intensifier is coupled to a television pickup tube. Three types of television tubes have been used for recording image-intensified fluoroscopy: the vidicon, plumbicon, and image orthicon. The *image orthicon* has never been widely used because of its cost and temperature sensitivity. The *vidicon* has been the least expensive and most

The **vidicon** *has been the least expensive and most widely used TV camera for fluoroscopy.*

widely used TV camera for fluoroscopy, although the *plumbicon* has had the advantage of better contrast and less image lag. In recent years, electronic advances in the design of the vidicon have increased its contrast and reduced the image lag to the point that the vidicon rivals the plumbicon camera.

The television pickup tube has a light-sensitive target plate composed of a thin film of photoconductive material. When light strikes the photoconductive material, it produces an electronic image, much like the photoconductive layer of the image intensifier. An electron beam scans the electronic image in 525 horizontal lines 30 times a second. This electronic scanning converts the image to an electronic signal, which is transmitted to a television monitor. The television monitor has an electron gun that repeats the 525-line scanning pattern on the fluorescent screen of the TV monitor's picture tube. Areas with greater electric charges on the TV pickup tube's photoconductive layer are reproduced on the TV monitor's picture tube, resulting in a corresponding bright spot on the fluorescent screen. The pattern of bright spots along the 525-line screen results in a visible television picture.

The major advantage of television monitoring of the fluoroscopic image is that brightness and contrast are electronically controlled. Additionally, the television monitor permits viewing by more than one person, which is extremely useful in teaching situations. Television monitoring also allows for recording the image on one of several electronic media. Disadvantages of television systems include lower resolution of detail than mirror optics, although this may be offset by the gains in contrast and brightness. Also, some television monitoring equipment uses a greater number of lines per inch to increase resolution. The other disadvantages are related to the cost of purchasing and maintaining the TV-monitored system.

Television monitoring allows the recording of electronic information produced by the television pickup camera on magnetic media. The most familiar method of accomplishing this is through the use of the videotape recorder. In recent years, the videotape recorder has gained widespread acceptance in the home and in medical imaging. Its price has also decreased while its reliability has substantially increased. The major advantages of videotape recording of images include (1) no additional exposure to the patient, (2) instant playback, (3) no processing of film, and (4) ease of operation. Its major disadvantages center around its lower resolution. However, high-resolution systems are available that produce excellent images, although they are far more expensive.

Other methods of recording images from the television monitoring system include magnetic disk recorders, laser disk recorders, and multiformat cameras. A magnetic disk recorder functions much as a videotape recorder, only it uses a rigid magnetic disk and usually records single television frames. The laser disk also functions similar to a magnetic disk recorder, except the image is recorded and read from a reflective metallic disk sealed in plastic. The laser disk has the disadvantage of not being able to record over previous recordings. Once a disk is recorded, the images are permanent. The multiformat camera is simply a television monitor with a single lens or series of lenses that allow photographing of the TV image on single-emulsion film. Multiformat cameras can record multiple images on a single sheet of film. Common formats are 6, 9, and 12 images on a single sheet of film, although some cameras allow for more.

Chapter 5—Review Questions

1. What is one of the major drawbacks of conventional fluoroscopy?
   a. the cost of the equipment
   b. the low-light level of the image
   c. the use of photopic vision
   d. two of the above
   e. all of the above
2. Which of the following devices revolutionized fluoroscopy in the 1950s?
   a. fluorescent screen
   b. image intensifier
   c. cine
   d. television
   e. spot-film cameras
3. The input phosphor of second-generation image intensifiers is composed of what phosphor?
   a. calcium tungstate
   b. zinc cadmium sulfide
   c. cesium iodide
   d. none of the above
4. What is the function of the input phosphor of an image intensifier?
   a. to convert x-ray energy to electrons
   b. to convert light to electrons
   c. to convert electrons to x-rays
   d. to convert x-rays to light
5. What is the function of the photocathode of an image intensifier?
   a. to convert x-ray energy to electrons
   b. to convert light to electrons
   c. to convert electrons to x-rays
   d. to convert x-rays to light
6. The photocathode is:
   a. composed of cesium iodide
   b. referred to as the photoemissive layer
   c. the cathode of the image intensifier
   d. two of the above
   e. all of the above

7. What part of the image intensifier draws the electrons away from the photocathode?
   a. electrostatic focusing lenses
   b. output phosphor
   c. accelerating anode
   d. flux gain
   e. photocathode

8. The output phosphor of an image intensifier:
   a. converts electrons to light
   b. is smaller in diameter than the input phosphor
   c. is composed of zinc cadmium sulfide
   d. two of the above
   e. all of the above

9. The increased brightness achieved with an image intensifier is the result of what two phenomena?
   a. acceleration gain and photoconductivity
   b. flux gain and acceleration gain
   c. minification gain and acceleration gain
   d. anode gain and cathode gain
   e. none of the above

10. When comparing conventional fluoroscopy with image-intensified fluoroscopy, which of the following statements is not true?
    a. The radiologist uses scotopic vision with image-intensified fluoroscopy.
    b. Conventional fluoroscopy has better resolution of detail.
    c. The image-intensified image is brighter.
    d. The image-intensified image is distorted.
    e. none of the above

11. Vignetting is:
    a. distortion of the image
    b. a fall-off in brightness at the periphery of the field
    c. decreased resolution at the periphery of the field
    d. none of the above

12. Cine:
    a. is the recording of the dynamic image on film
    b. requires pulsing of the x-ray beam
    c. reduces patient exposure
    d. two of the above
    e. none of the above

13. Which of the following are major differences between cine and spot film cameras?
    a. film size
    b. frame rate
    c. patient dose
    d. two of the above
    e. all of the above
14. Which of the following is not a major disadvantage of spot-film cameras?
    a. improved resolution when compared to conventional films
    b. decreased film costs
    c. limited field size
    d. two of the above
    e. all of the above
15. Which of the following television tubes is most widely used for fluoroscopic imaging?
    a. orthicon
    b. plumbicon
    c. vidicon
16. When comparing mirror optics to a television system, which of the following is true?
    a. The TV system provides increased resolution and contrast.
    b. Mirror optics provide better resolution, and television provides better contrast.
    c. The two systems are equivalent in both resolution and contrast.
    d. none of the above
17. Which of the following is not a method of recording the television image?
    a. multiformat camera
    b. cine
    c. videotape recorder
    d. videodisk recorder
    e. none of the above
18. Which of the following is a disadvantage of both television systems and spot-film cameras?
    a. film cost
    b. maintenance costs
    c. decreased resolution
    d. two of the above
    e. none of the above

19. Which of the following imaging techniques places the greatest stress on the x-ray tube?
    a. conventional fluoroscopy
    b. image-intensified fluoroscopy
    c. cine
    d. spot-film cameras
    e. television systems

20. Which of the following methods does not record the dynamic nature of fluoroscopy?
    a. spot-film camera
    b. spot-film device
    c. multiformat camera
    d. magnetic disk recorder
    e. all of the above

6

X-Ray Films, Intensifying Screens, and Cassettes

OBJECTIVES

After completing Chapter 6, you should be able to:

1. Define the following terms:
   antihalation layer
   base
   emulsion
   intensification factor
   intensifying screens
   intrinsic efficiency
   latent image
   parallax
   phosphorescence
   screen efficiency
   sensitivity speck
   system speed
2. Discuss the use of intensifying screens.
3. Discuss the processes of radiographic duplication and subtraction.
4. Discuss technique considerations and radiation protection as they relate to the use of intensifying screens.

The most common method of receiving and storing the radiographic image is through the use of photographic film. All photographic film is sensitive to both light and x-radiation. X-ray film is photographic film modified to better meet the needs of medical radiography.

X-Ray Film Construction

X-ray film consists of a transparent base on which the light-sensitive *emulsion* is coated. X-ray film used for most purposes has emulsion coated on both sides of the base. The double emulsion reduces the amount of radiation required to produce a satisfactory image. The emulsion is bound tightly to the base by an adhesive layer. An overcoat or supercoat protects the emulsion from mechanical damage. Figure 6-1 illustrates a cross section of x-ray film construction.

X-ray film consists of a transparent base on which the light-sensitive **emulsion** *is coated.*

The x-ray film *base* is a transparent plastic that provides support for the photographic emulsion. The x-ray film base must be strong and flat and have the right degree

The x-ray film **base** *is a transparent plastic that provides support for the photographic emulsion.*

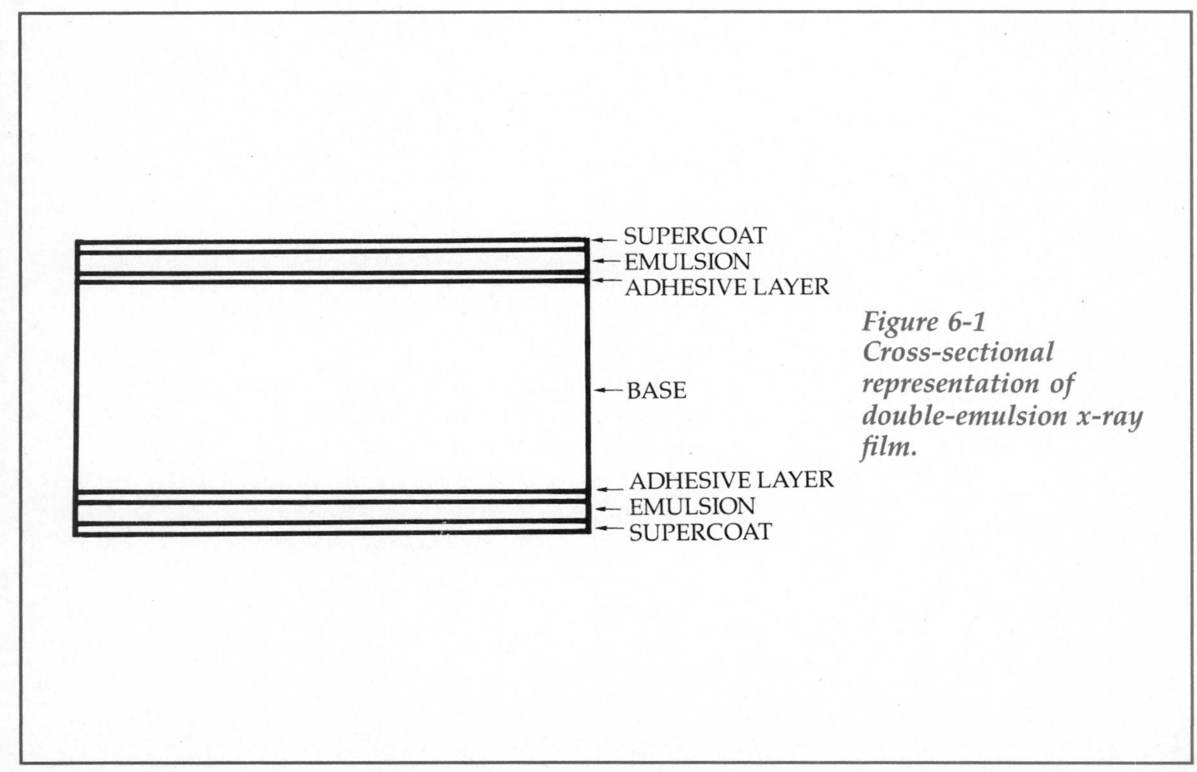

Figure 6-1 Cross-sectional representation of double-emulsion x-ray film.

of stiffness for handling and processing. The base also must absorb little water and maintain its size and shape during processing. X-ray film base is usually tinted blue, although many special-application films have no tint in the base. Tint is eliminated from the base when it would interfere with density or contrast, such as with image-camera films.

The **gelatin** *keeps the silver halide crystals well dispersed and gives permanence to the emulsion.*

The two most important components of x-ray film emulsion are gelatin and silver halide. The *gelatin,* made from cattle bone, must meet several important requirements. The gelatin keeps the silver halide crystals well dispersed and gives permanence to the emulsion. The gelatin emulsion also allows rapid processing because developing solutions easily penetrate it.

The **silver halide crystals** *are the light-sensitive portion of the emulsion.*

Silver halide is in the form of tiny crystals dispersed throughout the emulsion. The silver halide crystals are the light-sensitive portion of the emulsion. Silver halide is primarily silver bromide, although a small amount of silver iodide is present.

Latent-Image Production

When a light photon strikes a silver halide crystal, its energy removes an electron from a halogen atom. The free electron or photoelectron is caught by a trap in the crystal. The trap may be an imperfection in the crystal or an added chemical. Sulfur compounds are often added to the emulsion, and they react with the silver halide, creating silver sulfide. Silver sulfide usually forms on the surface of a crystal and is referred to as the sensitivity speck. The *sensitivity speck* provides the location for the formation of the latent image.

The **sensitivity speck** *provides the location for the formation of the latent image.*

When light strikes a silver halide crystal, the photoelectrons begin to collect at the sensitivity speck. The electrons have a negative charge and attract positive silver ions. This change is not visible, but it is the basis for the image produced by film development. The metallic silver serves as a development center when the film is developed. This invisible deposition of metallic silver is the *latent image.*

The invisible deposition of metallic silver is the **latent image.**

When developing the x-ray film, the metallic silver at the sensitivity speck serves as a catalyst for development of the entire crystal. Only those silver halide grains that absorb enough light to form development centers will change to elemental silver.

The tiny particles of black metallic silver that form in the emulsion are too small to be seen. However, the accumulation of the particles in the emulsion attenuates light and results in radiographic density. More radiation interacting with the silver halide would produce greater silver deposition. The more silver deposited in the emulsion, the greater is the radiographic density.

Types of X-Ray Film

Several types of x-ray film are available for use today. Film intended for exposure with x-rays and not light from intensifying screens is *direct-exposure film*. The use of direct-exposure film is for studies such as extremities, where radiation exposure risk is low and high resolution is required. True direct-exposure film has a thick emulsion to absorb more x-rays from the beam and reduce the exposure required. True direct exposure cannot be processed in automatic processors.

Film intended for exposure with x-rays and not light from intensifying screens is **direct-exposure film.**

Screen-type films are designed for exposure with the light from intensifying screens. Their thinner emulsions are not as sensitive to x-rays but are sensitive to the light of the screens. Most film used in medical radiography is screen-type film due to the small amount of radiation required for exposure. The use of screens and screen-film requires from 35 to several hundred times less exposure to produce a given density. This decrease in exposure requirement reduces patient dose and allows short exposure times, reducing blurring from motion.

Screen-type films *are designed for exposure with the light from intensifying screens.*

Several different screen-type films are available. Most screen-type film is double emulsion. *Double-emulsion film* has emulsion on both sides of the base. This increases its speed or response to radiation.

Double-emulsion film *has emulsion on both sides of the base.*

Double-emulsion film is affected by the physical phenomenon known as parallax. *Parallax* is the result of light entering the film emulsion on an angle, passing through the base, and affecting the emulsion on the opposite side of the film. This causes density to be recorded on both sides of the film, but not in the exact same location. These slightly discrepant images cause a loss of detail on the radiograph. Figure 6-2 illustrates the parallax phenomenon. In most cases, the decrease in detail is far outweighed by the reduction in patient exposure.

Parallax *is the result of light entering the film emulsion on an angle, passing through the base, and affecting the emulsion on the opposite side of the film.*

Single-emulsion film has a lower speed, but when used with a single screen, it can produce radiographs with excellent detail. Some screen-type film is sensitive to certain colors of light produced by special screens. In some cases, light-absorbing dyes added to the emulsion can reduce diffracted light from striking nearby crystals. Density caused

Single-emulsion film *has a lower speed, but when used with a single screen, it can produce radiographs with excellent detail.*

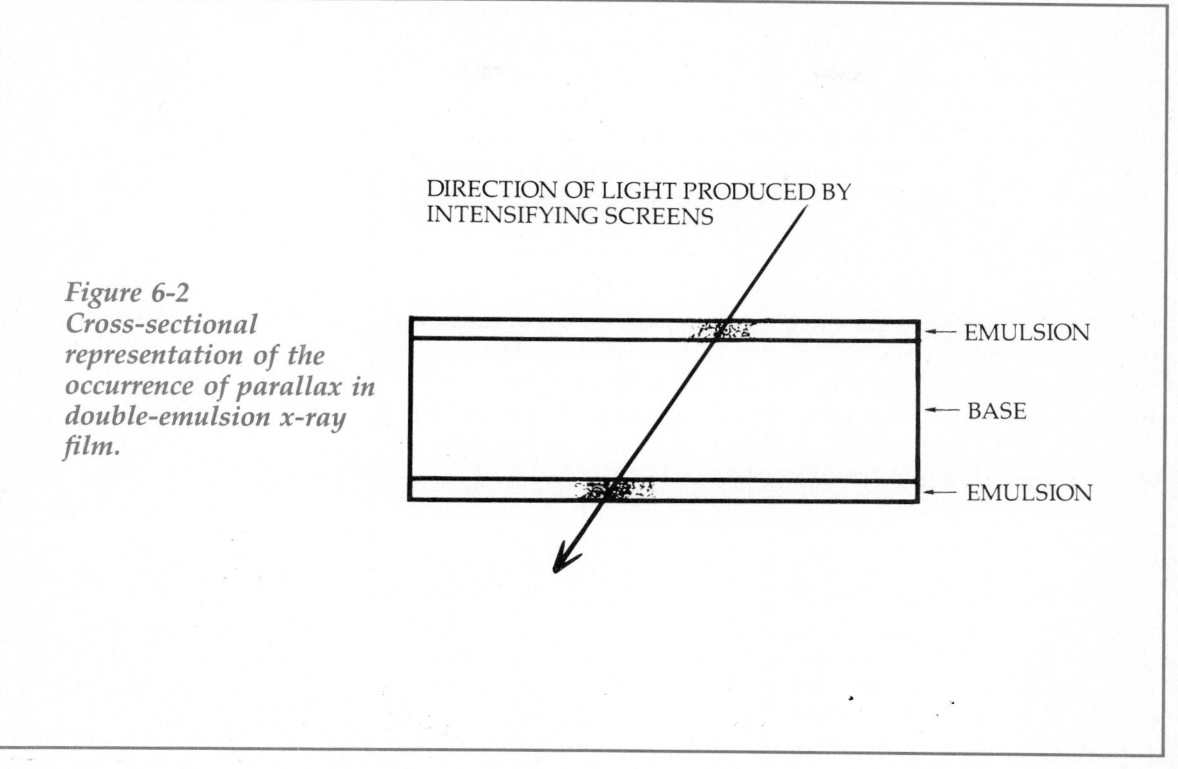

Figure 6-2
Cross-sectional representation of the occurrence of parallax in double-emulsion x-ray film.

The **antihalation layer** *is a type of light-absorbing coating.*

In **tabular-grain films** *the silver halide crystals are tabular or flat in shape.*

by this phenomenon would reduce detail. In addition, some single-emulsion films have a light-absorbent layer on the nonemulsion side of the base. This prevents light exiting the base from being reflected back into the film. This type of light-absorbent coating is an *antihalation layer.* Both light-absorbing dyes in the emulsion and antihalation layers are washed from the film during processing. Single-emulsion film is commonly used in studies of the extremities and the breasts, where the need to resolve fine structures such as bony trabeculation or microcalcifications is critical.

Tabular-grain films differ from conventional films in the shape of the silver halide crystals. In conventional film, the silver halide crystals are essentially round in shape. In tabular films, the silver halide crystals are tabular or flat in shape. Tabular-grain film provides better resolution than conventional films.

Other films are made for special applications. *Duplicating* or *copy film,* manufactured for the duplication of radiographs, is one example. Duplicating film is unique in that it is completely exposed if taken from the box and processed. Exposure to light causes the film to lose density instead of gaining it. Duplicating film is solarized, which means it is exposed to the point that any additional exposure results in loss of density. Duplicating film has an inherent contrast that will neither increase nor decrease from the contrast of the copied film. Duplicating film is single emulsion since detail and not exposure is the primary concern.

Duplicating film *is solarized, which means it is exposed to the point that any additional exposure results in loss of density.*

Subtraction mask film and *subtraction print film* are two types of film used to produce subtractions of angiographic films. Subtraction mask film is a single-emulsion film designed to produce an exact opposite of the angiographic film. Subtraction print film is a single-emulsion film designed to produce a high-contrast opposite of the mask and angiographic film combination.

Subtraction mask film *and* **subtraction print film** *are two types of film used to produce subtractions of angiographic films.*

Fluorescent Intensifying Screens

X-rays can cause materials called phosphors to fluoresce or give off light. *Fluorescent intensifying screens* produce a light image to which screen-type x-ray film is sensitive. For many years, the phosphor in intensifying screens was calcium tungstate ($CaWO_4$) (see next section). When exposed to x-rays, calcium tungstate emits light in the blue and ultraviolet range of the spectrum. The natural sensitivity of silver halide to this portion of the spectrum is high.

Fluorescent intensifying screens *produce a light image to which screen-type x-ray film is sensitive.*

Phosphors used in intensifying screens must possess certain characteristics. One very important characteristic is minimal afterglow or phosphorescence. *Phosphorescence* or *afterglow* is the tendency of a phosphor to continue to give off light after the x-ray exposure has stopped. Excessive phosphorescence would render a screen useless for radiography.

Phosphorescence *or* **afterglow** *is the tendency of a phosphor to continue to give off light after the x-ray exposure has stopped.*

Intensifying screens normally have four layers. The first layer is the base, constructed of plastic or cardboard; the second, the reflective layer; the third, the phosphor layer; and the fourth, the protective layer. Figure 6-3 illustrates the construction of an intensifying screen.

The *base* of an intensifying screen is a high-grade cardboard or plastic. The base layer serves to provide support for the other layers of the screen.

The **base layer** *serves to provide support for the other layers of the screen.*

The *reflective layer* is a white reflective substance such as titanium dioxide (TiO_2). It is applied to the base in a very thin layer. Light generated in the phosphor layer travels in all directions. The reflective layer reflects light moving toward the base back toward the film. Although this

The **reflective layer** *reflects light moving toward the base back toward the film.*

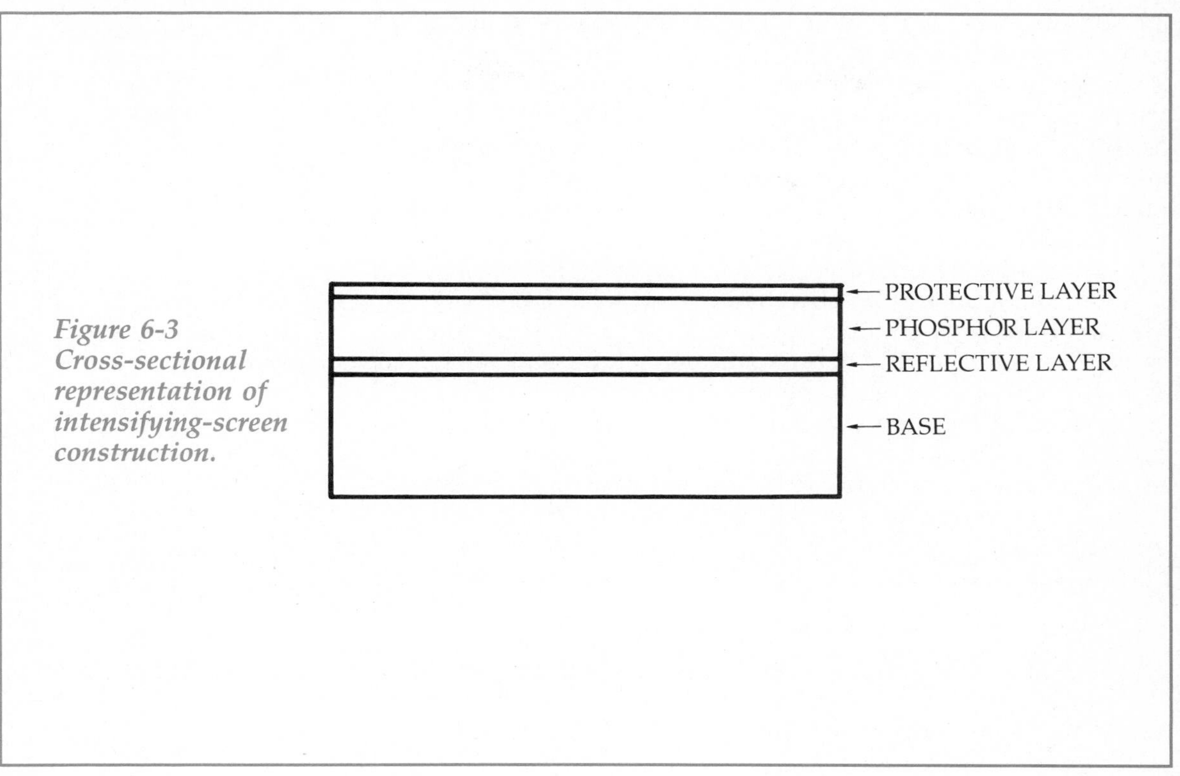

Figure 6-3 Cross-sectional representation of intensifying-screen construction.

helps to increase screen speed, it reduces detail somewhat due to diffusion of the light. For this reason, not all screens have a reflective layer. Screens designed to produce detail often have no reflective layers.

The *phosphor layer* is a plastic substance that contains the phosphor crystals. A more detailed discussion of the phosphor layer follows.

The **protective layer** *is composed of cellulose.*

The *protective layer,* composed of cellulose, serves three functions: (1) it provides protection for the phosphor layer, (2) it provides a surface durable enough to tolerate cleaning, and (3) it helps prevent the production of static electricity.

Intensifying-Screen Phosphors

As stated earlier, calcium tungstate was widely used as an intensifying-screen phosphor. Calcium tungstate emits light in the blue-ultraviolet range of the spectrum, with a peak wavelength of 4300 angstroms or 430 nanometers (a nanometer is one-billionth of a meter). The use of intensifying screens converts a few x-ray photons to many light photons. The ability of a given phosphor to convert x-ray photons to light photons is the *intrinsic efficiency* of the phosphor. Calcium tungstate has an intrinsic efficiency of approximately 5 percent. Later in this section we discuss newer phosphors with intrinsic efficiencies of approximately 20 percent.

The ability of a given phosphor to convert x-ray photons to light photons is the **intrinsic efficiency** *of the phosphor.*

Once excited by x-rays, the light produced by the phosphor must escape the phosphor layer of the screen. Some of the light will be absorbed by the screen and lost. The ability of light emitted by the phosphor to escape the screen is *screen efficiency*. A typical screen allows only about half the light to ever reach the film.

The ability of light emitted by the phosphor to escape the screen is **screen efficiency.**

A useful measure of screen speed is the intensification factor of the screens. The *intensification factor* is the ratio of the exposure needed to produce a density on a film using screens compared to the exposure required to produce the density without screens. Intensification factor is typically expressed as:

The **intensification factor** *is the ratio of the exposure needed to produce a density on a film using screens compared to the exposure required to produce the density without screens.*

$$\text{Intensification factor} = \frac{\text{Exposure without screens}}{\text{Exposure with screens}}$$

Three factors determine the speed of a calcium tungstate screen:

1. The thickness of the phosphor layer influences speed. Thicker layers produce more light and therefore are faster. However, the thicker phosphor layer reduces detail.
2. The size of the phosphor crystals affects speed because larger crystals give off more light. Again, the larger crystals reduce detail.
3. The presence or absence of light-absorbing dyes in the screen influences speed. Light-absorbing dyes are added to decrease light from the phosphor crystals that is not traveling directly toward the film. This helps increase detail, but it decreases speed.

It should be evident that *the relationship between screen speed and detail is inverse.* Faster screens have poorer detail, and slower screens produce better detail.

The relationship between screen speed and detail is inverse.

Three classifications of calcium tungstate screens are slow, medium, and fast. Slow- or detail-speed screens have an intensification factor of 35. Detail-speed screens have thin phosphor layers with smaller phosphor crystals. Medium- or par-speed screens have an intensification factor of 50. High- or fast-speed screens have an intensifica-

Rare earth phosphors *convert x-rays to light approximately four times more efficiently than calcium tungstate.*

tion factor of 100. Fast-speed screens have thicker phosphor layers with larger phosphor crystals.

Since 1973, new phosphors have been available in intensifying screens, including terbium-activated gadolinium oxysulfide (Gd_2O_2S:Tb), terbium-activated lanthanum oxysulfide (La_2O_2S:Tb), terbium-activated yttrium oxysulfide (Y_2O_2S:Tb), and lanthanum oxybromide (LaOBr). These new phosphors are referred to as rare earth phosphors. The term "rare earth" indicates that these elements are difficult to separate from the earth, not because they are particularly rare. *Rare earth phosphors* convert x-rays to light approximately four times more efficiently than calcium tungstate. This means that rare earth phosphors have an intrinsic efficiency of 20 percent compared with calcium tungstate's 5 percent.

Rare earth screens' principal advantage over other screens is their speed. Rare earth screens are manufactured at different speed levels, but each is approximately twice as fast as a similar calcium tungstate screen. This doubling of speed occurs without sacrificing detail.

Rare earth screens emit light in the green region of the visible spectrum, with a peak wavelength of 5400 angstroms or 540 nanometers. Conventional x-ray film is not particularly sensitive to this region of the visible spectrum. Therefore, to recognize the speed of rare earth screens, they must be used with film sensitive to green light. A wide variety of green-sensitive films for use with rare earth screens have characteristics suitable for radiographic applications.

Green light-sensitive films are rather quickly fogged by the safelights used for blue-light sensitive films. Green-light sensitive films require a safelight that is colored more to the red portion of the visible spectrum. Safelights and safelight filters are available that are suitable for both blue- and green-sensitive films.

The advantages of using rare earth screens are obvious:

1. They require less exposure to produce a given density on a radiographic film.
2. Since less exposure is required for a given density, patient exposure is reduced.
3. The ability to use shorter exposure times can reduce lack of sharpness due to patient motion.
4. The lower techniques required will likely result in increased x-ray tube life.

The relationship between the type and speed of a film and the type and intensification factor of a screen is what actually determines the response of a film-screen combination to radiation exposure. For this reason, *relative speed* is normally used to describe the response of a particular film-screen combination. Relative speed is not an absolute measure and it does not represent any particular unit; however, it does allow the comparison of the speed of one film-screen combination with the speed of another. Medium-speed calcium tungstate screens used with medium-speed blue-sensitive film is arbitrarily assigned a relative speed of 100. This was the film-screen combination that was referred to as *medium speed* or *par speed.*

Relative speed can be used to calculate technique changes from one film-screen combination to another. A film-screen combination with a relative speed of 400 requires approximately one-fourth the mAs to produce a given density in a film-screen combination with a relative value of 100. Relative speed is established in the 70 to 80 kVp range. When kVp of less than 60 or greater than 100 is used, relative speed may be less accurate in technique conversion. Additionally, each manufacturer establishes relative speed based on their own brand of calcium tungstate medium-speed screens, and there may be some variation between different manufacturers' relative speed values. Relative speeds of contemporary imaging films range from a low range of 20 to 30 to a high range of 1200 to 1600.

Radiographic Cassettes

Since x-ray film is sensitive to light, it requires protection from room light during handling. In addition, when used with intensifying screens, the film must be in intimate contact with both sets of screens, or detail loss will occur. The x-ray cassette serves both of these functions (Figure 6-4).

The cassette usually has a steel frame for rigidity. The front of the cassette is made of a radiolucent material, such as plastic, aluminum, or graphite, to allow the x-rays to pass through to the screens and film. The material on the back of the cassette varies depending on whether it is a phototiming cassette or not.

Nonphototiming cassettes have lead-lined steel backs. The lead lining prevents backscatter from affecting the film. Backscatter occurs when x-rays exit the back of the cassette, and scatter radiation is generated back toward the cassette. With high-kilovolt techniques, backscatter can fog the film in the cassette.

Phototiming cassettes must allow radiation to pass

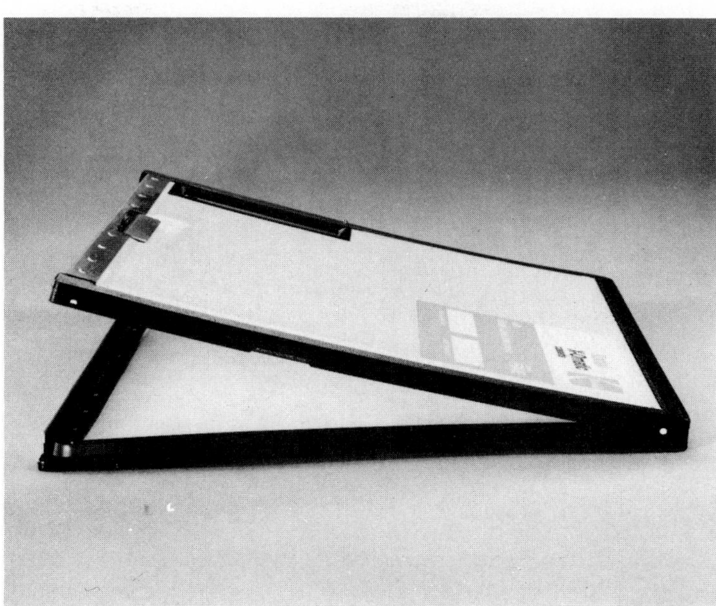

Figure 6-4
An X-Omatic Cassette. (Courtesy of Eastman Kodak Co.)

through the cassette to strike the phototimer. Phototiming cassettes have a layer of thin lead foil on the back of the cassette. The foil is thin enough to allow most of the x-rays to exit the cassette. However, it is thick enough to prevent backscatter from fogging the film.

The intensifying screen or screens are mounted inside the cassette facing each other. The film is placed between the screens and the cassette is closed. The use of spring clips or a slight curve at the rear of the cassette causes the two sides to press tightly against each other when locked. This pressure produces intimate screen-film contact. "Light baffles" or felt seals around the edges of the cassette keep light out.

Cassettes for use with single-emulsion film have a single screen mounted in them. It is important to place the film emulsion so that it faces, and is in contact with, the screen. Failure to correctly position a single-emulsion film will result in loss of detail and possibly density. Common examples of single-screen cassettes are extremity and mammography cassettes. Imaging camera cassettes use single-emulsion film but have no screens, since the film is exposed by photographing a monitor image or by laser light from a laser camera.

Most cassettes have a shielded area that permits identification of the patient depicted on the film. Grid-front cassettes have radiographic grids permanently attached.

Technique Considerations

The use of fluorescent intensifying screens reduces the amount of exposure required by a factor of 35 or greater. The *lower the intensification factor of the screens, the greater is the exposure required to produce a given density.* Conversely, intensifying screens with a higher intensification factor require less exposure to produce the same density.

The lower the intensification factor, the greater is the exposure required to produce a given density.

Screen speed also affects radiographic detail or resolution. In general, *the higher the speed of the screens, the lower is the resolution.* With calcium tungstate screens, slow-speed screens produce the best radiographic detail, and high-speed screens produce less radiographic detail.

The higher the speed of the screens, the lower is the resolution.

Radiography requiring high resolution of detail usually demanded the use of nonscreen film. However, since most nonscreen film cannot be rapidly processed, its use has declined. Today, the use of special single-emulsion cassettes and film allows the performance of high-resolution radiography.

Radiation Protection

Fluorescent intensifying screens significantly reduce patient exposure. The higher the intensification factor of the screens, the greater is the reduction in patient exposure. However, there are trade-offs with intensifying screens. With a given phosphor, as screen speed increases, detail decreases. The technologist is responsible for carefully weighing the relationship of detail and patient dose when selecting a screen-film combination for an examination. This decision must include the requirements for high resolution and the radiation sensitivity of the body part being examined.

Chapter 6—Review Questions

1. What are the two most important components of x-ray film emulsion?
   a. silver halide and gelatin
   b. silver bromide and silver iodide
   c. silver halide and the base
   d. gelatin and the base
   e. none of the above
2. What provides the location for the formation of the latent image?
   a. the base
   b. the gelatin
   c. the sensitivity speck
   d. the emulsion
   e. none of the above
3. What causes the latent image to become visible?
   a. exposure to light
   b. exposure to x-rays
   c. both of the above
   d. none of the above
4. What comprises the density visible on the film?
   a. the gelatin
   b. metallic silver
   c. silver halide
   d. the base
   e. none of the above
5. What is the loss of detail resulting from a slight discrepancy in the images on double-emulsion film termed?
   a. parallel
   b. direct exposure
   c. parallax
   d. none of the above
6. Which of the following types of film has the highest speed?
   a. direct-exposure film
   b. double-emulsion screen-type film
   c. single-emulsion screen-type film

7. What is the light-absorbent layer on film called?
   a. parallax layer
   b. reflective layer
   c. solarization layer
   d. antihalation layer
8. What is the most significant difference between conventional radiographic film and duplicating film?
   a. the contrast
   b. the base
   c. the emulsion
   d. none of the above
9. What is the primary purpose of intensifying screens?
   a. to protect the radiographic film from damage
   b. to prevent fogging of the film
   c. to convert x-rays to light
   d. two of the above
   e. all of the above
10. Which of the following materials is used to construct the base layer of intensifying screens?
    a. cardboard
    b. polyester
    c. plastic
    d. two of the above
    e. all of the above
11. What is the primary purpose of the reflective layer?
    a. to improve detail
    b. to protect the phosphor layer
    c. to increase screen speed
    d. two of the above
    e. all of the above
12. Which of the following phosphors emits light in the blue-ultraviolet spectrum?
    a. calcium tungstate
    b. titanium oxide
    c. rare earth phosphors
    d. two of the above
    e. all of the above

13. What is the tendency of a phosphor to continue to give off light after the x-ray exposure has stopped?
    a. afterglow
    b. fluorescence
    c. phosphorescence
    d. two of the above
    e. all of the above
14. Which of the following is not a function of the protective layer of an intensifying screen?
    a. to provide protection for the phosphor layer
    b. to provide a surface durable enough for cleaning
    c. to prevent the production of scatter radiation
    d. two of the above
    e. all of the above
15. What is the term used to describe the ability of a given phosphor to convert x-ray photons to light?
    a. intensification factor
    b. screen efficiency
    c. intrinsic efficiency
    d. phosphor efficiency
    e. none of the above
16. What is the term used to describe the ability of light emitted by the phosphor to escape the screen?
    a. intensification factor
    b. screen efficiency
    c. intrinsic efficiency
    d. phosphor efficiency
    e. none of the above
17. What is the ratio of the exposure needed to produce a density on a radiograph using screens compared to the exposure required to produce the density without screens?
    a. intensification factor
    b. screen efficiency
    c. intrinsic efficiency
    d. phosphor efficiency
    e. none of the above
18. In general, as screen speed increases:
    a. patient dose increases
    b. density increases
    c. detail increases
    d. two of the above
    e. all of the above

19. Which of the following is not a function of the radiographic cassette?
    a. to protect the film from exposure to room light
    b. to maintain intimate contact between the film and screens
    c. to provide a vacuum for the production of light through fluorescence
    d. two of the above
    e. all of the above

20. Which of the following facts is true concerning the speed of a calcium tungstate screen?
    a. Thicker phosphor layers produce more light and are faster.
    b. The larger the crystals, the faster is the screen.
    c. The presence of light-absorbing dyes in the phosphor layer increases the speed of the screen.
    d. two of the above
    e. all of the above

7

Sensitometry

OBJECTIVES

After completing Chapter 7, you should be able to:

1. Define the following terms:
   characteristic curve
   densitometer
   film speed
   fog
   radiographic contrast
   radiographic density
   sensitometry
2. Discuss the relationships between density and contrast.
3. Identify the various portions of the characteristic curve, and discuss the relationship of the characteristic curve to density and contrast.

It is important for the technologist to understand how changes in technique and processing will affect the radiographic image recorded on film. The study of the response of film to changes in technique and processing is called *sensitometry*. Before explaining sensitometry, it is necessary to define certain terms relating to radiographic film: exposure, density, contrast, film speed, and fog.

Exposure

Technologists frequently use the term "exposure." The use of the terms "overexposed" or "underexposed," in reference to radiographs, is intuitively understood. One speaks of "patient exposure," and again the meaning is understood. Exposure refers to the amount of energy that interacts with a given material.

In radiography, *exposure* or *technique* normally defines the kilovoltage peak (kVp), milliamperes, and time used to produce a radiograph. When discussing sensitometry, exposure refers to the amount of radiation or light reaching the film and producing a certain radiographic density after processing. For the purpose of discussing sensitometry, exposure is expressed as:

In radiography, ***exposure*** *or* ***technique*** *normally defines the kilovoltage peak (kVp), milliamperes, and time used to produce a radiograph.*

$$\text{Exposure} = \text{Intensity} \times \text{Time}$$

Exposure = Intensity × Time

The measurement of exposure can be in either absolute or relative units. Expressing the measurement of exposure in ergs per square centimeter for light or roentgens for x-rays would be *absolute units*. Measurement can also be in *relative units* in which one exposure is the basis for comparison of all others. Relative units are frequently more convenient and just as useful as absolute units of measurement.

Radiographic Density

Radiographic density *is the black metallic silver deposited in the emulsion of x-ray film after exposure to light or radiation and processing. Milliampere-seconds, or mAs, is the primary controlling factor for radiographic density.*

Radiographic density is the black metallic silver deposited in the emulsion of x-ray film after exposure to light or radiation and processing. Milliampere-seconds, or mAs, is the primary controlling factor for radiographic density. However, both kVp and source-to-image receptor distance have pronounced effects on density. Other factors that influence radiographic density include scatter radiation, base fog or light fog, intensifying screens, radiographic grids, beam-restricting devices, filtration, and processing.

A ***densitometer*** *is an instrument that measures density.*

Density *is the ratio of the logarithm of the incident light striking the radiograph and the logarithm of the light transmitted through the film.*

A *densitometer* is an instrument that measures density. *Density* is the ratio of the logarithm of the incident light striking the radiograph and the logarithm of the light

$$Density = \frac{Log\ I_0}{Log\ I_t}$$

The numerical range of perceptible densities in radiology is from 0.25 to 2.5.

transmitted through the film. Density is algebraically expressed by the following equation:

$$\text{Density} = \frac{\text{Log } I_0 \text{ (Incident intensity)}}{\text{Log } I_t \text{ (Transmitted intensity)}}$$

The human eye and available light sources limit the useful density range for diagnostic radiology. The numerical range of perceptible densities in radiology is from 0.25 to 2.5. One must remember that the measurement of density is a logarithmic function, as indicated by the density equation. An increase of 1.0 in the numerical density value translates into a tenfold increase in density. An increase of 0.3 in the numerical density value represents a doubling of the radiographic density.

Radiographic Contrast

Radiographic contrast *exists when comparing two or more radiographic densities on an x-ray film.*

$$C = \frac{(Log\ I_0)_2}{(Log\ I_t)_2} - \frac{(Log\ I_0)_1}{(Log\ I_t)_1}$$

The kVp is the primary controlling factor for contrast.

Radiographic contrast exists when comparing two or more radiographic densities on an x-ray film. Algebraically, radiographic contrast is expressed by the following equation:

$$\text{Contrast} = \frac{(\text{Log } I_0)_2}{(\text{Log } I_t)_2} - \frac{(\text{Log } I_0)_1}{(\text{Log } I_t)_1}$$

The kVp is the primary controlling factor for contrast. Other factors affecting contrast include radiographic grids, beam-restricting devices, filtration, intensifying screens, film type, and processing.

With **long-scale contrast** *or* **low contrast** *present, the range of densities is wide and large in numbers.*

Long-scale or low contrast is usually the result of higher kVp and has a wide exposure latitude.

The two general types of contrast seen in medical radiography are long scale and short scale. When *long-scale contrast* or *low contrast* is present, a radiograph of a step wedge or penetrameter (an absorber that increases in thickness in uniform steps) has gradual change in density between steps. The range of densities is wide and large in number. The densities begin with no density, progress through a large number of grays, and end in black. This is often the more desirable contrast in medical radiography. Long-scale or low contrast is usually the result of higher kVp and has a wide exposure latitude.

With **short-scale contrast** *or* **high contrast** *present, the range of densities is small and few in numbers.*

Short-scale or high contrast is usually the product of low kVp and has a narrow exposure latitude.

When *short-scale contrast* or *high contrast* is present, a radiograph of a step wedge has more significant change in density between steps. The range of image densities is small and few in number. The densities progress through a small number of grays and end in black. Its main use is in demonstrating tissues with little subject contrast. Short-scale or high contrast is usually the product of low kVp and has a narrow exposure latitude.

Film Speed

Film speed is the sensitivity of film to exposure. Film speed is inversely related to exposure. The lower the exposure required to produce a given density on a particular film, the higher is the film speed. Conversely, films requiring large exposures to produce a given density have lower film speeds.

Film speed is an important consideration in the selection of radiographic films. Higher-speed films require less exposure to produce a given density and result in less radiation dose to the patient.

Film speed *is the sensitivity of film to exposure.*

Fog

Fog is density on film that is not a result of radiation carrying the desired image. The term "gross fog" describes density that is inherent in the base and emulsion. The base, film tint, and emulsion all produce some small amount of density. Film emulsion will have some silver halide crystals develop even without exposure. Development of silver halide crystals without exposure can result from many factors, including background radiation, heat, humidity, and chemical fumes.

Many other factors can cause fogging of the radiograph, including safelight, room light, and chemistry contamination. Regardless of the cause, fog increases density and decreases contrast on the radiograph.

Fog *is density on film that is not a result of radiation carrying the desired image.*

Characteristic Curve

The principal factors measured in sensitometry are the exposure to the film and the light transmitted through the film after processing. The plotting of the relationship between measurements of exposure and density is the *characteristic curve*. The characteristic curve is also known as an H & D curve after Hurter and Driffield, who first described it. Figure 7-1 illustrates a typical characteristic curve. The characteristic curve is plotted on a graph. The vertical axis is the density, and the horizontal axis is the logarithm of the relative exposure. The characteristic curve has three portions: the toe, straight-line portion, and shoulder.

The plotting of the relationship between measurements of exposure and density is the **characteristic curve.**

The characteristic curve has three portions: the toe, straight-line portion, and shoulder.

The *toe* of the curve represents the area of exposure that is below the film's ability to respond to exposure. Fairly large changes in exposure result in only small changes in density in the toe portion. Note that the toe of the characteristic curve does not begin at zero, since density caused by gross fog occurs even without exposure.

The **toe** *of the curve represents the area of exposure that is below the film's ability to respond to exposure.*

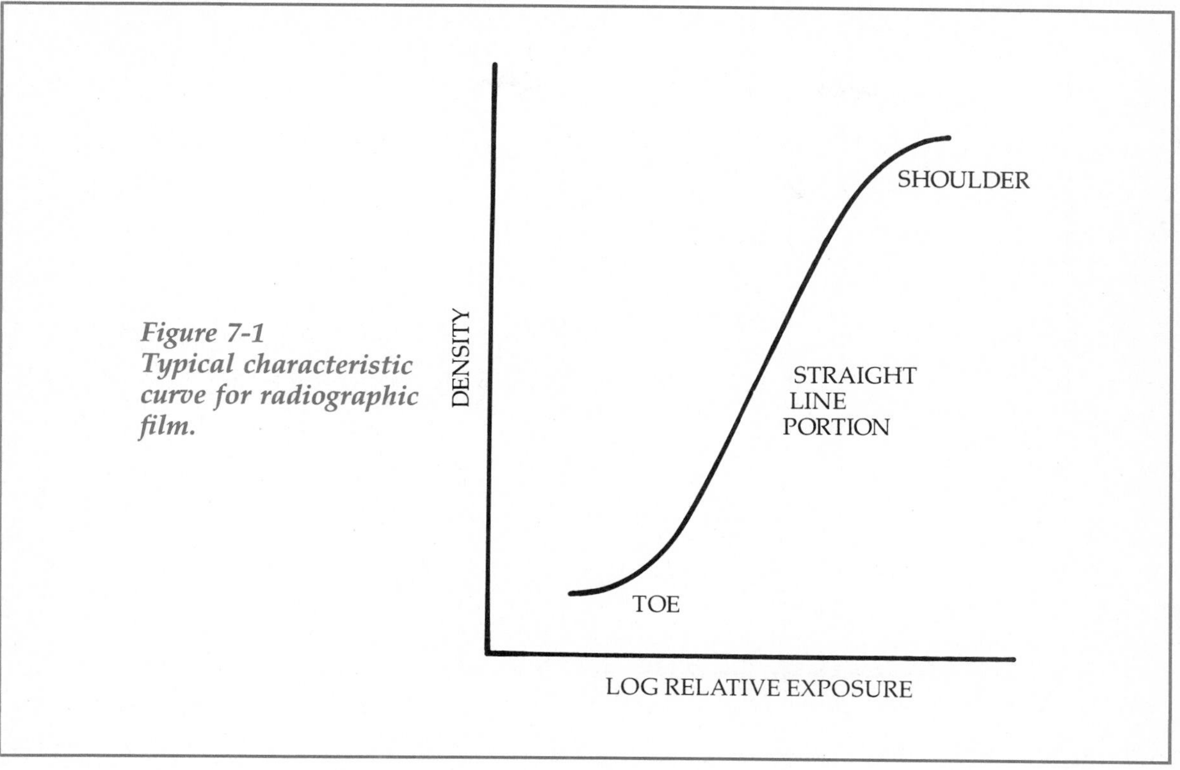

Figure 7-1
Typical characteristic curve for radiographic film.

The **straight-line portion** *of the curve represents the area of film response where increases in exposure produce corresponding increases in density on the film.*

The **shoulder** *of the curve represents the area where the film is reaching its maximum exposure. In the shoulder portion, large increases in exposure do not produce significant increases in density.*

When comparing the characteristic curves of films, those closer to the left side of the graph are faster whereas those lying to the right are slower.

The next part of the characteristic curve, the *straight-line portion,* represents the area of film response where increases in exposure produce corresponding increases in density on the film. The straight-line portion of the characteristic curve is the useful exposure range for diagnostic radiology.

The *shoulder* of the curve represents the area where the film is reaching its maximum exposure. In the shoulder portion, large increases in exposure do not produce significant increases in density.

Examination of the characteristic curve reveals much about the properties of a given film. The location on the horizontal axis, the logarithm of the relative exposure, easily determines the speed of a film. Higher-speed films require less exposure to produce a given density and are closer to the density axis. Lower-speed films require more exposure to produce a given density and lie farther from the density axis. When comparing the characteristic curves of films, those closer to the left side of the graph are faster, whereas those lying to the right are slower. The two characteristic curves in Figure 7-2 illustrate this point.

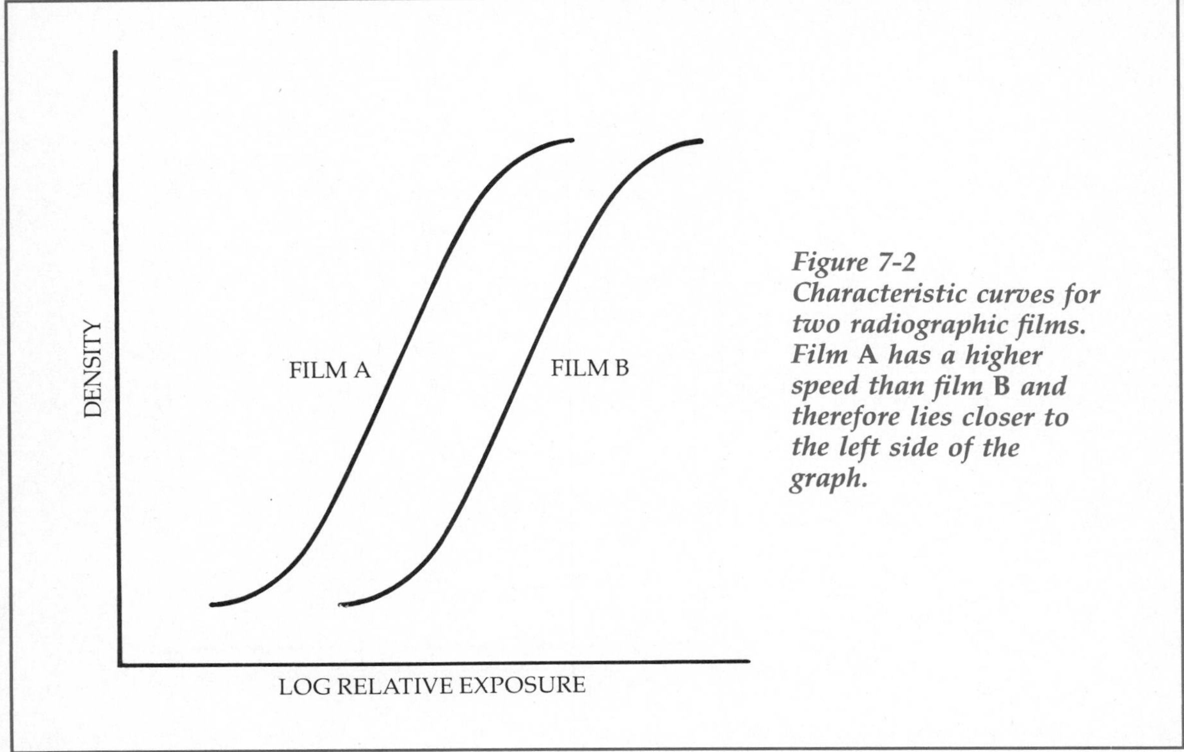

Figure 7-2
Characteristic curves for two radiographic films. Film **A** *has a higher speed than film* **B** *and therefore lies closer to the left side of the graph.*

The characteristic curve also identifies the contrast of a film. The slope of the straight-line portion identifies the contrast. *Slope* is the rise over run of the straight-line portion. High-contrast films go from low- to high-density quickly and have steep straight-line portions. The straight-line portion is nearer vertical, since small exposure increases (short run) produce significant density increases (high rise). Low-contrast films have less steep, or more horizontal, straight-line portions. With low-contrast films, increasing the density requires more exposure (long run) to produce less density (low rise). Figure 7-3 illustrates the characteristic curves of two films with differing contrast levels.

The **slope** *of the straight-line portion identifies the contrast.*

Average gradient is a method used to express film contrast numerically. Average gradient is the slope of the straight line drawn between the density levels 0.25 and 2.0 above gross fog. Average gradient is calculated by the following equation:

Average gradient *is a method used to express film contrast numerically.*

$$AG = \frac{\text{Density}_2 - \text{Density}_1}{\text{Log relative exposure}_2 - \text{Log relative exposure}_1}$$

$$AG = \frac{D_2 - D_1}{LRE_2 - LRE_1}$$

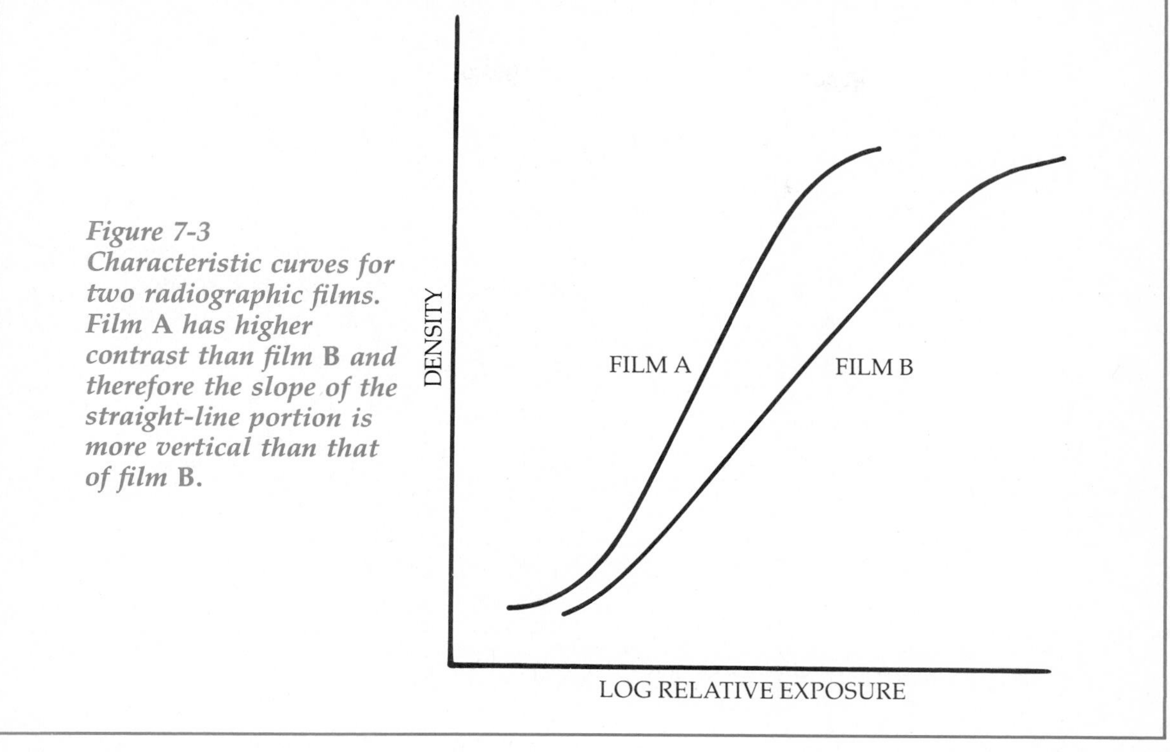

Figure 7-3
*Characteristic curves for two radiographic films. Film **A** has higher contrast than film **B** and therefore the slope of the straight-line portion is more vertical than that of film **B**.*

Average gradient is a useful measurement of contrast. If the average gradient of a film is greater than 1, the film will enhance contrast. If the average gradient is less than 1, the film will detract from contrast. If the average gradient is 1, the film will not alter subject contrast.

Characteristic curves also provide information on the exposure latitude of a film.

Characteristic curves also provide information on the exposure latitude of a film. Film that allows greater errors in exposure to produce a given technique has wide exposure latitude. Films with wide exposure latitude have characteristic curves, with a low rise in density for a long run of exposure. In other words, these films have characteristic curves that do not have steep slopes. Films with steep slopes to their characteristic curves have narrow exposure latitude. It should be evident that contrast and exposure latitude are inversely related. High-contrast films have narrow exposure latitude, and low-contrast films have wide exposure latitude.

The overall shape of the characteristic curve also identifies its response to exposure throughout its range of densities. The characteristic curve in Figure 7-4 shows a typical appearance of film designed to provide normal contrast

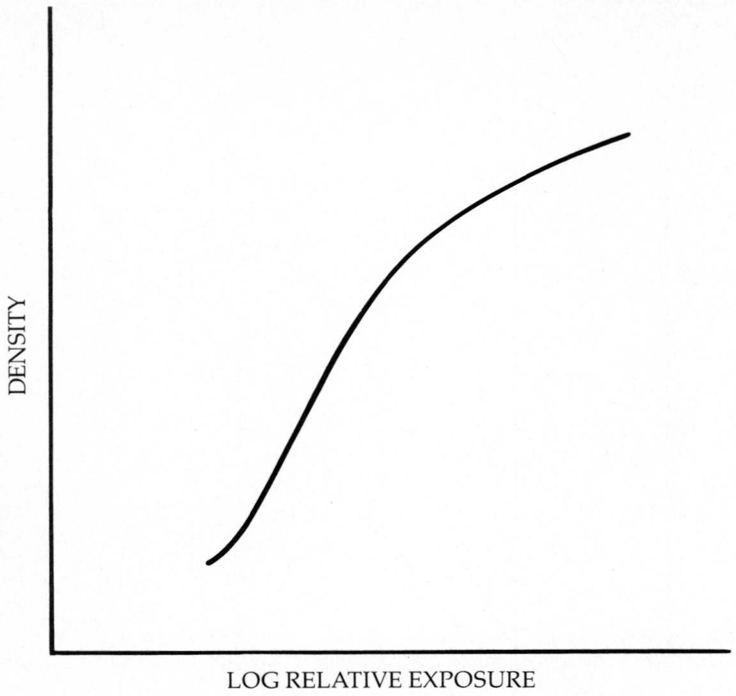

DENSITY

LOG RELATIVE EXPOSURE

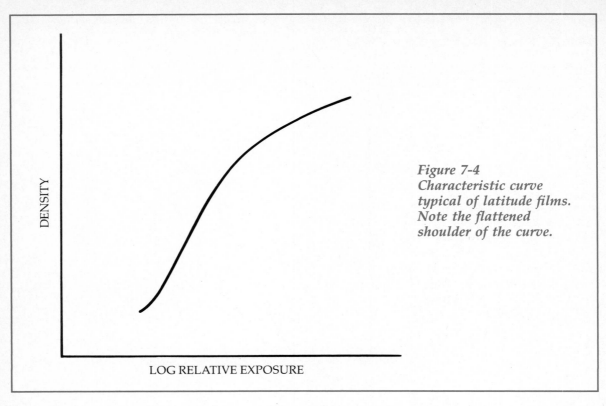

Figure 7-4
Characteristic curve typical of latitude films. Note the flattened shoulder of the curve.

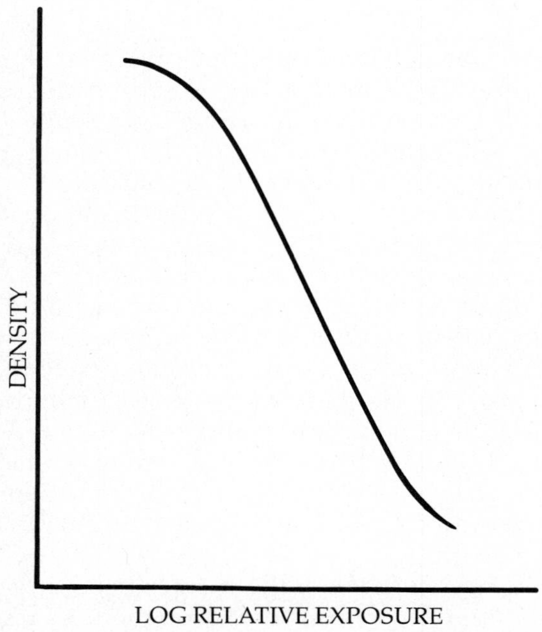

DENSITY

LOG RELATIVE EXPOSURE

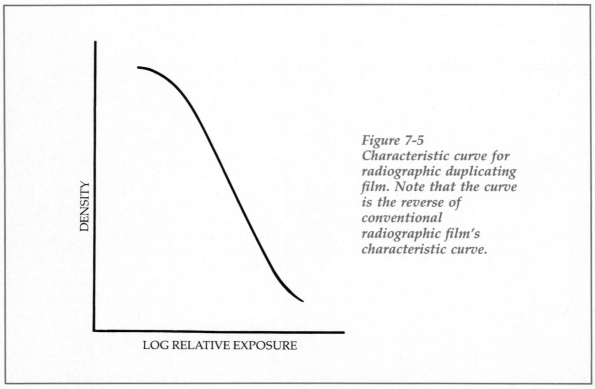

Figure 7-5
Characteristic curve for radiographic duplicating film. Note that the curve is the reverse of conventional radiographic film's characteristic curve.

with greater latitude in the higher-density region. The shoulder of the film is flatter, representing a decrease in density per unit of exposure. Latitude films often have characteristic curves similar to this.

The characteristic curve in Figure 7-5 is exactly the opposite of the others we have been discussing. This characteristic curve is representative of duplicating or copy film. Since unexposed copy film is completely black at development, its characteristic curve starts at maximum density. As the logarithm of relative exposure increases, the density of the film decreases. Duplicating film has an average gradient close to 1. Duplicating film neither enhances nor detracts from the contrast of the original radiograph.

Chapter 7—Review Questions

1. What is the term used to describe the black metallic silver deposited in the emulsion of the x-ray film after exposure to light or radiation and processing?
   a. contrast
   b. density
   c. exposure
   d. film speed
   e. none of the above
2. What term is used to describe the comparison of two or more radiographic densities?
   a. contrast
   b. density
   c. exposure
   d. film speed
   e. none of the above
3. What term refers to the amount of energy that interacts with a given material?
   a. contrast
   b. density
   c. exposure
   d. film speed
   e. none of the above
4. What term refers to the study of the response of film to changes in technique and processing?
   a. contrast
   b. density
   c. exposure
   d. film speed
   e. none of the above
5. What term describes the ratio of the logarithm of the incident light striking the radiograph and the logarithm of the light transmitted through the film?
   a. contrast
   b. density
   c. exposure
   d. film speed
   e. none of the above

6. What is the primary controlling factor of contrast?
   a. mAs
   b. kVp
   c. filtration
   d. subject contrast
   e. none of the above
7. What is the primary controlling factor of density?
   a. mAs
   b. kVp
   c. filtration
   d. subject contrast
   e. none of the above
8. What is the useful density range in diagnostic radiology?
   a. 0 - 3.0
   b. 0.25 - 2.0
   c. 0.25 - 2.5
   d. 1.0
9. What increase in the numerical density value corresponds to a doubling of the radiographic density?
   a. a twofold increase in the numerical value
   b. 0.25
   c. 0.3
   d. 1.0
   e. 2.0
10. Which of the following radiographic conditions is consistent with high-kVp techniques?
    a. short-scale contrast
    b. low contrast
    c. narrow latitude
    d. two of the above
    e. none of the above
11. Which of the following radiographic conditions is consistent with low-kVp techniques?
    a. short-scale contrast
    b. low contrast
    c. narrow latitude
    d. two of the above
    e. none of the above

12. What term is used to describe the sensitivity of film to exposure?
    a. film sensitivity
    b. sensitometry
    c. film speed
    d. contrast
    e. none of the above
13. What is the impact of fog on the radiograph?
    a. increased density and increased contrast
    b. increased density and decreased contrast
    c. decreased density and increased contrast
    d. decreased density and decreased contrast
14. Which portion or aspect of the characteristic curve represents the area where the film is reaching its maximum exposure?
    a. toe
    b. straight-line portion
    c. slope of the straight-line portion
    d. average gradient
    e. shoulder
15. Which portion or aspect of the characteristic curve represents the area of the exposure that is below the film's ability to respond to exposure?
    a. toe
    b. straight-line portion
    c. slope of the straight-line portion
    d. average gradient
    e. shoulder
16. Which portion or aspect of the characteristic curve represents the area of film response where an increase in exposure produces corresponding increases in density on the film?
    a. toe
    b. straight-line portion
    c. slope of the straight-line portion
    d. average gradient
    e. shoulder
17. What portion or aspect of the characteristic curve identifies the contrast?
    a. toe
    b. straight-line portion
    c. slope of the straight-line portion
    d. average gradient
    e. shoulder

18. What portion or aspect of the characteristic curve numerically expresses film contrast?
    a. toe
    b. straight-line portion
    c. slope of the straight-line portion
    d. average gradient
    e. shoulder

19. Given two characteristic curves, which one would represent the faster- or higher-speed film?
    a. film with the steepest slope in the straight-line portion
    b. film with the highest shoulder
    c. film whose curve lies farthest to the left
    d. film whose curve lies farthest to the right
    e. film with the lowest average gradient

20. Given two characteristic curves, which one would represent the film with the highest contrast?
    a. film with the steepest slope in the straight-line portion
    b. film with the highest shoulder
    c. film whose curve lies farthest to the left
    d. film whose curve lies farthest to the right
    e. film with the lowest average gradient

8

Processing and Processor Monitoring

OBJECTIVES

After completing Chapter 8, you should be able to:

1. Discuss the four major steps in processing x-ray film.
2. Discuss the time-temperature relationship.
3. Explain replenishment.
4. Describe the eight major sections of an automatic processor.
5. Discuss processor quality control.

X-Ray Film Processing

The processing of x-ray film is an important part of the overall radiographic process. The major steps in processing of x-ray film are developing, fixing, washing, and drying.

Developing is the step during which the latent or invisible image becomes manifest or visible and the reduction of exposed silver halide crystals to metallic silver occurs. The developer used for x-ray film has six major components: (1) a solvent, (2) a developing agent, (3) activators, (4) restrainers, (5) a preservative, and (6) a hardener.

Developing *is the step during which the latent or invisible image becomes manifest or visible and the reduction of exposed silver halide crystals to metallic silver occurs.*

The solvent for the developer is water, which dissolves and ionizes the developer chemicals. Water also serves to soften the emulsion, permitting the chemicals to come in contact with the emulsion. The developing agent is a reducer; it gives up an electron to the silver halide, reducing it to metallic silver. Common developing agents are hydroquinone, phenidone, and metol. The activators or accelerators are potassium carbonate or sodium carbonate and potassium hydroxide or sodium hydroxide. The activators are alkaline in pH (the logarithm of the reciprocal of the hydrogen in concentration) and increase the activity of the developers. The restrainers are potassium bromide and potassium iodide. The restrainers serve to retard the development of unexposed silver halide crystals, controlling chemical fog. A preservative, usually sodium sulfite, prevents oxidation of the developer. Finally, the hardener, glutaraldehyde, serves to harden the emulsion, reducing artifacts and film transport problems in the processor.

The next step in processing is *fixing* of the film. The fixer has six major components: (1) a solvent, (2) a clearing agent, (3) a preservative, (4) a hardener, (5) an acidifier, and (6) a buffer.

Fixing *is the step during which the undeveloped silver halide is removed from the emulsion.*

The solvent is water, which serves to dissolve the other ingredients and carry them into the emulsion of the film. The clearing agent removes undeveloped silver halide from the emulsion, putting silver into the solution. The clearing agent is often called hypo, and the two most common clearing agents are sodium thiosulfate and ammonium thiosulfate. The preservative is usually sodium sulfite, which prevents the decomposition of the clearing agents. The acidifier is usually acetic acid, which accelerates the action of the other chemicals and neutralizes any remaining alkaline developer. Buffers are added to maintain the desired acidity or alkalinity and prevent the development of sludge in the fixer.

Washing and *drying* are also important steps in the processing of x-ray film. During the wash, the water removes all the fixer in the emulsion. Failure to wash the fixer from the emulsion will result in a film with poor archival or storage qualities. The drying process removes the water from the emulsion. While the emulsion is wet, it is soft and subject to damage. Drying the film hardens the emulsion and protects it from handling damage.

Time-Temperature Relationship

Two factors, **time** *and* **temperature,** *control the rate of film development.*

As developer temperature increases, development time decreases.

Two factors, time and temperature, control the rate of film development. These two controlling factors have an inverse relationship. As one increases, the other must decrease to maintain the same rate of development. In general, *as developer temperature increases, development time decreases.* This is a very important relationship that controls the actual development of the radiograph. Development of the film must be a standardized factor in the radiographic process.

Replenishment

Replenishment *maintains constant levels of chemical activity.*

As one processes multiple films, the chemicals in the processing solutions are depleted. As depletion occurs, less development and fixing take place. To maintain constant levels of chemical activity, fresh chemistry is added to the working solution. The amount of replenishment is based on the number and size of films processed. As one adds replenisher, it is important that the solution is properly mixed. This prevents layering and uneven processing of the film. The developer replenisher is identical to the working solution, with the exception of restrainers. This is intentional because restrainer, potassium bromide, is a byproduct of development. When restarting a processor and filling the tanks with fresh replenisher, the addition of starter or potassium bromide is necessary to prevent overdevelopment. Fixer replenisher is also identical to the working solution, with the exception of the silver in solution in the fixing tank.

The Automatic Processor

The automatic processor has revolutionized the radiology darkroom in many ways (Figure 8-1). Twenty-five years ago, a 90-second dry-to-dry processing method was

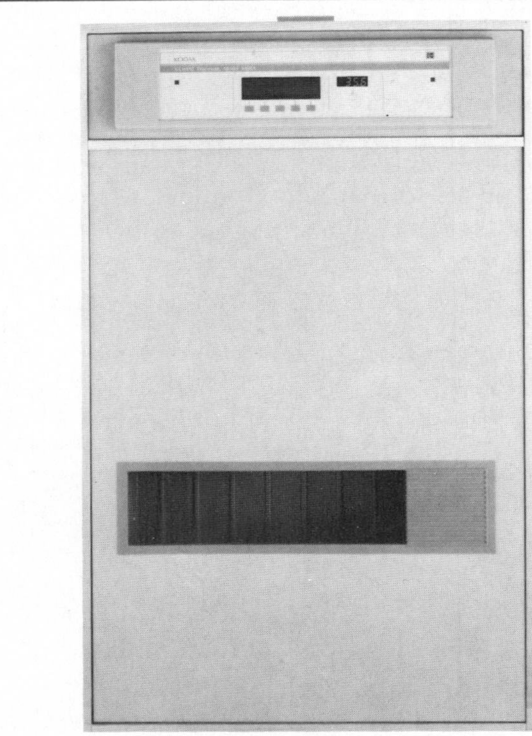

Figure 8-1
Automatic radiographic film processor. (Courtesy Eastman Kodak Co.)

nonexistent. Emergency reading of films required removing the films from the wash and carrying them to the radiologist while they were still wet. The term "wet reading" is still commonly used to request an immediate interpretation.

The typical automatic processor has eight major sections: (1) transport, (2) development, (3) fixing, (4) washing, (5) drying, (6) replenishment, (7) recirculation, and (8) temperature control.

The purpose of the transport system is to transport film through the processor. This system also provides agitation of the chemistry near the surface of the film. The transport system typically is composed of a series of rollers contained in racks, turnarounds, and crossovers (Figure 8-2). The transport system controls the amount of time the film is in contact with the developer and thus controls development time.

The development and fixing sections contain the chemicals for developing and fixing the radiograph. These usually consist of stainless-steel or plastic tanks in which

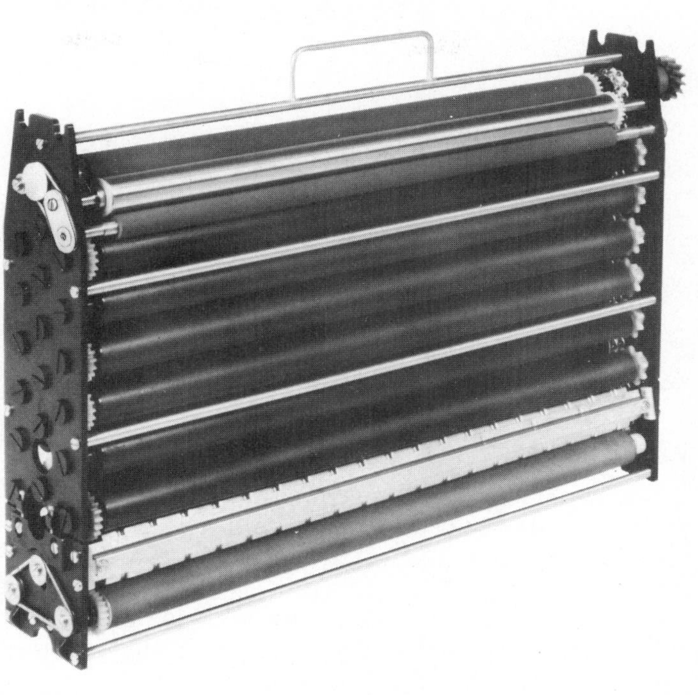

Figure 8-2
Developer rack from an automatic radiographic film processor. (Courtesy Eastman Kodak Co.)

the racks of transport rollers are found. The replenishment, recirculation, and temperature-control systems all are incorporated into these sections.

The wash section is also a stainless-steel or plastic tank in which transport rollers are found. The wash system uses a large volume of water, which is either tempered or cold. Tempered-water processors sometimes pass the developer through tubing in the wash tank to cool the developer and help regulate its temperature. Cold-water processors are becoming more widely used due to the significant energy savings when compared to hot-water use.

The dryer section serves to dry the film. This is important because the wet film has a soft emulsion and is susceptible to damage. The dryer temperature should be high enough to dry the film and no higher. This conserves energy and minimizes the heat generated in the work area.

The replenisher system functions to maintain the chemical activity in the solutions. Replenishment rates are established, and as film is fed into the processor, fresh chemistry is added to the working solutions in both the developer and the fixer tanks. Replenishment rates depend on the type of film used, the type of imaging being performed, and the volume. One consults the film manufacturer's guidelines when determining replenishment rates.

The recirculation system mixes the chemistry to ensure uniformity throughout the developer and fixer tanks. This system prevents layering and unequal processing of the radiograph.

The temperature-control system regulates developer temperature. As discussed earlier, the temperature of the developer can have a significant impact on development. This system usually consists of a thermostat, a heater, and a method of cooling the developer. The cooling or heat-exchanger system may be air or water cooled.

Processor Quality Control

Daily evaluation of the processor is an important quality control measure. Variations in processing can result in an increased repeat rate and associated costs, as well as problems in the archival quality of radiographs. Evaluation of the processor is more important in the small department with a low volume because of the increased likelihood of chemistry problems. The daily evaluation should include sensitometric evaluation; determination of developer temperature, replenishment, replenisher levels, dryer temperature, and proper function of the time-delay relay; and maintenance of cleanliness in the darkroom area.

The daily evaluation of the processor should include sensitometric evaluation; determination of developer temperature, replenishment, replenisher levels, dryer temperature, and proper function of the time-delay relay; and maintenance of cleanliness in the darkroom area.

Daily sensitometric evaluation of the processor involves determination of the speed, contrast, and base plus fog or gross fog. The two pieces of equipment required to carry out sensitometry are the sensitometer and the densitometer.

Daily sensitometric evaluation of the processor involves determination of the speed, contrast, and base plus fog or gross fog.

The *sensitometer* is a device that uses light to make an exposure on film (Figure 8-3). The sensitometer is capable of producing a consistent exposure from day to day for comparison. The exposure must be of a wavelength to which the film is sensitive. Typically, the exposure produces a series of several densities, as illustrated in Figure 8-4. The film used to record the densities should be the type normally used in the department.

The **sensitometer** *is a device that uses light to make an exposure on film.*

The technologist processes one sensitometrically exposed film in each processor, then monitors and records other parameters at this time. This usually works out well because the film is in the processor for 90 seconds or more. One checks built-in thermometers and replenishment rate devices regularly to ensure accuracy.

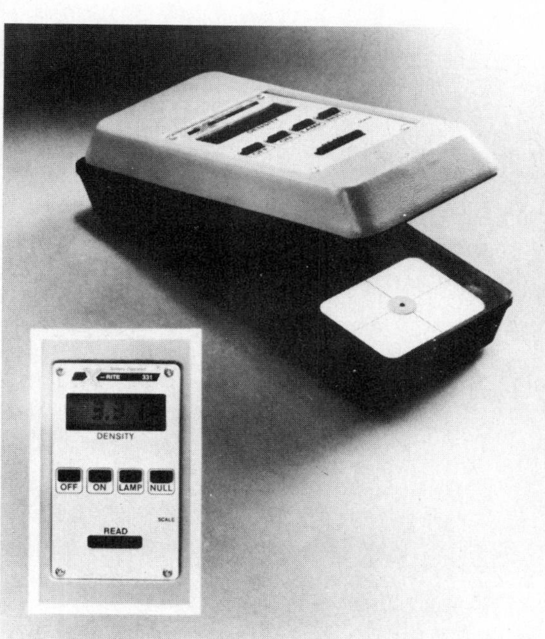

Figure 8-3
Sensitometer. (Courtesy X-Rite Co.)

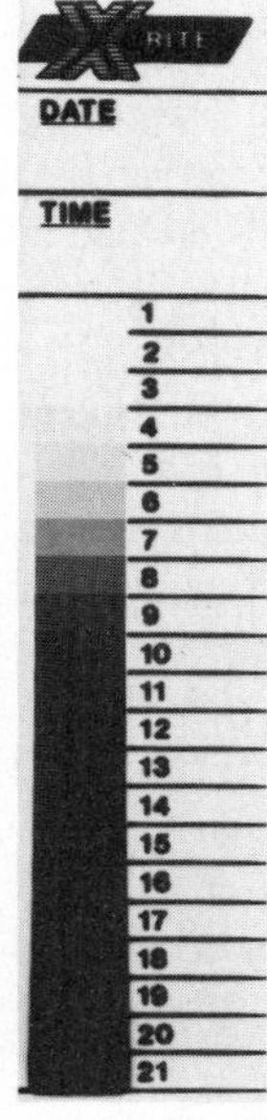

Figure 8-4
Example of the step wedge produced on a radiograph using a sensitometer. (Courtesy X-Rite Co.)

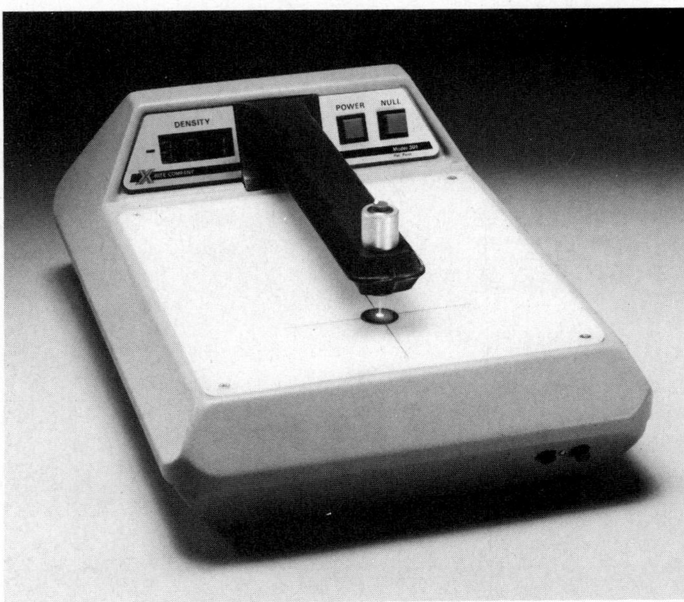

Figure 8-5
Densitometer. (Courtesy X-Rite Co.)

After processing, a *densitometer* is used to evaluate the film (Figure 8-5). The densitometer reads the density by comparing the incident light to the transmitted light. Included in the evaluation are the base plus fog, the speed, and the contrast. One should consult the film manufacturer's guidelines for recommendations in this area.

*A **densitometer** is a device that reads the density by comparing the incident light to the transmitted light.*

Another quality control measure that must be monitored in the darkroom is illumination. Steps must be taken to ensure that the safelight filter is appropriate for the film being used. Periodic evaluation of the safelight is done to monitor safelight fog. Fog from the safelight or light leaks in the darkroom can have a detrimental effect on film quality. The safelight test is performed in the following manner:

1. Use a piece of exposed film, since exposed film is approximately eight times as sensitive to light as unexposed film.
2. After placing the film in a cassette and exposing it very slightly, take the film into the darkroom and remove it from the cassette in total darkness.

Exposed film is approximately eight times as sensitive to light as unexposed film.

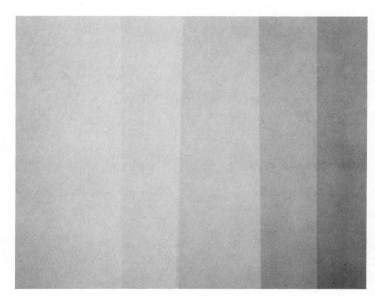

Figure 8-6
Example of a darkroom safelight test film.

3. Place the film on the loading bench, covering all but one section of the film.
4. Turn on all the safelights typically used in the darkroom.
5. After each minute of safelight exposure, slide the covering material back, exposing a little more of the film. Repeat this process for a total of 6 minutes.
6. Leave one section of the film unexposed to the safelight.
7. Turn off the safelights and process the film.
8. Examine the film to determine the maximum time for handling films in the darkroom (Figure 8-6).

Chapter 8—Review Questions

1. During which step of film processing does the latent image become visible?
   a. development
   b. fixing
   c. washing
   d. drying
2. Which of the following are solvents for the developer?
   a. hydroquinone
   b. phenidone
   c. glutaraldehyde
   d. two of the above
   e. none of the above
3. What is the function of potassium bromide in the developer?
   a. a reducer
   b. an activator
   c. a preservative
   d. a restrainer
   e. none of the above
4. Which of the following is the hardener in the developer?
   a. hydroquinone
   b. phenidone
   c. glutaraldehyde
   d. two of the above
   e. none of the above
5. Which of the following is not a major component of the fixer?
   a. reducer
   b. clearing agent
   c. preservative
   d. buffer
   e. hardener
6. Sodium sulfite is the preservative for which of the following solutions?
   a. developer
   b. fixer
   c. both of the above

7. What is the purpose of the clearing agent?
   a. to reduce the silver halide crystals in the emulsion
   b. to remove undeveloped silver halide crystals from the emulsion
   c. to maintain the desired acidity or alkalinity of the fixer
   d. to accelerate the chemical action in the fixer
   e. none of the above
8. What is the primary purpose of the wash?
   a. to remove the emulsion from the film
   b. to remove fixer from the emulsion
   c. to remove undeveloped silver halide from the emulsion
   d. to soften the emulsion
   e. none of the above
9. Time and temperature share which type of relationship in the development of film?
   a. direct
   b. inverse
10. What is the primary purpose of replenishment?
    a. to maintain constant levels of chemical activity
    b. to prevent layering and uneven processing of the film
    c. to deplete the processing chemistry
    d. two of the above
    e. all of the above
11. What is the difference between working developer solution and developer replenisher?
    a. silver in solution
    b. sodium sulfite
    c. restrainer
    d. preservative
    e. none of the above
12. How often should the processor be evaluated?
    a. daily
    b. weekly
    c. biweekly
    d. monthly
13. What device is used to expose the film to produce a series of several different densities?
    a. a densitometer
    b. a sensitometer
    c. a penetrameter

14. Which of the following is *not* a part of the sensitometric evaluation?
    a. speed
    b. density
    c. contrast
    d. base plus fog
    e. none of the above
15. Which of the following statements is true concerning the safelight test?
    a. The film should be removed from the box in total darkness.
    b. The film should be unexposed to determine actual fog.
    c. One portion of the film is left unexposed.
    d. two of the above
    e. all of the above

9

Controlling Factors of the Radiographic Process

OBJECTIVES

After completing Chapter 9, you should be able to:

1. Define the following terms:
   exposure latitude
   15 percent rule
   milliampere-seconds
   rule of thumb
2. Discuss the four primary controlling factors of the radiographic process.
3. Discuss the interrelationships between density and contrast.

Four primary factors control the production of a radiograph: kilovoltage, milliamperage, time, and distance. All other variable factors, such as processing, grids, cones, and screens, are secondary factors.

Kilovoltage

Kilovoltage, or kilovoltage peak (kVp), is the factor that has the greatest effect on the radiographic image. Kilovoltage affects both contrast and density of the image. *Kilovoltage is a controlling factor of the quality of the radiation produced.* Increasing the kilovoltage of the x-ray tube increases the potential difference across the tube. This causes an increase in the speed with which the electrons cross the tube and strike the target. The increase in the kinetic energy of the electrons results in production of x-rays with shorter wavelengths or higher energy. X-rays produced with high kilovoltage are more energetic and therefore more penetrating. In addition, high-kilovoltage x-rays are an important factor in the production of scatter radiation, which is detrimental to the overall quality of the radiograph and necessitates the use of beam-restricting devices and grids.

Kilovoltage *is a controlling factor of the quality of the radiation produced.*

Kilovoltage has a pronounced effect on the density of a radiograph. Increasing the kilovoltage without increasing the quantity of radiation will result in a greater photographic effect on the film, and the resultant radiograph will have more density. The relationship between kilovoltage and radiographic density is not linear. At low-kilovoltage ranges, small changes in kilovoltage will have a pronounced effect on the density of the radiograph. At higher-kilovoltage ranges, greater changes in kilovoltage are required to effect the same change in density. Two "rules" attempt to define the kilovoltage-density relationship and allow the technologist to use kilovoltage to control density.

The relationship between kilovoltage and radiographic density is not linear.

The *rule of thumb* states that to maintain the same density on a radiograph, one may cut the milliampere-seconds (mAs) in half and add 12 kVp (see later section on milliampere-seconds). Conversely, one may double the mAs and subtract 12 kVp. The rule of thumb is of limited value to the technologist. It works in a fairly narrow range, from about 70 to 90 kVp.

The **rule of thumb** *states that to maintain the same density on a radiograph, one may cut the milliampere-seconds (mAs) in half and add 12 kVp.*

The *15 percent rule* states that to maintain the same density on a radiograph, one may cut the mAs in half and increase the kVp by 15 percent. Conversely, one may double the mAs and decrease the kVp by 15 percent. The 15

The **15 percent rule** *states that to maintain the same density on a radiograph, one may cut the mAs in half and increase the kVp by 15 percent.*

percent rule is probably more accurate over a wider range of kilovoltage than the rule of thumb. It should be emphasized, however, that both rules are a quick, easy guide for the technologist rather than a scientific prediction of the effect of kilovoltage changes on density.

Low kilovoltage will produce an image that is high in contrast.

Kilovoltage also affects radiographic contrast. The use of low kVp will produce an image that is high in contrast. A high-contrast image has a short range of densities, going quickly from white to black with few intermediate shades of gray. A high-contrast image possesses short-scale contrast. The number of different densities is few, and a high-contrast image of a step wedge produces a short scale of densities. High-contrast images result in dense structures such as bones having virtually no density, whereas less dense structures, such as the soft tissues, have high density. This results in the bones appearing very white against a black background of soft tissue.

High kilovoltage will produce an image that is low in contrast.

Higher kilovoltage will produce an image that is low in contrast. A low-contrast image has a long range of densities, going gradually from white to black with many intermediate shades of gray. A low-contrast image possesses long-scale contrast. Many different densities exist, and a low-contrast image of a step wedge produces a long scale of densities. Low-contrast or long-scale images result in dense structures, such as bones, having some density on a radiograph, whereas less dense structures, such as the soft tissues, have more density, but less than air density. This results in a grayer image, with light-gray to white densities in the bone and darker-gray to black densities in the soft tissues. Figure 9-1 shows step wedge radiographs with high and low contrast.

Exposure latitude *can be defined as the range between the minimum and maximum exposure that will produce an acceptable density on the radiograph.*

High-kilovoltage techniques result in wide exposure latitude, which allows considerable error in mAs selection. Lower-kilovoltage techniques result in narrow exposure latitude, which does not allow for much error in mAs selection.

Kilovoltage also influences exposure latitude. *Exposure latitude* can be defined as the range between the minimum and maximum exposure that will produce an acceptable density on the radiograph. In simpler terms, it is the technologist's margin for error. High-kilovoltage techniques result in wide exposure latitude, which allows considerable error in mAs selection. Lower-kilovoltage techniques result in narrow exposure latitude, which does not allow for much error in mAs selection. In general, the higher the kVp and longer the scale of contrast, the wider is the exposure latitude. The lower the kVp and shorter the scale of contrast, the narrower is the exposure latitude.

Higher-kilovoltage techniques have several advantages over lower-kilovoltage ones and are said to have a higher radiographic efficiency.

Higher-kilovoltage techniques have several advantages over lower-kilovoltage ones and are said to have a higher radiographic efficiency. Higher kilovoltage produces low- or long-scale contrast, which gives some den-

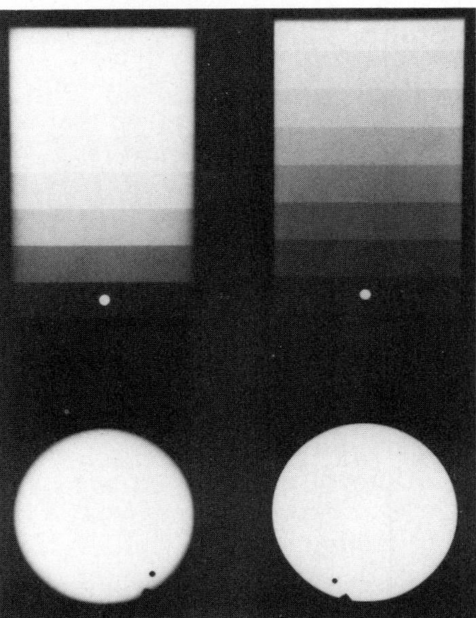

Figure 9-1
Radiographs of a step wedge, obtained at 60 kVp (left) *and 120 kVp* (right), *demonstrating high contrast and low contrast, respectively.*

sity to more tissues, making them visible on the radiograph. Higher kilovoltage can produce increased image sharpness because it reduces the heat load on the x-ray tube, allowing the use of shorter exposure times and smaller focal spots. *Shorter exposure times help prevent patient motion, which is the single greatest factor in radiographic unsharpness* (Figure 9-2). The reduction in heat produced extends the x-ray tube life. Higher kilovoltage also reduces the radiation exposure to the patient, since high-energy radiation is less attenuated by the patient and the amount of radiation required to produce a given density is smaller. Finally, the increase in exposure latitude with high kilovoltage reduces repeat procedures, with subsequent savings in film and processing costs.

Shorter exposure times help prevent patient motion, which is the single greatest factor in radiographic unsharpness.

It might appear that high-kilovoltage techniques are best for every radiographic examination; however, this is not the case. Many indications exist for lower-kilovoltage techniques, including iodinated contrast media studies, mammography, and soft tissue examinations. Even in the same body part, the area of interest may mandate different

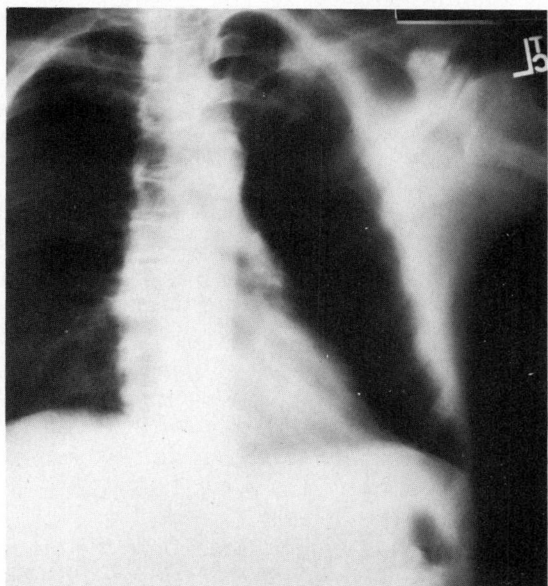

Figure 9-2
Radiograph demonstrating motion unsharpness.

An optimum kilovoltage exists for every type of examination.

kilovoltage techniques. Most institutions use high kilovoltage for chest examinations to record radiographically the wide range of densities in the chest. When the area of interest is the ribs, however, using a lower kilovoltage is necessary. Remember: an optimum kilovoltage exists for every type of examination. The optimum kVp depends on the body part and the anatomy of interest. This will be discussed further in Chapter 14.

Contrast has an effect on the perceived resolution or detail of the radiograph. As the difference between the densities of two objects increases, the more readily the eye can perceive the objects. The presence of high contrast appears to improve resolution. However, it is the *perception* of resolution and not the resolution that increases. Therefore, as contrast decreases, the differences between the densities of two objects also decrease, making detail more difficult for the eye to perceive.

In summary, high-kilovoltage techniques produce (1) low contrast, (2) many shades of gray in the radiographic image, (3) long-scale contrast, (4) wide exposure latitude, and (5) higher radiographic efficiency. Low-kilovoltage techniques produce (1) high contrast, (2) black and white images with few shades of gray, (3) short-scale contrast, (4) narrow exposure latitude, and (5) lower radiographic efficiency.

Milliamperage

Milliamperage (mA) is another controlling factor for the quantity of radiation produced by the x-ray tube. Increasing the milliamperage increases the number of electrons boiled off at the cathode of the x-ray tube. Increasing the quantity of electrons that strike the target of the x-ray tube increases the quantity of x-ray photons produced. Since milliamperage controls the quantity of radiation produced, it affects the density of a radiograph. The relationship of milliamperage to density is linear. In theory, *doubling the milliamperage should double the density,* when all other factors remain constant. Likewise, halving the milliamperage should halve the density.

The relationship of milliamperage to density is linear.

Changing the milliamperage affects only the quantity of radiation produced and does not affect the quality of the radiation produced. Therefore, milliamperage has no effect on contrast, assuming the density changes are within the limitations of the image receptor.

Time

Time, measured in seconds or fractions of seconds, is a quantity factor. Time represents the duration that a given quantity and quality of radiation interacts with the image receptor. Time has a linear relationship to density. *Doubling the time of exposure will double the density,* and halving the time of exposure will halve the density. Time has no effect on contrast, assuming the density changes are within the limits of the image receptor.

The relationship of time to density is linear.

Milliampere-Seconds

Milliampere-seconds (mAs) is a quantitative concept and is the most practical measure of the quantity of radiation. *Milliampere-seconds* is the product of milliamperage and time (mA × seconds = mAs). In theory and in practice, a given mAs will always produce the same density on a radiograph, regardless of the combination of mA and time used. In other words, to achieve a given radiographic density, the technologist may change the mA or time to fit

Milliampere-seconds *is the product of milliamperage and time (mA × seconds = mAs).*

The relationship of mAs to density is linear.

the radiologic need as long as the product, mAs, remains the same. The mAs-density relationship is linear. In theory, doubling the mAs will double the density of a radiograph, and halving the mAs will halve the density.

When altering mAs, the time station is the usual variable because the greater selection of time stations allows greater variability. However, some conditions make it more appropriate to change the mA station, including (1) the use of high mA to stop motion, (2) the use of lower mA to employ smaller focal spots, and (3) the use of low mA to overcome generator limitations when using techniques at very high mAs.

It requires a 35 percent change in mAs to produce an effect on density.

A few guidelines can predict the effect of mAs changes on the density of a radiograph. One must realize that it requires at least a 35 percent change in mAs to produce a significant effect on density (Figure 9-3). If a radiograph is seriously underexposed, the technologist should double the mAs. Conversely, if a film is seriously overexposed, the technologist should halve the mAs. The mA for a given radiographic density is inversely proportional to

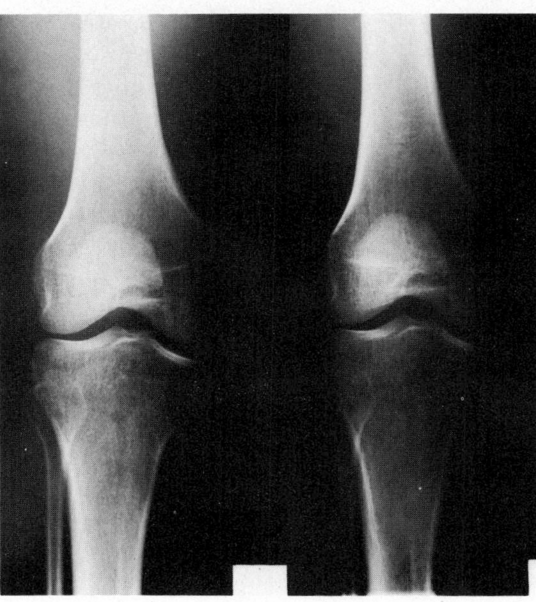

Figure 9-3 Radiographs demonstrating the effect of a 35 percent change in mAs. The film on the right-hand side was obtained using an increase of 35 percent of the original mAs.

the time of exposure when all other factors remain constant. Algebraically, this is expressed as:

$$\frac{\text{Original mA}}{\text{New mA}} = \frac{\text{New time}}{\text{Original time}}$$

Distance

Distance is usually described in one of the four following terms:

1. Focal film distance (FFD)
2. Anode film distance (AFD)
3. Target film distance (TFD)
4. Source-to-image receptor distance (SID)

All four terms refer to the distance between the source of x-rays and the recording medium for the image, and all four are commonly used. The term "source-to-image receptor distance" is probably the most appropriate, however, since it does not limit the image-recording medium to film only. The SID has three important influences on the radiographic image: influences on (1) radiographic density, (2) size and shape of the image recorded, and (3) sharpness of the image detail. At this point we will discuss only the influence on radiographic density.

X-rays travel in diverging lines from the target of the tube. As the distance from the target of the tube increases, the number of x-ray photons per unit of area decreases, as illustrated in Figure 9-4. This phenomenon is the same as the laws governing the intensity of light generated from a point source and is referred to as the *inverse square law*. If an x-ray beam covered exactly 4 square inches at a distance of 36 inches, the x-ray beam would cover 16 square inches at a distance of 72 inches. In other words, if one doubles the distance from the source of x-rays, the quantity of x-rays per unit of area decreases by one fourth. Conversely, if one halves the distance from the source, the quantity of x-rays per unit of area increases four times. One can compensate for a change in distance by altering the mAs. The following equation allows one to calculate the mAs-distance relationship:

$$\frac{\text{Original mAs}}{\text{New mAs}} = \frac{\text{Original SID}^2}{\text{New SID}^2}$$

Density is inversely proportional to the square of the distance and is a quantity factor.

Density is inversely proportional to the square of the distance and is a quantity factor.

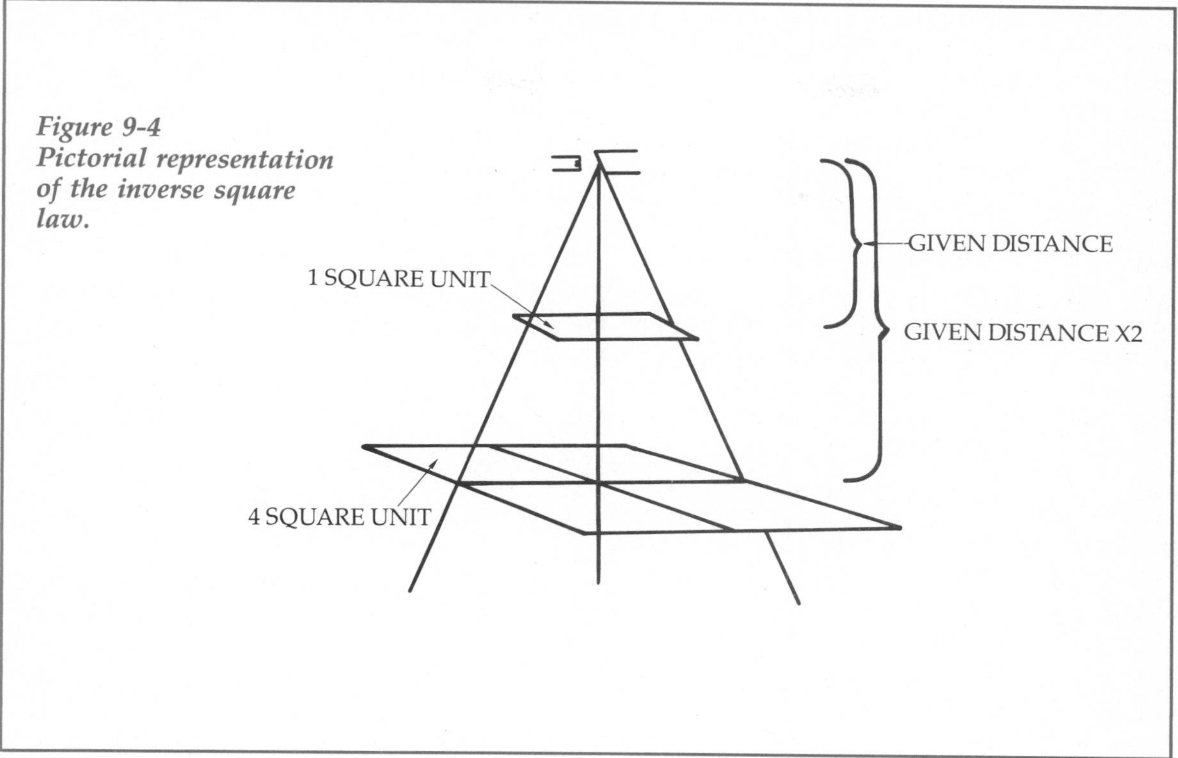

Figure 9-4
Pictorial representation of the inverse square law.

The concept of **photographic effect** *states that the quantity and quality of radiation have a predictable effect on film.*

$$PE = \frac{mA \times T \times kVp^2}{D^2}$$

Photographic Effect

The concept of *photographic effect* states that the quantity and quality of radiation have a predictable effect on film. The photographic effect is a numerical value and has a direct linear relationship to density. If one doubles the photographic effect, one doubles the density on the film. Halving the photographic effect halves the density. Photographic effect (PE) is algebraically expressed as:

$$\mathrm{PE} = \frac{\mathrm{mA} \times \mathrm{T} \times \mathrm{kVp}^2}{\mathrm{D}^2}$$

where T is time and D is distance.

Interrelationship Between Density and Contrast

The technologist must understand an important relationship between density and contrast. Contrast cannot exist without density because contrast is the relationship between two or more densities. Throughout this chapter, we have assumed that changing the mAs increases or decreases density without affecting contrast. This assumption is true within the limitations of the image receptor. Film as an image receptor has certain limitations. A level of exposure exists below which the film cannot respond, and a level of exposure exists above which the film cannot respond. If the technologist uses too little mAs to expose a film, this will affect contrast. The scale of contrast will be shortened by the elimination of densities at the minimum-density end of the scale. Conversely, if the technologist uses too much mAs to expose a film, the scale of contrast will be shortened by the elimination of densities on the maximum-density end of the scale.

Chapter 9—Review Questions

1. Which of the following is considered to be a primary controlling factor for contrast?
   a. kilovoltage
   b. milliamperage
   c. time
   d. distance
   e. two of the above
   f. three of the above
   g. all of the above
   h. none of the above
2. Which of the following is considered to be a primary controlling factor for density?
   a. kilovoltage
   b. milliamperage
   c. time
   d. distance
   e. two of the above
   f. three of the above
   g. all of the above
   h. none of the above
3. Which of the following is considered to be a primary controlling factor for density *and* contrast?
   a. kilovoltage
   b. milliamperage
   c. time
   d. distance
   e. two of the above
   f. three of the above
   g. all of the above
   h. none of the above
4. What is the relationship between density and SID?
   a. inverse relationship
   b. direct inverse relationship
   c. direct linear relationship
   d. inverse square relationship
   e. direct square relationship

5. Which of the following does not refer to the distance between the sources of x-rays and the recording medium for the image?
   a. FFD
   b. AFD
   c. OFD
   d. TFD
   e. SID

6. If a satisfactory radiograph is obtained at an SID of 72 inches, using 80 mAs at 80 kVp, what exposure factors will have to be used at 36 inches?
   a. 40 mAs at 80 kVp
   b. 20 mAs at 80 kVp
   c. 10 mAs at 80 kVp
   d. 160 mAs at 80 kVp
   e. none of the above

7. Which of the following formulas correctly represents the photographic effect?
   a. $PE = mA \times T \times kVp^2$
   b. $PE = \frac{mA \times T \times kVp}{D}$
   c. $PE = \frac{mA \times T \times kVp^2}{D}$
   d. $PE = \frac{mA \times T \times kVp^2}{D^2}$
   e. none of the above

8. What percentage change in mAs is required to make a noticeable change in density?
   a. 10 percent
   b. 25 percent
   c. 35 percent
   d. 50 percent
   e. none of the above

9. Which of the following is true concerning high-kVp technique?
   a. It produces high contrast and wide exposure latitude.
   b. It produces high contrast and narrow exposure latitude.
   c. It produces low contrast and wide exposure latitude.
   d. It produces low contrast and narrow exposure latitude.
   e. none of the above

10. Which of the following is true concerning low-kVp technique?
    a. It produces high contrast and wide exposure latitude.
    b. It produces high contrast and narrow exposure latitude.
    c. It produces low contrast and wide exposure latitude.
    d. It produces low contrast and narrow exposure latitude.
    e. none of the above

11. Which of the following radiographic factors is a quality factor?
    a. kilovoltage
    b. milliamperage
    c. time
    d. distance
    e. two of the above
    f. three of the above
    g. all of the above
    h. none of the above

12. Which of the following radiographic factors is a quantity factor?
    a. kilovoltage
    b. milliamperage
    c. time
    d. distance
    e. two of the above
    f. three of the above
    g. all of the above
    h. none of the above

13. At higher-kVp ranges, what effect will a small increase in kVp have on density when compared to a low-kVp range?
    a. a large increase in density
    b. a moderate increase in density
    c. a small increase in density

14. If 80 mAs at 100 kVp produced a satisfactory density on a radiograph, but patient motion was evident, requiring the time to be cut by 50 percent (40 mAs), what kVp should be used according to the 15 percent rule?
    a. 85 kVp
    b. 100 kVp
    c. 115 kVp
    d. 130 kVp
    e. none of the above

15. If 80 mAs at 100 kVp produced a satisfactory density on a radiograph, but patient motion was evident, requiring the time to be cut by 50 percent (40 mAs), what kVp should be used according to the rule of thumb?
    a. 88 kVp
    b. 100 kVp
    c. 112 kVp
    d. 115 kVp
    e. none of the above

16. Using the factors in problem 15, what would the new kVp be using the 15 percent rule?
    a. 88 kVp
    b. 100 kVp
    c. 112 kVp
    d. 115 kVp
    e. none of the above

17. Using the 15 percent rule, which of the following techniques would produce the greatest radiographic density?
    a. 60 kVp at 600 mAs
    b. 85 kVp at 150 mAs
    c. 90 kVp at 75 mAs
    d. 92 kVp at 300 mAs

18. Using the rule of thumb to equalize mAs, which of the following techniques would produce the greatest radiographic contrast?
    a. 60 kVp at 600 mAs
    b. 79 kVp at 150 mAs
    c. 90 kVp at 75 mAs
    d. 102 kVp at 35 mAs

19. Using the rule of thumb, which of the following techniques would produce the greatest radiographic density?
    a. 80 kVp at 40 mAs at 36 inches SID
    b. 92 kVp at 80 mAs at 72 inches SID
    c. 68 kVp at 100 mAs at 36 inches SID
    d. 92 kVp at 20 mAs at 36 inches SID
20. Which of the following techniques would produce the least radiographic density?
    a. 83 kVp at 50 mAs at 72 inches SID
    b. 100 kVp at 100 mAs at 36 inches SID
    c. 115 kVp at 50 mAs at 36 inches SID
    d. 100 kVp at 25 mAs at 72 inches SID

10

Beam-Restricting Devices

OBJECTIVES

After completing Chapter 10, you should be able to:

1. Define the following terms:
   aperture diaphragm
   beam-restricting device
   collimator
   cylinder cone
   flare cone
2. Discuss the construction and function of collimators.
3. Describe the impact of field size on density and contrast.
4. Discuss the radiation protection implications of beam-restricting devices.

Beam-restricting devices control the size and shape of the primary beam. The main purpose of beam-restricting devices is the reduction of patient exposure to radiation. However, the use of these devices can also improve image quality. Beam restriction is an essential element in certain radiographic techniques and imaging modalities.

Beam-restricting devices control the size and shape of the primary beam. The main purpose of beam-restricting devices is the reduction of patient exposure to radiation.

The three major types of beam-restricting devices are aperture diaphragms, cones and cylinders, and collimators. Each type has certain advantages and disadvantages that determine its suitability for specific applications. The following discussions examine each of these beam-restricting devices in detail.

Aperture Diaphragms

Aperture diaphragms are the simplest type of beam-restricting device. They are usually constructed of a lead sheet of adequate thickness to ensure attenuation of the primary beam. An opening is cut in the center to allow the desired portion of the primary beam to pass through unattenuated. The opening may be of any shape but is usually round, square, or rectangular. The size of the opening depends on the desired field size, the source-to-image receptor distance (SID), and the distance of the aperture diaphragm from the focal spot of the x-ray source. If lead is used as the attenuating material, it is often enclosed between two sheets of another harder metal to protect the soft lead from damage during handling.

Aperture diaphragms are constructed of a lead sheet with an opening cut in the center.

The aperture diaphragm is the simplest and least expensive of all the beam-restricting devices, which are its most significant advantages. One disadvantage of using the aperture diaphragm is its ability to produce only one field size at a given SID. Its principal disadvantage is the large *penumbra,* or geometric unsharpness, produced at the periphery of the field. Mounting the aperture diaphragm at a greater distance from the x-ray source will reduce penumbra, as shown in Figure 10-1.

The principal disadvantage of the aperture diaphragm is the large penumbra produced at the edge of the field.

When using aperture diaphragms, one must take care to avoid inserting the device incorrectly. Although this is not a problem with circular or square apertures, it can result in diaphragm cutoff with rectangular apertures. Additionally, the projected field size should never exceed the size of the image receptor and ideally should be tailored to the area of interest.

The fixed field size produced by the aperture diaphragm limits its use to applications where the SID and the desired field size do not vary. Equipment dedicated to

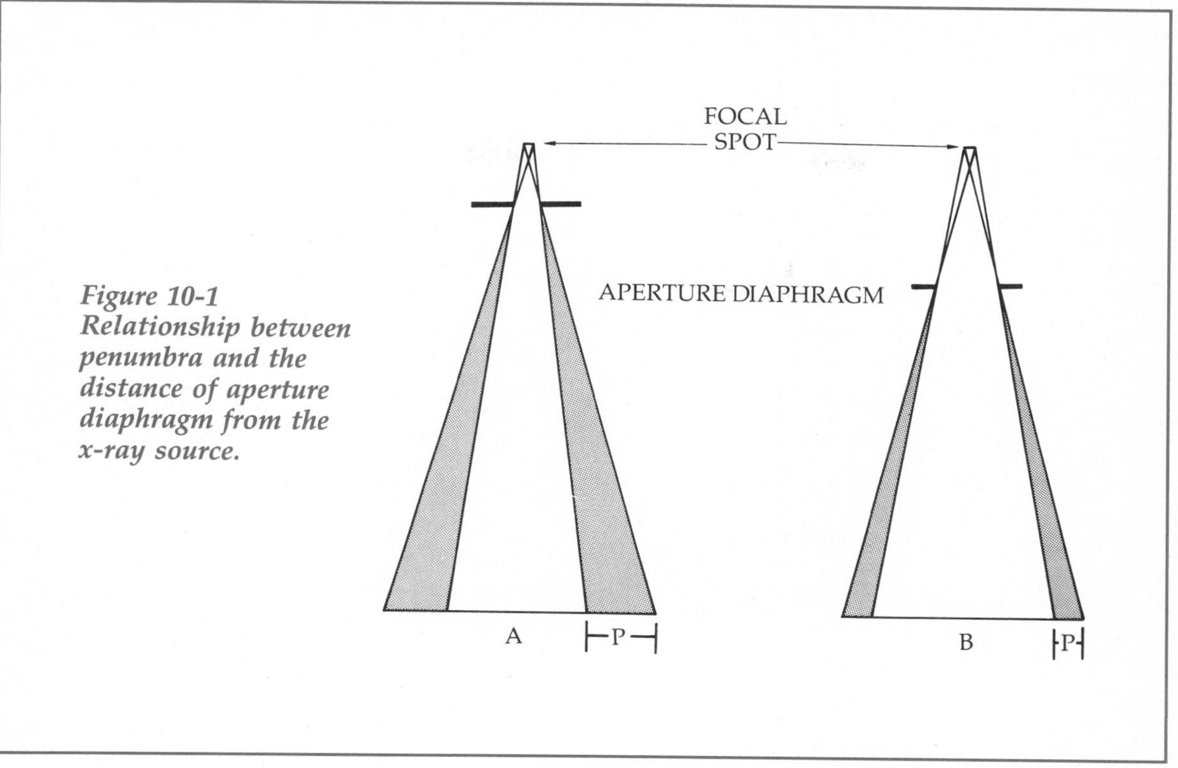

Figure 10-1 Relationship between penumbra and the distance of aperture diaphragm from the x-ray source.

chest radiography and tomographic studies often use aperture diaphragms. Some computed tomographic scanners also utilize a type of aperture diaphragm to produce a pencil or fan-shaped beam.

Cones

A **flare cone** *is essentially an aperture diaphragm with a conical extension that appears to match the divergence of the beam.*

The two major groups of cones are flare and cylinder cones. A *flare cone* is essentially an aperture diaphragm with a conical extension that appears to match the divergence of the beam. In reality, the flare of the cone is usually greater than the divergence of the beam and does not contribute to beam restriction. This renders the flare cone little more than an elaborate aperture diaphragm, as demonstrated in Figure 10-2.

A **cylinder cone** *is an aperture diaphragm with a cylindrical extension that restricts the beam at the distal end.*

A *cylinder cone* is an aperture diaphragm with a cylindrical extension that restricts the beam at the distal end. Since restriction of the beam takes place at an increased distance from the x-ray source, penumbra is reduced at the periphery of the field. This results in improved beam re-

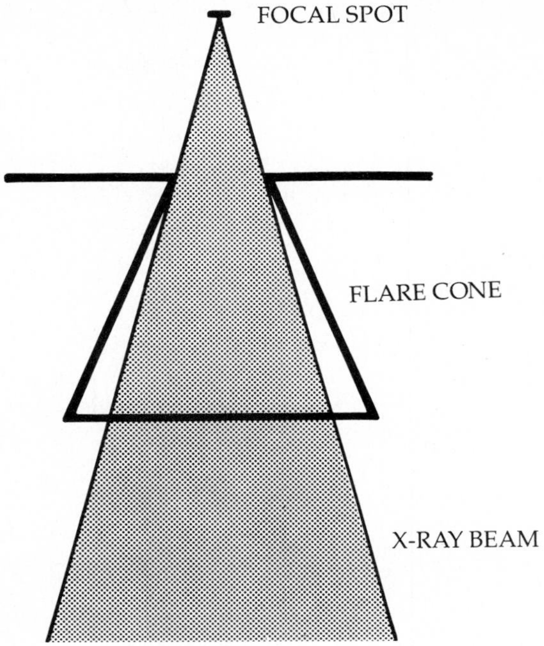

FOCAL SPOT

FLARE CONE

X-RAY BEAM

Figure 10-2
Flared portion of a flare cone does not contribute to beam restriction.

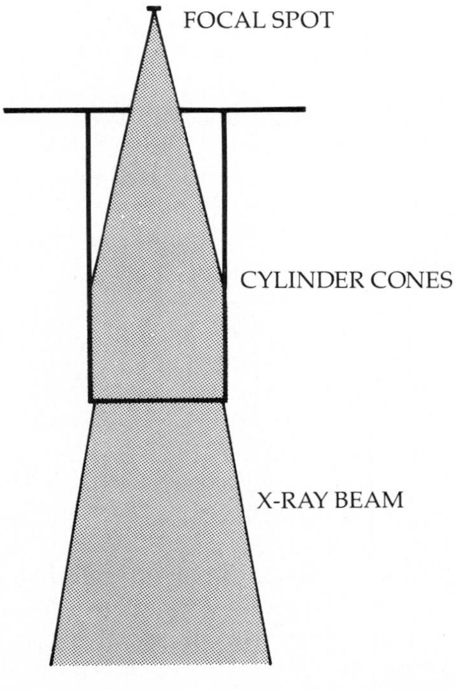

FOCAL SPOT

CYLINDER CONES

X-RAY BEAM

Figure 10-3
Increased beam restriction obtained with the use of a cylinder cone.

striction, as demonstrated in Figure 10-3. Cylinder cones are also available with extension sleeves and are called extension cylinders. This modification allows the beam restriction to occur at an even greater distance, further reducing penumbra.

Cones, as with aperture diaphragms, are inexpensive and simple to use. Also, cylinder cones provide better beam restriction when compared to aperture diaphragms. The physical weight of cones, however, makes them difficult to handle and can cause problems with tube locks. When used in the upright position, the weight of the cone may cause the tube to angle slightly, resulting in cone cutting. Cones also have the limitation of fixed field size, and flare cones fail to reduce penumbra further.

The major application of cones is in radiography of the skull and spine. Other applications include mammography, dental radiography, cholecystography, and applications that require small field size.

Collimators

The x-ray collimator is the most frequently employed beam-restricting device on contemporary radiographic equipment.

The x-ray collimator is the most frequently employed beam-restricting device on contemporary radiographic equipment. The construction of collimators is more complex than other beam-restricting devices. The collimator consists of at least two sets of shutters, one near the bottom of the collimator and one above. The two sets of shutters function as a variable aperture diaphragm in controlling the size of the field, as shown in Figure 10-4. Each set of shutters is composed of four lead vanes that move in opposing pairs, symmetrically from the center, as shown in Figure 10-5. This allows the selection of an infinite number of square and rectangular fields. Collimators designed for some special applications have two lead iris diaphragms and produce circular fields, whereas others provide both rectangular and circular fields.

The two sets of shutters in the collimator serve two functions other than regulating the size of the beam. The bottom set of shutters reduces penumbra at the periphery of the field because of its distance from the x-ray source. The upper set of shutters helps to control the escape of off-focus or stem radiation.

Collimators also provide a light field, which defines the center and margins of the radiation field.

Collimators also provide a light field, which defines the center and margins of the radiation field. To accomplish this, a mirror is mounted at a 45-degree angle in the x-ray beam where it passes through the collimator. A light source is then mounted in the collimator, opposite the mir-

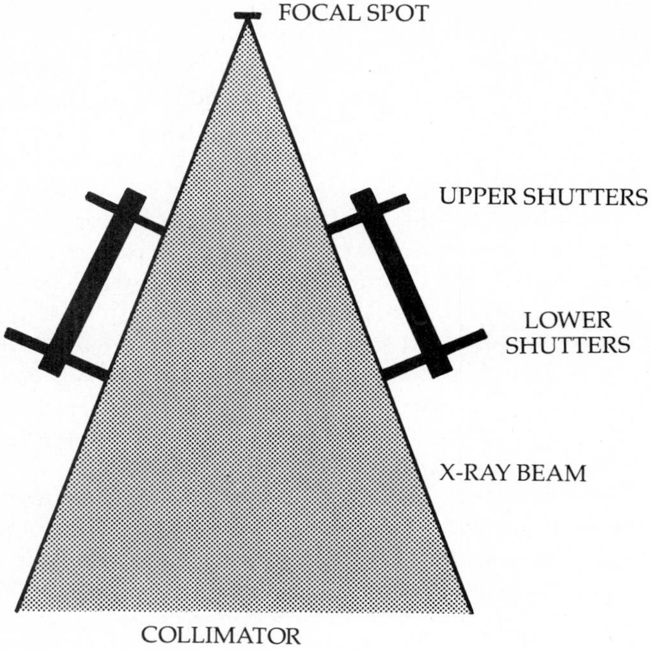

Figure 10-4
Relationship of the upper and lower shutters in a collimator.

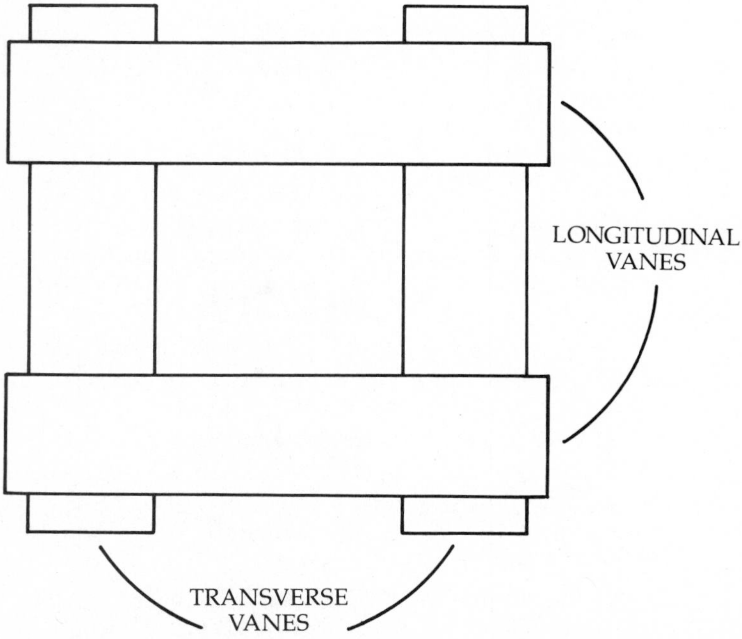

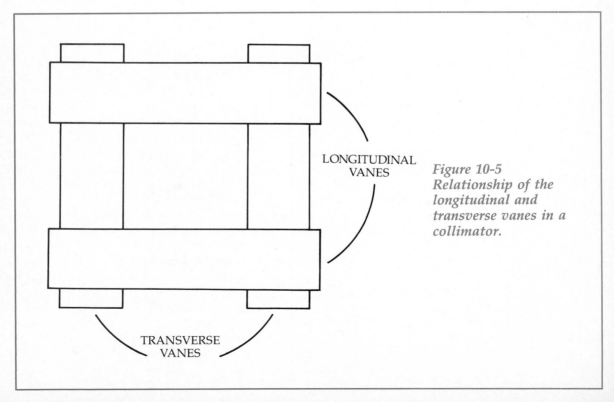

Figure 10-5
Relationship of the longitudinal and transverse vanes in a collimator.

ror, which projects both the margin of the beam and a cross hair. The light source and the radiation source must be equidistant from the mirror to ensure that the light and radiation field are equal in size. Improper positioning of the light source or mirror will result in improper alignment of the light-to-radiation field. Collimators usually incorporate a backup system of field-size determination in case of light source failure. This usually consists of a calibrated scale for various SIDs printed on the collimator adjustment mechanism.

A simple test can evaluate the congruence of the light-to-radiation field:

1. Project the light field on a film, and mark its margins with radiopaque indicators.
2. Place a left or right marker in the appropriate corner of the film so that direction can be easily ascertained later.
3. Make one exposure with the field collimated to the markers and a second covering the entire film.
4. Process the film and then inspect it to ensure that the radiation field is properly aligned with the opaque markers.

Figure 10-6 demonstrates an example of this test. Variations of up to 1.2 percent of the SID are acceptable.

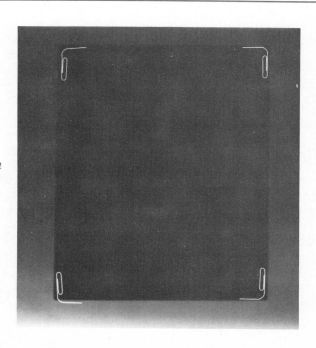

Figure 10-6
Example of a radiograph used to evaluate the congruence of the light and radiation fields.

Since 1974, federal law has required that all fixed radiographic equipment be equipped with automatic collimators, or *positive beam limitation* (PBL). The construction of these collimators is similar to the manual collimator, with the exception that electric motors drive the shutters. Sensors in the film tray detect the size of the film, and the electric motors then collimate to the proper field size. Some equipment, for special applications, is exempted from this regulation.

Since 1974, federal law has required that all fixed radiographic equipment be equipped with automatic collimators, or **positive beam limitation** *(PBL).*

The use of collimators, due to their construction, results in some filtration of the x-ray beam. This is because the mirror is situated in the primary beam. The collimator itself has about 1.0 mm aluminum equivalent filtration, and many collimators provide a means of adding additional filtration. The inherent filtration of the collimator may render it unacceptable for some low-kVp radiography, including mammography. Thus, some collimators are equipped with mirrors that can be removed from the primary beam for low-kVp examinations.

The advantages of the collimator are its ability to provide an infinite number of field sizes and to project the light field corresponding with the radiation field. This allows the technologist to tailor the radiation field to the part being examined, not just the size of the film. Disadvantages include the initial cost of the device, potential maintenance problems, and the inability to be used in some low-kVp applications.

The advantages of the collimator are its ability to provide an infinite number of field sizes and to project the light field corresponding with the radiation field.

Collimators have widespread application and few limitations. Contemporary radiographic and fluoroscopic equipment normally comes equipped with collimators on both overtable radiographic and undertable fluoroscopic tubes.

Calculation of Field Size

The technologist may find it necessary to calculate the size of an aperture necessary to produce a given field size at a given SID. This is especially true when designing a beam-restricting device for a special application. This is easily calculated by using the algebraic formula for determination of the length of the bases or the height of similar or isosceles triangles, as demonstrated in Figure 10-7. The ratio of the aperture diaphragm's diameter to the field's diameter equals the ratio of the distance between the x-ray source and the aperture diaphragm to the distance between the x-ray source and the source-to-image receptor.

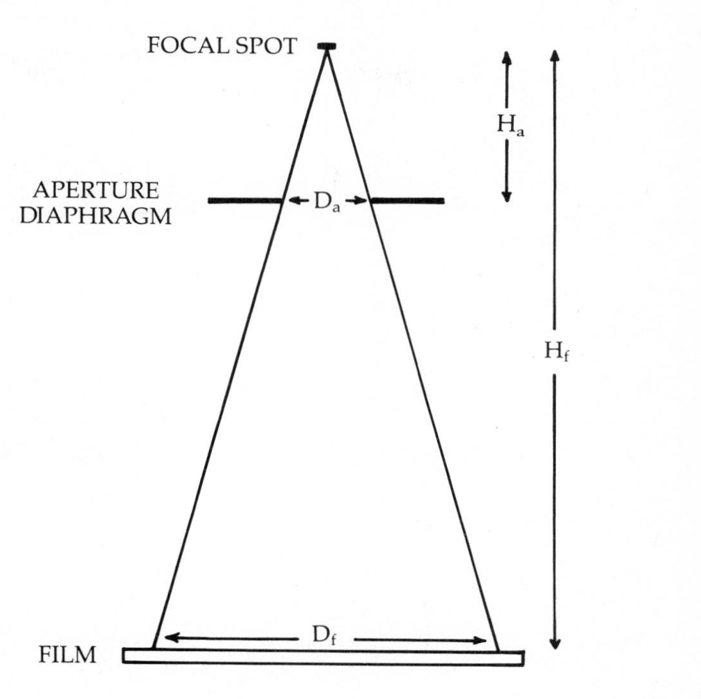

Figure 10-7
Relationship between aperture size and field size. D_a is the diameter of the aperture diaphragm, D_f is the diameter of the field, H_a is the distance from the x-ray source to the aperture diaphragm, and H_f is the distance from the x-ray source to the source-to-image receptor.

This is expressed as (see Figure 10-7 for explanation of variables):

$$\frac{D_a}{D_f} = \frac{H_a}{H_f}$$

Technique Considerations

Although the primary function of beam-restricting devices is patient protection, beam restrictors were used before the risks of radiation exposure were known. Early researchers discovered that using small fields improved the quality of the images produced on film. The reason for this is that larger fields produce greater amounts of scatter radiation. The increase of scatter radiation production is even more pronounced when radiographing thick body parts or using high-kVp techniques. Scatter radiation produces fog on the film, which increases the density and decreases the contrast of the image. Since a smaller field produces less scatter radiation, at a given technique, increased collimation or use of a smaller field will result in less density and more contrast on a film. Conversely, a less colli-

Increased collimation or use of a smaller field will result in less density and more contrast on a film.

mated or larger field will result in more density and less contrast. In general, *the larger the field size, the greater is the density and lower is the contrast;* the smaller the field, the lower the density and higher the contrast produced on a film. If the technologist wishes to maintain the same density on a film when reducing the size of a field, he or she must increase the technical factors by increasing the milliampere-seconds (mAs) or kVp.

Collimation has no direct effect on the detail recorded on the film. Since increased contrast enhances detail visibility, a small field appears to have greater detail than a large field used to produce a given radiograph. Accurate collimation and use of the smallest field size possible become even more important when the technologist is unable to use other means to reduce the amount of scatter radiation reaching the film.

Radiation Protection

As stated earlier, patient protection is the primary purpose of beam-restricting devices. The effect of radiation exposure on an organism depends on the total amount of tissue irradiated. The benefit of collimation should be readily evident, since less tissue is irradiated, with less biological effect on the patient. Collimation is one of the primary means by which the operator can control patient dose.

Patient protection is the primary purpose of beam-restricting devices.

Changes in the size of the field produce corresponding changes in the volume of tissue irradiated in the patient. Even small reductions in the field size produce substantial reductions in the area of the field and corresponding decreases in the volume of tissue irradiated. A spot film of the lumbosacral junction obtained on an 8 × 10-inch film produces a field size of 80 square inches, if collimated to the size of the film. If the field size is reduced to 6 × 6 inches or 36 square inches, the tissue irradiated is reduced more than 50 percent. In this example, the field size is adequate for the part examined, film quality is improved, and patient dose is significantly reduced.

Even small reductions in the field size produce substantial reductions in the area of the field and corresponding decreases in the volume of tissue irradiated.

Collimation is the responsibility of the operator, not the equipment. *The field size should never exceed the size of the image receptor.* In addition, the operator should not depend on automatic collimation, but rather should tailor the field to the part being examined. This is especially true during fluoroscopic examinations, where personnel as well as patient dose is higher. Minimizing the amount of scatter radiation by decreasing the field size will reduce patient dose, improve fluoroscopic image quality, and reduce personnel dose.

Collimation is the responsibility of the operator, not the equipment. **The field size should never exceed the size of the image receptor.**

Chapter 10—Review Questions

1. What is the primary purpose of beam-restricting devices?
   a. the control of off-focus radiation
   b. the reduction of patient exposure to radiation
   c. the improvement of image quality
   d. the control of radiographic contrast
2. What is the simplest type of beam-restricting device?
   a. the aperture diaphragm
   b. the cone
   c. the collimator
   d. the mask
3. Ideally, what should determine the field size?
   a. the image receptor
   b. the part being examined
   c. the collimator
   d. the SID
   e. none of the above
4. Which of the following devices provides the best control of penumbra?
   a. the aperture diaphragm
   b. the flare cone
   c. the extension cone
   d. the collimator
5. Which of the following devices provides the best control of off-focus radiation?
   a. the aperture diaphragm
   b. the flare cone
   c. the extension cone
   d. the collimator
6. What impact does increased collimation have on a radiograph?
   a. increased density and increased contrast
   b. increased density and decreased contrast
   c. decreased density and increased contrast
   d. decreased density and decreased contrast
7. The field size should never exceed the size of the:
   a. primary barrier
   b. secondary barrier
   c. image receptor
   d. none of the above

8. What is the major advantage of the collimator as a beam-restricting device?
   a. the initial cost of the device
   b. to provide an infinite number of field sizes
   c. the projection of a light field corresponding to the radiation field
   d. two of the above
   e. all of the above

9. What is the purpose of positive beam limitation?
   a. to simplify the radiographic process for the technologist
   b. to prevent the field size from exceeding the size of the image receptor
   c. to improve the reproducibility of collimation
   d. to prevent collimation to other than the film size
   e. none of the above

10. What is the primary purpose of the mirror in the collimator?
   a. to increase the filtration of the collimator
   b. to provide a light field that corresponds to the radiation field
   c. to defract radiation from the x-ray tube through the collimator
   d. two of the above
   e. all of the above

11

Radiographic Grids

OBJECTIVES

After completing Chapter 11, you should be able to:

1. Define the following terms:
   Bucky factor
   contrast improvement factor
   grid ratio
   grid selectivity
   radiographic grid
2. Discuss grid construction in general and as it pertains to linear, crossed, and focused grids.
3. Describe the measurement of grid performance.
4. Discuss the use of grids, including the following:
   air-gap technique
   considerations for grid selection
   grid-positioning errors
   moving grids
   radiation protection
   technique considerations

Radiographic grids are devices that reduce the amount of secondary or scatter radiation reaching the film. When the primary x-ray beam interacts with the patient, scatter radiation is generated in all directions. Although scatter radiation is of lower energy than the primary beam, it will produce additional density on a radiograph. This density is termed "fog," and it does not contribute diagnostic information to the radiograph. Fog detracts from the contrast in the image.

Radiographic grids *are devices that reduce the amount of secondary or scatter radiation reaching the film.*

Fog detracts from the contrast in the image.

The radiographic grid was invented by Dr. Gustav Bucky in 1913, and even though it has undergone several refinements, the basic principle behind its function remains unchanged. Essentially, the grid is constructed of a series of lead-foil strips, separated by radiolucent material. The alignment of the lead strips corresponds to the direction of the primary radiation emitted from the x-ray tube, as illustrated in Figure 11-1. Most of the scatter radiation generated by the patient is not traveling in the same direction as the primary beam. Thus, scatter radiation will strike the lead-foil strips on an angle and be absorbed, as illustrated in Figure 11-2. Only a small amount of scatter radia-

The grid is constructed of a series of lead-foil strips, separated by radiolucent material.

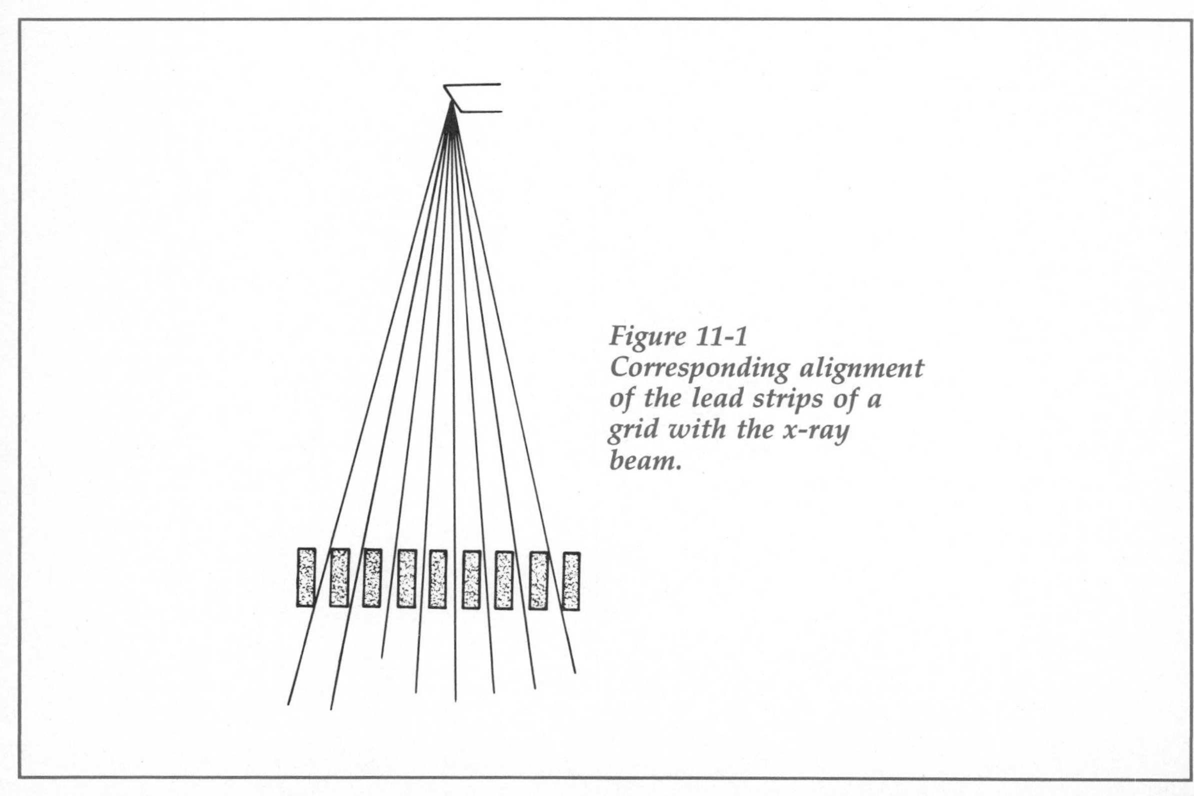

Figure 11-1
Corresponding alignment of the lead strips of a grid with the x-ray beam.

tion will pass through the grid and strike the film. Although the radiographic grid effectively removes most of the scatter radiation, it allows most of the primary radiation to pass through the lead strips unattenuated. This reduces film fog and improves contrast.

Grid Construction

Contemporary radiographic grids are delicate devices built to exacting standards. The lead strips are approximately 0.05 mm thick and are separated by radiolucent interspace material, which may be aluminum or an organic material. Aluminum interspace grids can be more precisely manufactured, but the aluminum absorbs more primary radiation. This results in a higher patient exposure for a given radiographic density, particularly at lower kVp. Aluminum also absorbs more secondary radiation, so aluminum interspace grids produce more contrast than organic ones. Since there is a trade-off between increased contrast and patient exposure, it is unclear whether one interspace material is preferable to the other, and both are in use.

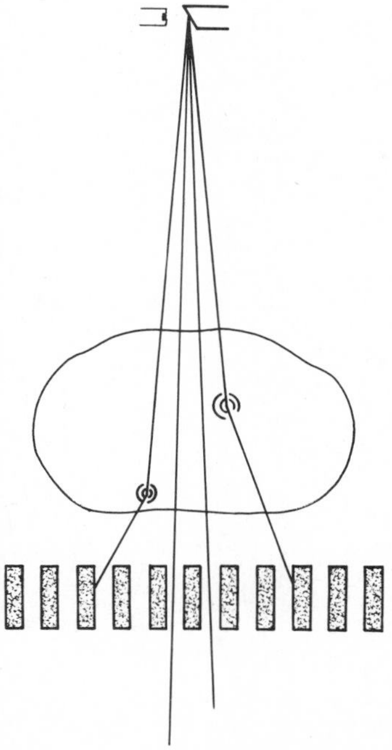

Figure 11-2
Absorption of scatter radiation produced in a patient by the lead strips of a grid. Note that the primary radiation is not absorbed.

However, the use of aluminum as an interspace material may result in the grid being somewhat more durable.

One of the most important characteristics of grid construction is the grid ratio. *Grid ratio* is the ratio of the height of the lead strips to the distance between the lead strips. This can be expressed by the following algebraic equation:

Grid ratio *is the ratio of the height of the lead strips to the distance between the lead strips.*

$$\text{Grid ratio} = \frac{\text{Height of lead strips}}{\text{Distance between lead strips}}$$

Grid ratios usually range from 4:1 to 16:1. In general, the higher the grid ratio, the more effective is the grid's ability to remove scatter radiation. This is due to the decrease in the angle that scatter radiation may be deviated before it is attenuated by the lead strips, as illustrated in Figure 11-3.

The higher the grid ratio, the more effective is the grid's ability to remove scatter radiation.

Another important consideration in the construction of grids is the *grid frequency* or the number of lead strips per inch or per centimeter. The greater the number of lead lines per inch in a grid, the less obvious the grid lines will appear on the film. This is because the grid lines are thinner and closer together, rendering them less obvious to the

Grid frequency *is the number of lead strips per inch or per centimeter.*

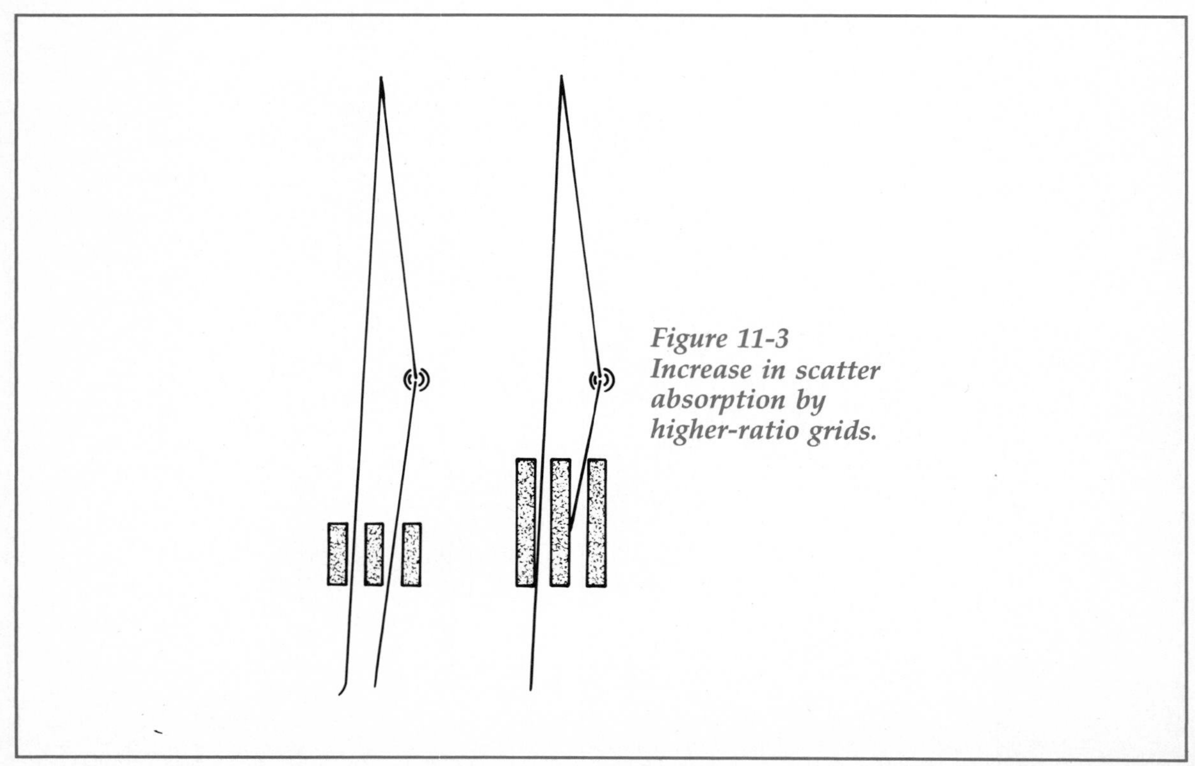

Figure 11-3
Increase in scatter absorption by higher-ratio grids.

human eye. Grids usually have between 60 and 150 lines per inch. Increasing the grid frequency or number of lines per inch reduces the visibility of grid lines but requires an increase in exposure to produce a given density. Therefore, high grid frequencies increase the exposure dose to the patient.

Linear Grids

In the **linear grid,** *all the lead strips are parallel to each other and oriented in the direction of the grid's longest dimension.*

The simplest type of grid is the linear grid. In the linear grid, all the lead strips are parallel to each other and oriented in the direction of the grid's longest dimension. The linear orientation of their lead strips allows angulation of the tube along the length of the grid without attenuation of the primary beam. The ability to angle the x-ray tube is a major advantage of the linear grid. A disadvantage occurs with decreased source-to-image receptor distance (SID). With short SID, there is decreasing density at the edges of the film. The divergence of the x-ray beam results in absorption of the primary beam by the lead strips at the edges of the grid, as illustrated in Figure 11-4. This unde-

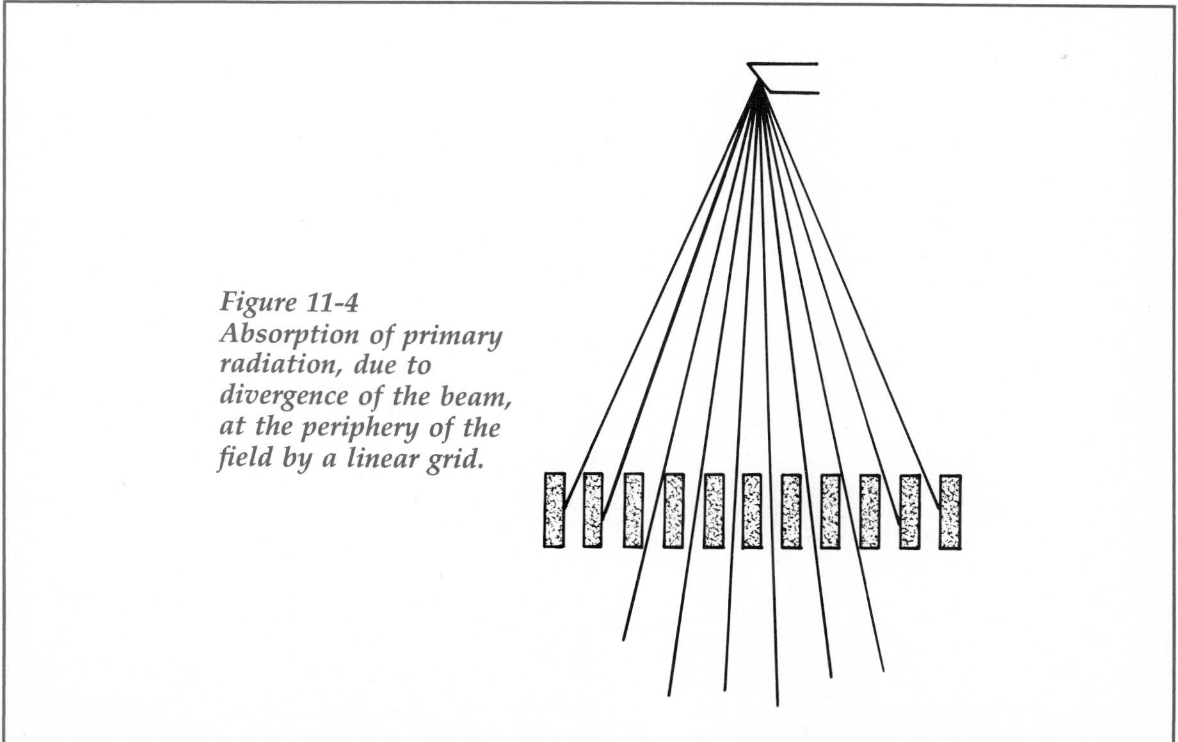

Figure 11-4
Absorption of primary radiation, due to divergence of the beam, at the periphery of the field by a linear grid.

sirable attenuation of the primary beam is called *grid cutoff*. This phenomenon can occur with any type of grid that is improperly aligned. However, it occurs most often with linear grids. Because of the potential of grid cutoff, linear grids are used only in applications involving a small radiation field or a great SID.

Grid cutoff *is the undesirable attenuation of the primary beam.*

Crossed Grids

A crossed grid, or *crosshatch grid*, is composed of two linear grids with their grid lines perpendicular to each other, as illustrated in Figure 11-5. A 6:1 crossed grid is composed of two 6:1 linear grids. However, a 6:1 crossed grid has an effective grid ratio of greater than 12:1. The major advantage of crossed grids is their excellent "clean-up" of scatter radiation. Crossed grids have the disadvantages of requiring accurate alignment of the central ray to the center of the grid and not allowing techniques that use angled central rays. Crossed grids are frequently used in simultaneous biplane angiography due to the high levels of scatter radiation produced.

A **crossed grid** *is composed of two linear grids with their grid lines perpendicular to each other.*

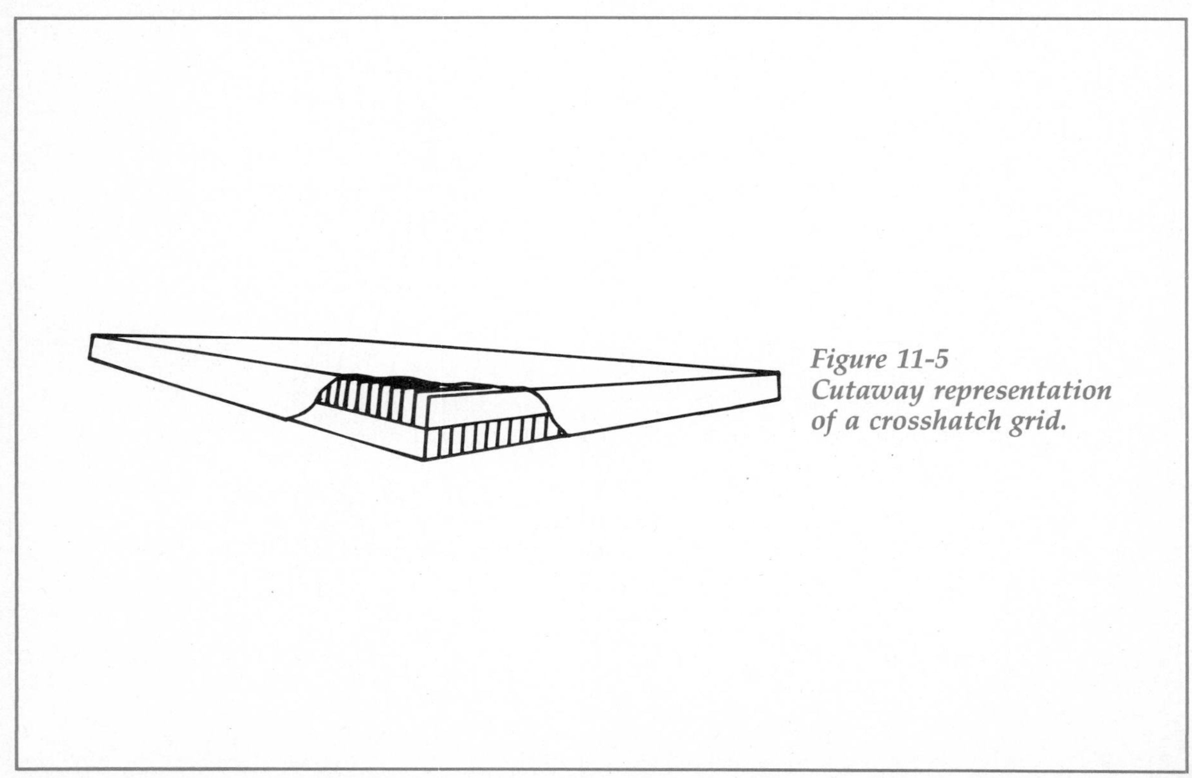

Figure 11-5 Cutaway representation of a crosshatch grid.

Focused Grids

In a **focused grid,** *the lead strips are at an angle that conforms to the diverging pattern of the x-ray beam.*

In a focused grid, the lead strips are at an angle that conforms to the diverging pattern of the x-ray beam, as illustrated in Figure 11-6. The angulation of the lead strips greatly reduces the grid cutoff at the edges that occurs with parallel linear and crossed grids. Since focused grids conform to the diverging x-ray beam, their use is limited to a specific SID range. This range, which is normally indicated on the front of a focused grid, is referred to as the *focal distance* or *grid radius.* The range of distance through which the technologist can use a focused grid is the *focal range.* The focal range is greater for low-ratio focused grids and smaller for high-ratio focused grids. Focused linear and focused crossed grids are available, and most grids in use today are focused.

The **focal distance** *or* **grid radius** *is the range of distance through which a technologist can use a focused grid.*

Measurement of Grid Performance

Since the primary function of a grid is to improve contrast, the ideal grid would remove all scatter radiation without absorbing any of the primary radiation. Unfortu-

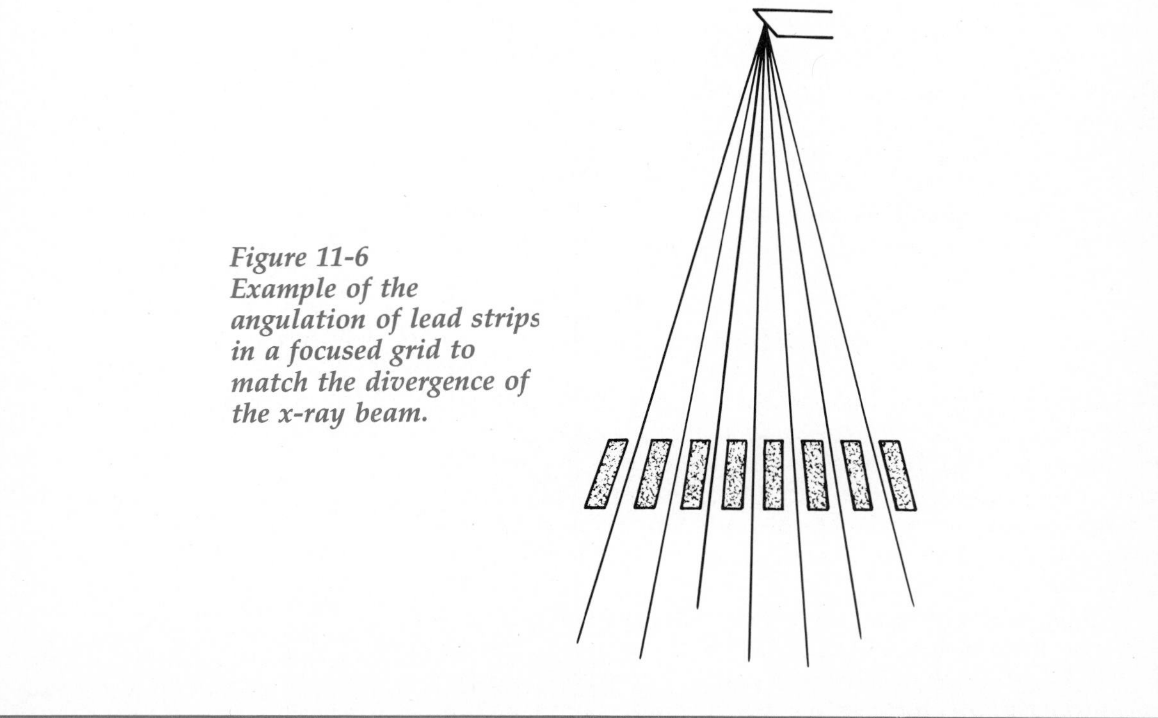

Figure 11-6
Example of the angulation of lead strips in a focused grid to match the divergence of the x-ray beam.

nately, no such grid exists. To evaluate the performance of a given grid, three factors must be considered:

1. How well the grid improves contrast
2. The relationship between primary radiation and secondary radiation attenuation
3. The exposure increase necessary to maintain a satisfactory density on the radiograph

The *contrast improvement factor (K)* measures a grid's ability to improve contrast. The contrast improvement factor is the ratio of the contrast of a radiograph taken with a grid to the contrast of a radiograph taken without a grid. Contrast improvement factor is mathematically expressed as follows:

The **contrast improvement factor (K)** *measures a grid's ability to improve contrast.*

$$K = \frac{\text{Radiographic contrast with a grid}}{\text{Radiographic contrast without a grid}}$$

The contrast improvement factor is usually measured at 100 kVp with a large field size and a 20-cm phantom (simulated patient). In general, higher-ratio grids have higher contrast improvement factors, and lower-ratio grids have lower contrast improvement factors. However, contrast improvement factor depends on several values, and the grid ratio alone is not an accurate indicator of this factor. Contrast improvement factor may be the most important measure of a grid's function, since it identifies how well a grid performs its primary purpose: improving contrast on the radiograph.

The ratio of the amount of primary radiation transmitted through a grid to the amount of scatter radiation transmitted through a grid is referred to as the *selectivity* of a grid (Σ). This is mathematically expressed as follows:

The **selectivity** *of a grid (Σ) is the ratio of the amount of primary radiation transmitted through a grid to the amount of scatter radiation transmitted through a grid.*

$$\Sigma = \frac{\text{Transmitted primary radiation}}{\text{Transmitted secondary radiation}}$$

Selectivity is a function of the construction of a grid. It is primarily influenced by the lead content of the grid, although the grid ratio also has an effect. In general, the heavier the grid, the more lead it contains and the more effective it is at cleaning up scatter radiation. This assumes it is correctly constructed. An efficient grid will have a high selectivity.

The last important consideration in the evaluation of a grid's performance is the *Bucky factor (B)* or *grid factor*. The Bucky factor represents the increase in exposure necessary to compensate for the loss of primary and secondary radi-

The **Bucky factor** *represents the increase in exposure necessary to compensate for the loss of primary and secondary radiation reaching the film.*

ation reaching the film. Mathematically, the Bucky factor is expressed as follows:

$$B = \frac{\text{Incident radiation}}{\text{Transmitted radiation}}$$

In general, the higher the grid ratio, the higher is the Bucky factor; conversely, the lower the grid ratio, the lower is the Bucky factor. Although a high Bucky factor might be desirable because it indicates good cleanup of scatter radiation, it also indicates the need for a larger exposure to produce a given radiographic density. This subsequently results in a greater radiation exposure to the patient.

Moving Grids

The images of the lead strips are called **grid lines.**

One problem with the use of grids is the image of the lead strips projected on the radiograph (Figure 11-7). The images of the lead strips are called *grid lines.* Grid lines are a result of the lead strips attenuating the primary radiation that strikes them. Grid lines tend to be less obvious with

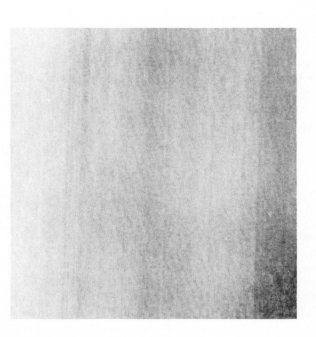

Figure 11-7
Radiograph showing the prominent grid lines produced by early grids.

high-frequency grids (those having a high number of lines per inch), although the width of the lead strips in the grid has a significant impact on the visibility of grid lines.

In 1920, Hollis E. Potter, MD, developed a mechanism to eliminate grid lines by moving the grid during the exposure. Since the grid moves in relation to the film, the grid lines are blurred. The image of the patient is unaffected, and the scatter radiation is still cleaned up. The moving grid is still sometimes referred to as a "Potter-Bucky diaphragm." Terms such as "Bucky diaphragm," "Bucky grid," "reciprocating grid," or "oscillating grid" are also frequently used.

The *moving grid* has found widespread use in radiographic equipment. Although the moving grid effectively removes grid lines from the radiograph, it does have certain disadvantages. The moving grid is an electromechanical device that is expensive and subject to failure. It may also cause motion on the radiograph due to vibrations transmitted to the film. Moving grids must be designed so the pulses of radiation produced by single-phase equipment do not correspond to the pausing of the grid as it changes direction. If this occurs, the grid lines will become evident on the radiograph. Also, very short exposure times may photographically "freeze" the moving grid lines and record them on the film. To accommodate the moving grid mechanism, an increase in the film-to-tabletop distance may be necessary. This results in an increased object-to-film distance, with subsequent magnification and loss of detail on the radiograph. Finally, a moving grid requires slightly more exposure than a stationary grid, since the grid is continuously off center because of its motion. The effect of off-centering a grid is discussed in the next section.

The **moving grid** *eliminates grid lines by moving the grid during the exposure and blurring the grid lines.*

Grid-Positioning Errors

To prevent unnecessary grid cutoff when using a grid, the grid must be positioned properly. Four major types of grid-positioning errors will result in grid cutoff.

The first of these errors is *positioning a focused grid upside-down.* Focused grids have a tube side, indicated on the grid, which must face the x-ray tube. When a focused grid is positioned upside-down, the center portion of the grid, where the lead strips are nearly parallel, allows radiation to pass through to the film. The edges of the upside-down grid, where the lead strips no longer correspond to the divergence of the x-ray beam, will stop virtually all the radi-

Focused grids have a tube side, indicated on the grid, which must face the x-ray tube.

ation from reaching the film, as illustrated in Figure 11-8. A radiograph produced with an upside-down focused grid will have complete grid cutoff on the edges of the film and a strip of density running down the center of the film. Positioning a focused crossed grid upside-down results in a square of density in the center of the radiograph, with grid cutoff on all sides of the film.

Grid design requires the central ray to be perpendicular to the plane of the grid.

The second positioning error is *using an off-level grid.* Grid design requires the central ray to be perpendicular to the plane of the grid. If the grid is not perpendicular to the central ray, uniform grid cutoff exists across the entire radiograph, as illustrated in Figure 11-9. Depending on the degree of tilt of the grid, the cutoff can be complete or result only in pronounced grid lines. Off-level grids can result from the x-ray tube being angled incorrectly across the grid. This problem is most often encountered when positioning grid cassettes during portable radiography.

Failure to direct the central ray toward the center line of a focused grid will result in grid cutoff.

The third positioning error is *lateral decentering of the grid.* Failure to direct the central ray toward the center line of a focused grid will result in grid cutoff, as illustrated in Figure 11-10. Lateral decentering also results in a uniform

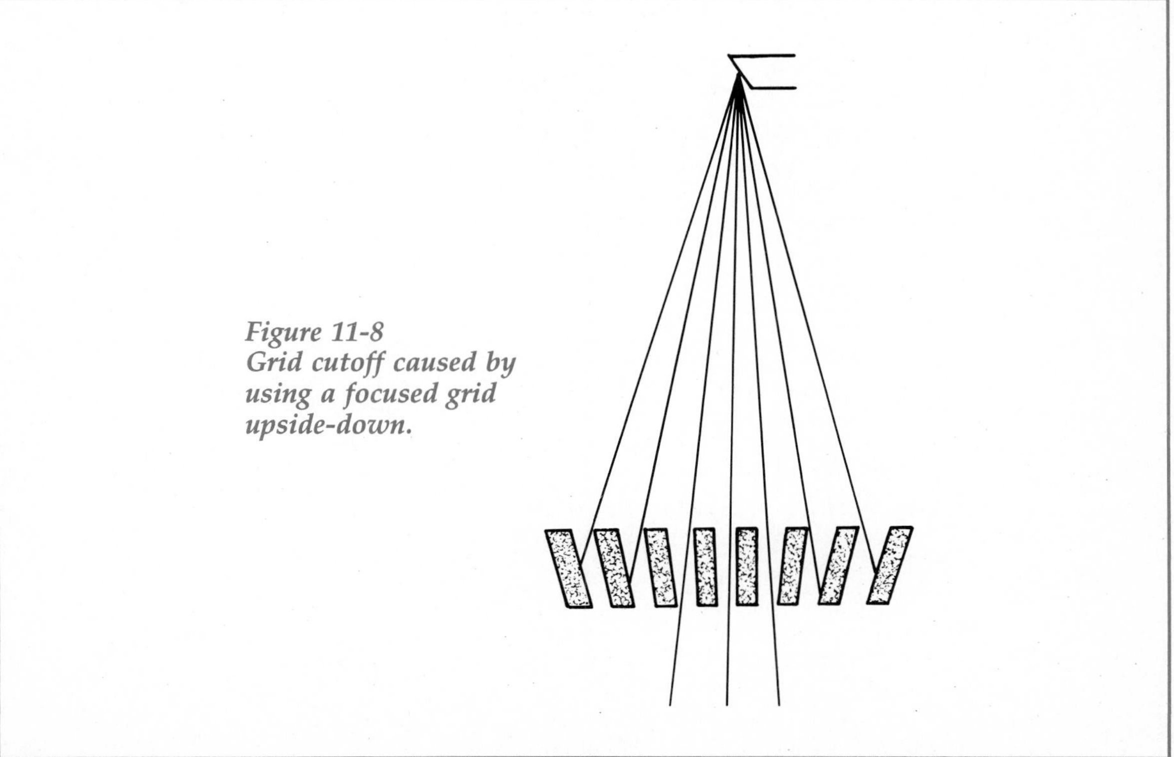

Figure 11-8
Grid cutoff caused by using a focused grid upside-down.

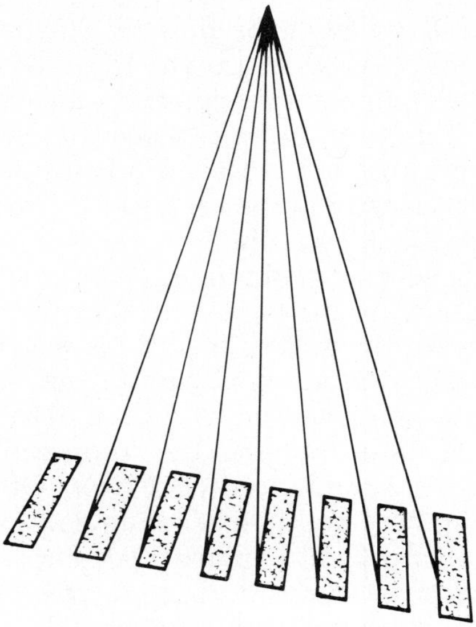

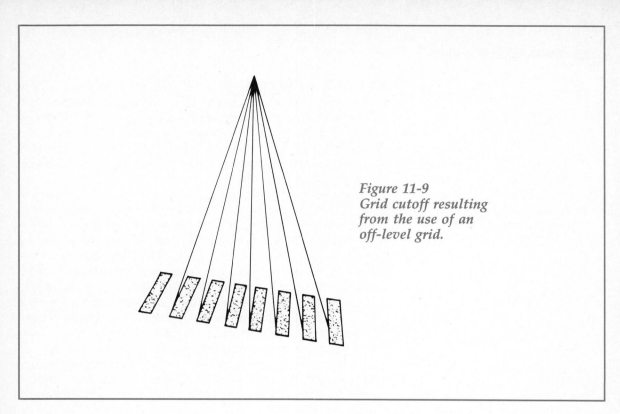

Figure 11-9
Grid cutoff resulting from the use of an off-level grid.

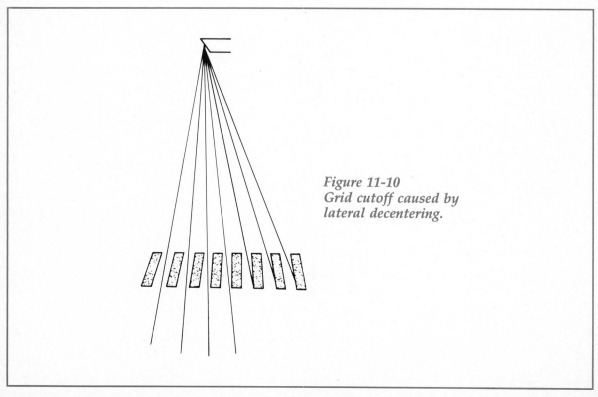

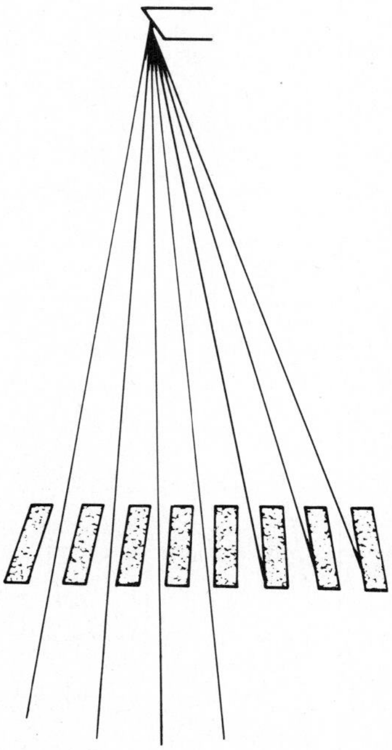

Figure 11-10
Grid cutoff caused by lateral decentering.

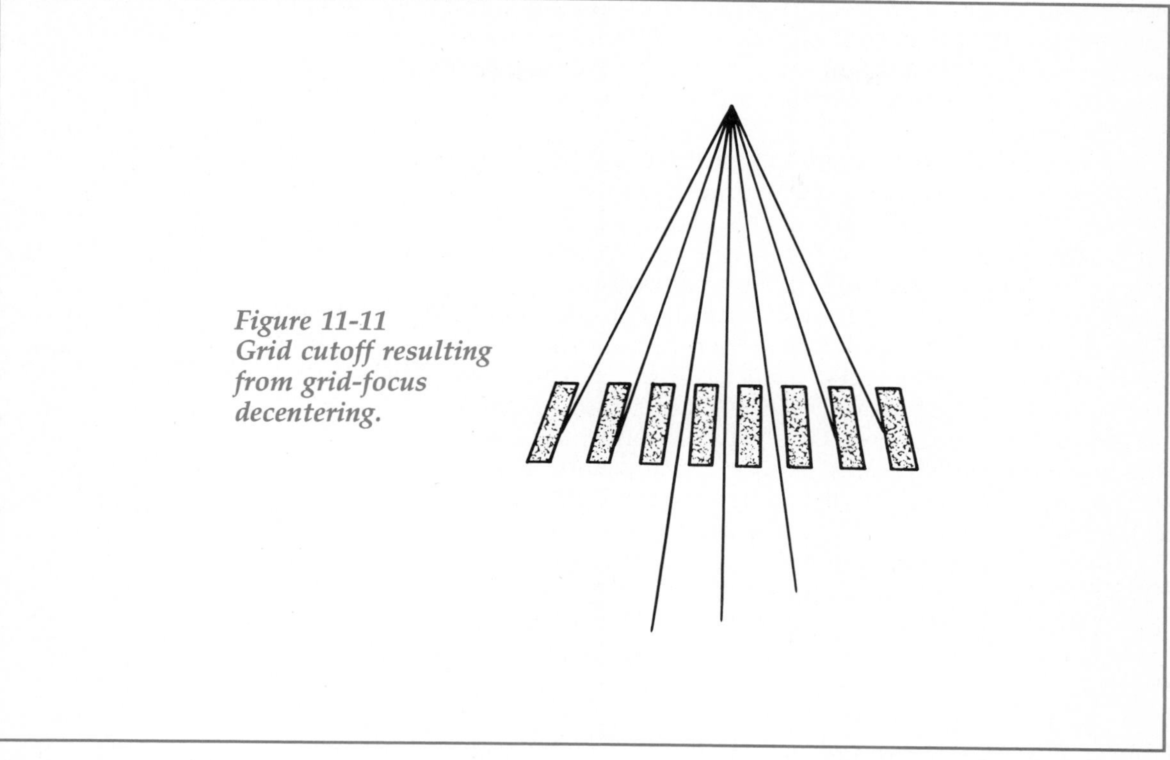

Figure 11-11
Grid cutoff resulting from grid-focus decentering.

When using a focused grid, the target of the x-ray tube must be within the specified focal distance or grid radius for that grid.

decrease in density on the radiograph. Lateral decentering is one of the major reasons why moving grids require slightly more exposure to produce the same radiographic density as a stationary grid.

The fourth positioning error is *grid-focus decentering.* When using a focused grid, the target of the x-ray tube must be within the specified focal distance or grid radius for that grid. If the x-ray tube is either too close or too far from the grid, the divergence of the x-ray beam will no longer correspond to the pattern of the lead strips in the grid. This will result in grid cutoff, as illustrated in Figure 11-11. With grid-focus decentering, the density in the center of the radiograph will appear normal, with increased grid cutoff toward the edges of the film.

Considerations for Grid Selection

Early grids produced objectionable grid lines on radiographs and necessitated the use of the moving grid. Contemporary high-frequency grids do not produce noticeable grid lines on the radiograph. Many radiologists prefer a stationary high-frequency grid over a moving grid. The use of a stationary grid eliminates the potential for detail loss caused by vibration induced by the Bucky device. This also eliminates the purchase and maintenance costs of a Bucky device.

Focused grids are generally more desirable than linear grids for routine work because they have no peripheral grid cutoff when using large fields. Focused grids do require accurate alignment to the x-ray beam, but this is usually easily accomplished in a fixed x-ray installation.

Focused grids are generally more desirable than linear grids for routine work because they have no peripheral grid cutoff when using large fields.

The kVp range used for most radiographic examinations determines the grid ratio. High-kVp techniques require the use of higher-ratio grids to clean up scatter radiation effectively. However, using higher-ratio grids increases patient exposure. One must carefully weigh the trade-off between increased scatter cleanup and increased patient exposure. A general rule of thumb for grid-ratio selection states: an 8:1 grid is satisfactory for techniques using 90 kVp or less, whereas techniques using higher than 90 kVp require a grid ratio higher than 8:1. The use of 16:1 ratio grids is limited to very-high-kVp techniques; 16:1 grids provide little additional cleanup compared with 12:1 grids, but they require a substantial increase in exposure. Crossed grids generally are used in examinations involving considerable scatter radiation, such as simultaneous-exposure biplane angiography.

The kVp range used for most radiographic examinations determines the grid ratio.

The use of grid ratios of less than 8:1 is uncommon with the exception of mammographic techniques. Since mammographic studies are usually performed at less than 30 kVp, scatter cleanup is easily accomplished with a low-ratio grid such as a 5:1 or 6:1 grid. The low-ratio grid easily enhances the low contrast of the soft tissues. It also requires less exposure to the patient than would a higher-ratio grid. The low-ratio grids used in mammography are usually high-frequency grids (100 lines per inch or more) and mounted in a reciprocating or Bucky device. This is done to prevent grid lines on the mammograms, which could obscure microcalcifications.

Air-Gap Technique

One alternative to the use of a grid is the air-gap technique. *Air-gap technique* is accomplished by moving the patient a short distance from the film. This causes a high percentage of the scatter radiation, which is generated in all directions, to miss the film (Figure 11-12).

***Air-gap technique** is accomplished by moving the patient a short distance from the film.*

In general, the first few inches from the film produce

the most significant effect, but distances from 4 to 10 inches have been reported as being the optimum air gap. The determination of optimum air gap must be based on several factors. First, the higher the kVp, the more forward is the direction of the scatter produced. Therefore, high-kVp techniques require greater air gaps to be effective. Increasing the air gap produces increased object-to-film distance, which results in magnification of the image and a decrease in resolution of fine detail. This can be overcome by increasing the SID; however, this requires increased exposure, as dictated by the inverse square law. Although increasing the SID and the technique used will not result in a substantial increase in patient exposure, it may require techniques exceeding the output of the equipment or may result in motion due to the increased time of exposure.

Air-gap techniques have been used for various examinations, especially in chest radiography and cerebral angiography. Although air-gap chest radiography has not been widely accepted, air-gap cerebral angiography is a common procedure.

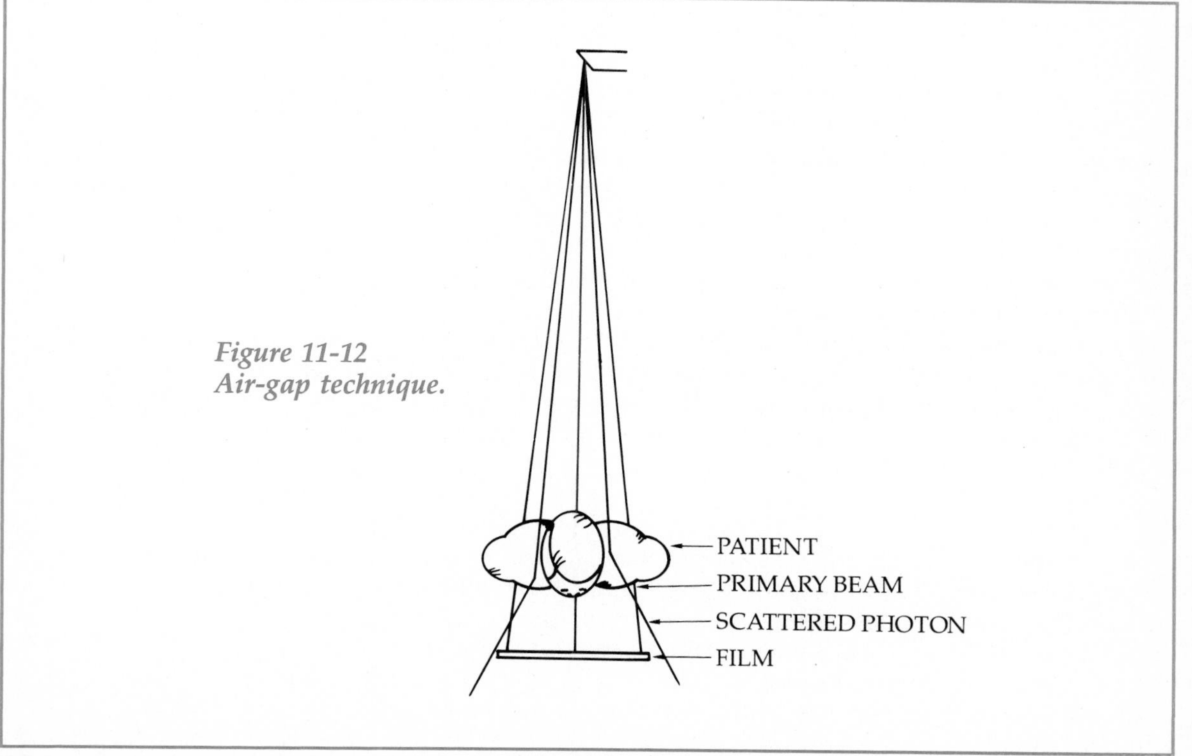

Figure 11-12
Air-gap technique.

Technique Considerations

The use of a grid requires additional exposure to maintain the same radiographic density as a nongrid technique. An efficient grid removes up to 90 percent of the scatter radiation that would otherwise contribute to the density on the radiograph. In general, *the higher the grid ratio, the greater is the exposure increase required to maintain density*. Although grid ratio is not the only determinant in exposure required, it is the most practical factor for the technologist to use. Interspace material may also influence technique consideration, especially with low-kVp techniques and aluminum interspace grids. This combination of low kVp techniques and aluminum interspace grids may require up to an additional 20 percent exposure. A moving grid also requires approximately 15 percent more exposure over a stationary grid.

The higher the grid ratio, the greater is the exposure increase required to maintain density.

Exposure increases for grid techniques can be accomplished by increasing either the milliampere-seconds (mAs) or the kVp. Grid techniques require substantial increases in mAs to maintain density. An 8:1 grid demands a threefold increase in the exposure compared with a nongrid technique. Higher-ratio grids and crossed grids may require up to eight times the exposure as a nongrid technique. It is usually preferable to use mAs as the factor to compensate for grid techniques, since increasing the kVp decreases contrast, which is contrary to the grid's purpose. When circumstances mandate the use of kVp to compensate for density changes, however, an increase of at least 20 kVp is necessary with an 8:1 grid. Higher-ratio grids require between 5 and 20 additional kVp to compensate. Incorrectly positioning a grid results in decreased density in some or all portions of the radiograph, for which compensation may be impossible.

Grid techniques require substantial increases in mAs to maintain density.

In general, *higher-ratio grids produce higher contrast on the radiograph but require more exposure to produce a given density*. Conversely, lower-ratio grids produce less contrast but require less exposure to produce a given density.

Higher-ratio grids produce higher contrast on the radiograph but require more exposure to produce a given density.

Radiation Protection

As stated frequently in this chapter, grids increase the exposure to the patient. Without the use of grids, however, the quality of many radiographic examinations would be so poor that they would yield little diagnostic information for the radiologist. Therefore, the benefit gained by the proper use of the grid far outweighs the risk of the additional radiation exposure.

The benefit gained by the proper use of the grid far outweighs the risk of the additional radiation exposure.

The technologist can minimize the additional exposure to the patient when using grid techniques by:

1. Ensuring that the grid used is appropriate for the kVp range and type of examination being performed
2. Making certain that the grid is correctly aligned and within the specified focal range
3. Providing proper collimation and shielding of the patient

Chapter 11—Review Questions

1. What is the primary purpose of the radiographic grid?
   a. the reduction of patient dose
   b. the reduction of the amount of scatter radiation generated in the patient
   c. the reduction of the amount of scatter radiation reaching the film
   d. two of the above
   e. none of the above
2. Which of the following materials is commonly used as interspace material for radiographic grids?
   a. aluminum
   b. lead
   c. organic material
   d. two of the above
   e. all of the above
3. Which of the following grid characteristics is the most important?
   a. grid frequency
   b. grid ratio
   c. Bucky factor
   d. selectivity
   e. contrast improvement factor
4. What is the definition of grid ratio?
   a. the ratio of the height of the lead strips to the width of the lead strips
   b. the ratio of the height of the lead strips to the distance between the lead strips
   c. the ratio of the distance between the lead strips to the width of the lead strips
   d. the ratio of the width of the lead strips to the height of the lead strips
5. What term describes the number of lead strips per inch or centimeter?
   a. grid frequency
   b. grid ratio
   c. Bucky factor
   d. selectivity
   e. contrast improvement factor

6. What term describes the undesirable attenuation of the primary beam?
   a. grid frequency
   b. grid ratio
   c. Bucky factor
   d. selectivity
   e. grid cutoff
7. What term describes the ratio of the amount of primary radiation transmitted through a grid to the amount of scatter radiation transmitted through a grid?
   a. grid frequency
   b. grid ratio
   c. Bucky factor
   d. selectivity
   e. contrast improvement factor
8. What term describes the increase in exposure necessary to compensate for the loss of primary and secondary radiation reaching the film?
   a. grid frequency
   b. grid ratio
   c. Bucky factor
   d. selectivity
   e. contrast improvement factor
9. What is the primary advantage of a moving grid?
   a. Grid lines tend to be less obvious.
   b. The pulsing of the radiation corresponds to the pausing of the grid.
   c. There is a slight reduction in patient dose when compared to stationary grids.
   d. It is an electromechanical device.
   e. It requires an increased object-to-film distance.
10. Which of the following statements is generally true concerning grid ratio?
    a. As grid ratio increases, the contrast improvement factor decreases.
    b. As grid ratio increases, the grid frequency increases.
    c. As grid ratio increases, the Bucky factor increases.
    d. two of the above
    e. all of the above

11. Which of the following grid-positioning errors results in a uniform decrease in density across the film?
    a. an off-level grid
    b. grid focus decentering
    c. lateral decentering
    d. two of the above
    e. all of the above
12. Which of the following grid-positioning errors results in a uniform decrease in density toward the edges of the film?
    a. an off-level grid
    b. grid-focus decentering
    c. lateral decentering
    d. two of the above
    e. all of the above
13. Which of the following is a reasonable alternative to using grid techniques for imaging large body parts?
    a. the use of less than 60 kVp
    b. the use of a Potter-Bucky diaphragm
    c. the use of air-gap techniques
    d. none of the above
14. What is a satisfactory grid ratio for techniques below 90 kVp?
    a. 8:1
    b. 10:1
    c. 12:1
    d. 16:1
    e. none of the above
15. Which of the following is an advantage of focused grids when compared to parallel grids?
    a. Focused grids can be used with either side facing the tube, thus reducing grid-positioning errors.
    b. Decreased peripheral grid cutoff occurs with large fields.
    c. Focused grids can be used with a wide range of SIDs.
    d. two of the above
    e. all of the above

12

Filtration of the X-Ray Beam

OBJECTIVES

After completing Chapter 12, you should be able to:

1. Define the following terms:
   added filtration
   compensating filter
   half-value layer
   inherent filtration
   total filtration
2. Describe the purpose, function, and technique considerations of filtration and the requirement defined by the National Council on Radiation Protection.
3. Discuss the half-value layer, its determination, and factors affecting it.
4. Discuss the purpose and use of compensating filters.

The primary purpose of *filtration* of the x-ray beam is to reduce patient dose. The photons produced by an x-ray tube have various energies (wavelengths), and therefore the x-ray beam is heterogeneous or polychromatic. The filter, usually constructed of aluminum, functions by absorbing low-energy (long-wavelength) x-rays from the beam, while allowing more energetic (short-wavelength) x-rays to pass through unattenuated. Without filtration, the low-energy x-rays would be absorbed by the patient, increasing the patient dose, but contributing nothing to the diagnostic image. Therefore, one can state that filtration "hardens" the x-ray beam since it increases the average energy of the beam by removing low-energy photons, as illustrated in Figure 12-1.

The primary purpose of ***filtration*** *of the x-ray beam is to reduce patient dose.*

Types of Filtration

Two types of filtration are present in most radiographic systems: inherent and added. *Inherent filtration* results from the construction of the x-ray tube and the collimator. In the x-ray tube, the glass envelope, or more specifically the port of the tube, filters the x-ray beam. In the

Inherent filtration *results from the construction of the x-ray tube and the collimator.*

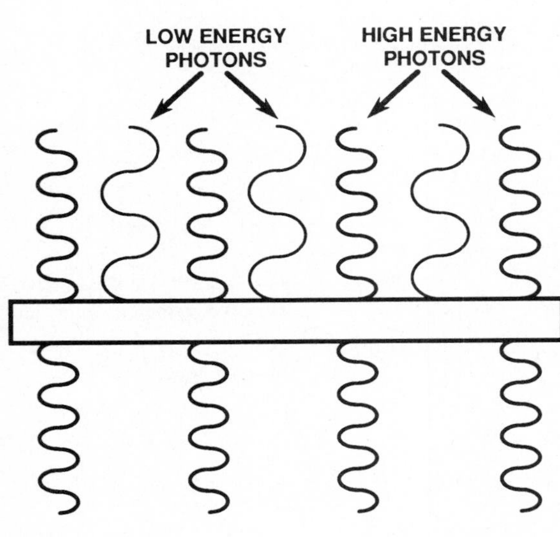

Figure 12-1
When both high- and low-energy incident photons strike filtration material, lower-energy photons are attenuated, whereas high-energy photons are not attenuated.

Added filtration *is filtration added to the beam.*

The amount of added filtration depends on the inherent filtration of the x-ray tube and collimator and the kVp range used on the equipment.

Total filtration *is the sum of the inherent and added filtration.*

Operating kVp	Total filtration
< 50 kVp	*0.5 mm aluminum*
50 to 70 kVp	*1.5 mm aluminum*
>70 kVp	*2.5 mm aluminum*

Filtration in excess of 3 mm offers no additional advantage and is even counterproductive, since it decreases the x-ray beam's intensity, requiring additional exposure to produce a given density.

collimator, both the mirror used to project the light field downward and the plastic cross-hair insert also filter the beam. The inherent filtration of the x-ray tube and collimator is usually indicated on the equipment in aluminum equivalents.

As its name implies, *added filtration* is filtration added to the beam. The presence and the amount of added filtration may or may not be under the technologist's control. As stated, filters are usually aluminum and range from 1 to 3 mm in thickness. Although yttrium and other heavy-metal filters have been used in diagnostic radiology to reduce patient dose, aluminum is still the material most frequently employed. The amount of added filtration depends on the inherent filtration of the x-ray tube and collimator and the kVp range used on the equipment.

Total filtration is the sum of the inherent and added filtration. The total filtration required for diagnostic radiology has been defined by the National Council on Radiation Protection as follows, based on the kVp used:

Operating kVp	Total filtration
Less than 50 kVp	0.5 mm aluminum
50 to 70 kVp	1.5 mm aluminum
Greater than 70 kVp	2.5 mm aluminum

A greater amount of filtration does not necessarily result in increased radiation protection for the patient. Filtration in excess of 3 mm offers no additional advantage and is even counterproductive, since it decreases the x-ray beam's intensity, requiring additional exposure to produce a given density.

In a few special x-ray examinations that use low kVp, it may be desirable to have as little total filtration as possible. Mammography is one such application where normal levels of filtration are undesirable. To achieve minimal total filtration, mammography x-ray tubes are designed with beryllium ports that have a low atomic number (4). This results in little filtration of the exiting beam. Mammography x-ray equipment usually has no added filtration and often uses cones to define the x-ray field; these cones have no mirrors to add filtration. Some mammographic units are equipped with collimators that have removable mirrors to reduce inherent filtration.

Technique Considerations with Filters

Although filters absorb low-energy photons, which do not contribute to the radiograph, they also absorb some higher-energy photons as well. This reduction of the higher-energy photons will result in less radiographic density and must be compensated for, usually by increasing milliampere-seconds (mAs). Filtration's effect on density is most pronounced when using low kVp and is negligible when using higher-kVp techniques.

Since filtration increases the average or mean energy of the x-ray beam, it results in lowered contrast on the radiograph. The effect is similar to increasing the kVp. Again, the reduction in contrast is most pronounced at low kVp and is least noticeable in the high-kVp ranges.

In general, increasing filtration reduces the density of a film and may require compensation to maintain the same density. Increasing filtration also reduces the contrast on a film. Both effects are most pronounced at low kVp and least pronounced with high-kVp techniques.

Radiation Protection

As stated earlier, the primary purpose of filtration is to reduce patient exposure. Since the x-ray beam is heterogeneous or polychromatic, an unfiltered beam will have a large percentage of very-low-energy photons. These low-energy photons do not possess enough energy to penetrate a patient's body; most are absorbed in the first few centimeters of tissue. Since these photons cannot reach the film, they contribute nothing to the radiograph but contribute substantially to the patient's skin dose. Filtration, both inherent and added, serves to increase the mean energy of the beam by removing the low-energy photons. This reduces the patient's skin dose. The effect of filtration on patient exposure is significant; 3 mm of total filtration can result in a skin exposure decrease of up to 80 percent.

The effect of filtration on patient exposure is significant; 3 mm of total filtration can result in a skin exposure decrease of up to 80 percent.

Half-Value Layer

The half-value layer (HVL) is that thickness of material that will reduce the intensity of a given beam of radiation by 50 percent. The HVL is a convenient measure of attenuation and is an indication of the quality of an x-ray beam. The *quality* of the x-ray beam is the ability to penetrate into various substances, including body tissue. Aluminum is a useful absorber in the 10 to 150 kVp range. It is useful in diagnostic radiology for determination of the HVL. A diagnostic x-ray beam usually has an HVL in the range of 1 to 5 mm of aluminum.

The half-value layer (HVL) is that thickness of material that will reduce the intensity of a given beam of radiation by 50 percent.

Determination of HVL

Determination of the HVL involves three principal parts: (1) the x-ray tube, (2) a radiation detector, and (3) graded thickness of an absorber, usually aluminum (Figure 12-2). The HVL is determined experimentally in the following manner.

An initial exposure is made with no attenuating material between the x-ray tube and the radiation-detecting device. The reading of the radiation-detecting device is recorded on a graph. Subsequent exposures use the same technical factors, and the recorded readings add absorbing material, between exposures, in millimeter increments. This is continued until the intensity of the initial exposure is reduced by at least 50 percent.

The intensity of the initial exposure is then divided by two. This x-ray quantity is found on the appropriate axis of the graph. A line *(A)*, parallel to the opposing axis, is drawn to the point that it intersects the curve. Line *B* is then drawn, perpendicular to *A* and intersecting the opposing axis. This point of intersection is the HVL in millimeters of absorbing material (Figure 12-3).

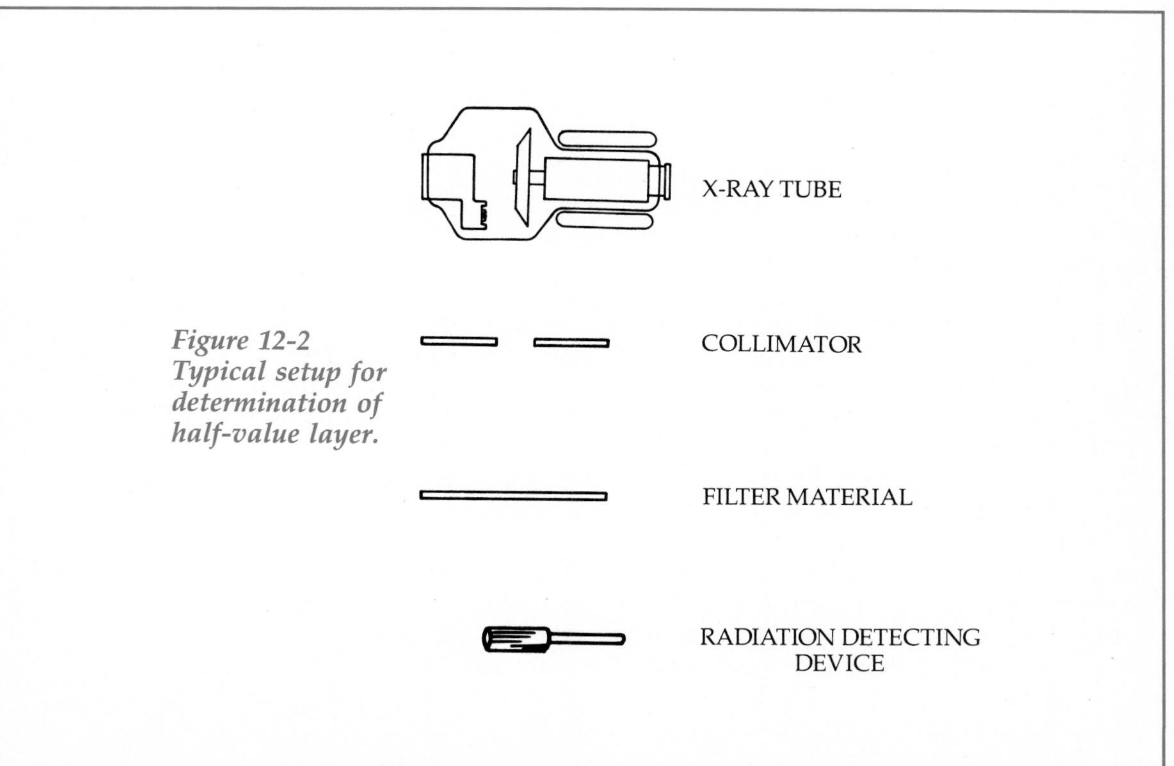

Figure 12-2 Typical setup for determination of half-value layer.

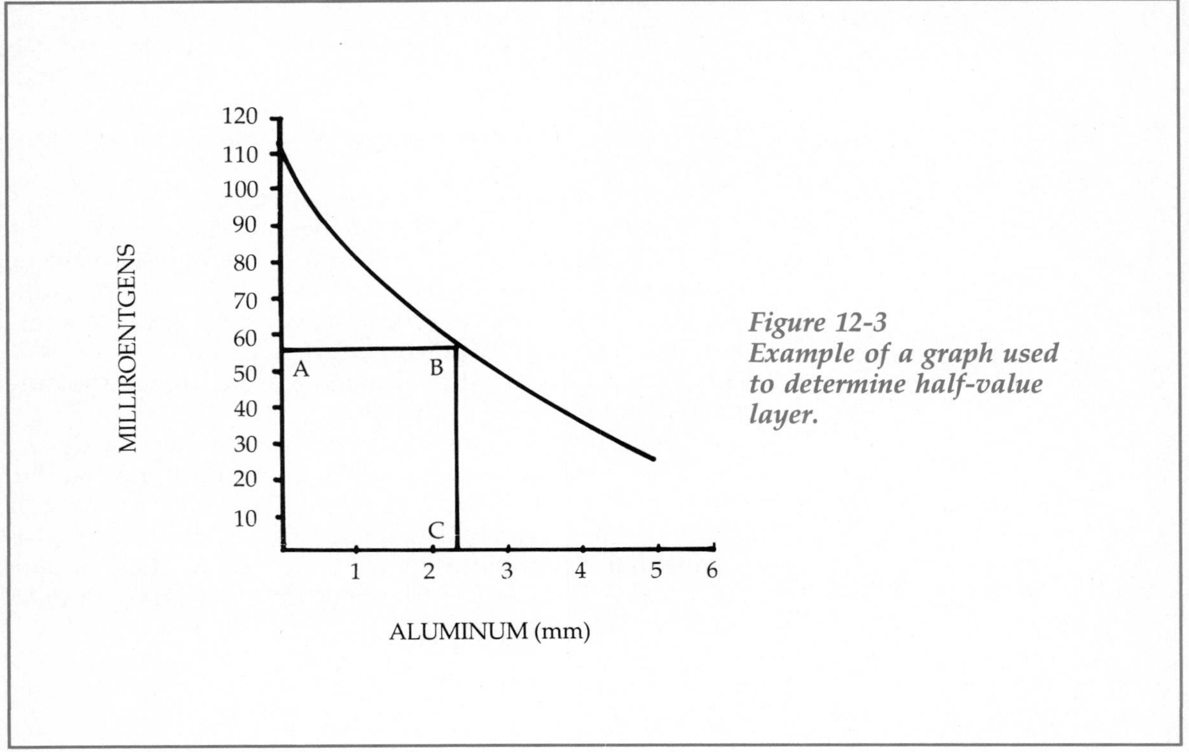

Figure 12-3
Example of a graph used to determine half-value layer.

Factors Affecting HVL

Two main factors affect the HVL for a given radiographic unit: the actual kVp output and the total filtration. As either one of these factors increases, the penetrating ability of the x-ray beam also increases. In turn, as the penetrating ability of the x-ray beam increases, the HVL increases as well. Therefore, the higher the kVp or the greater the filtration, the higher is the HVL for a given radiographic unit. The mAs used has no effect on HVL since it is a quantity, not a quality, factor.

The higher the kVp or the greater the filtration, the higher is the HVL for a given radiographic unit.

One factor that may result in an increase in a given radiographic unit's HVL is the deposit of tungsten on the inside of the x-ray tube. Tungsten can be deposited on the inside of the glass envelope following abuse or correct but long-term use of the equipment. The tungsten layer absorbs lower-energy photons, increasing inherent filtration and raising the mean energy of the beam. Tungsten deposits can substantially increase the HVL and may render an x-ray tube unsuitable for certain applications. An evaluation of HVL should be conducted annually.

Tungsten deposits can substantially increase the HVL and may render an x-ray tube unsuitable for certain applications.

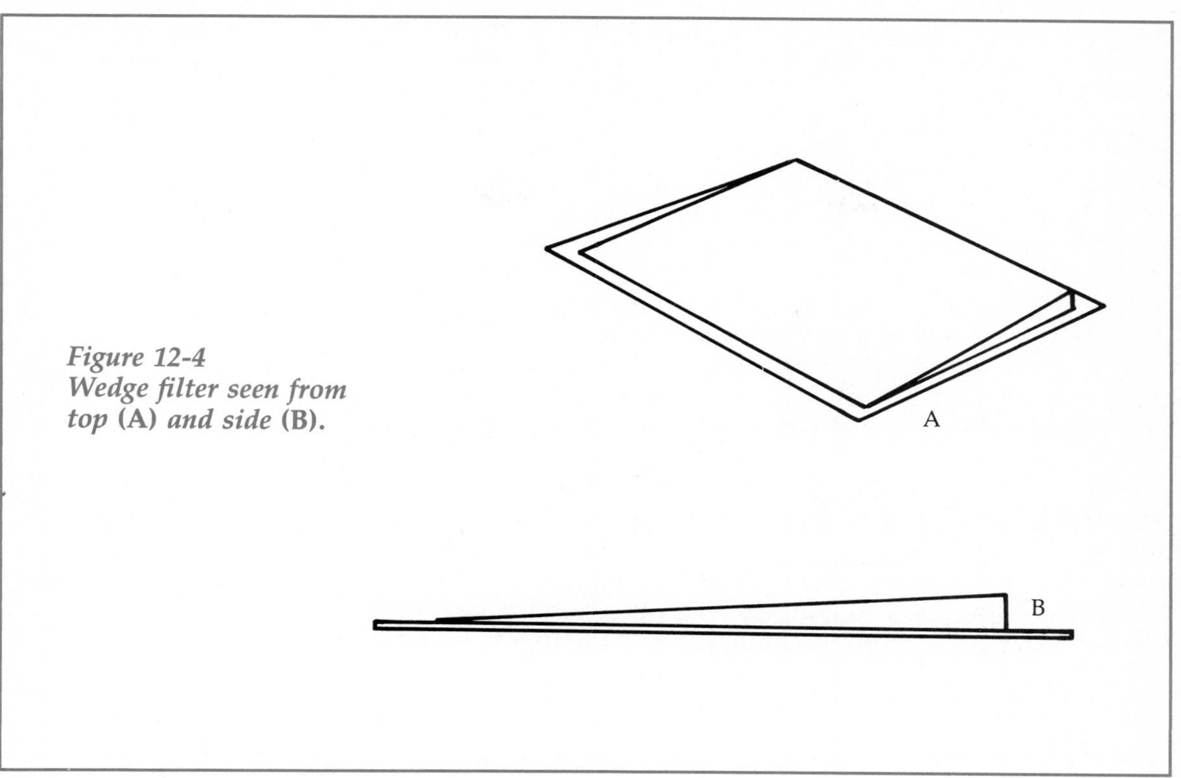

Figure 12-4
Wedge filter seen from top (A) *and side* (B).

Compensating filters are a special type of filter occasionally used in diagnostic radiology when the body part being examined changes in thickness or density from one area to another.

Compensating Filters

Compensating filters are a special type of filter occasionally used in diagnostic radiology when the body part being examined changes in thickness or density from one area to another. The most common example of a compensating filter is the *wedge filter* (Figure 12-4). A wedge filter, usually composed of aluminum, attenuates some of the radiation exiting the x-ray tube. Because of its shape, the wedge filter attenuates a greater percentage of radiation on its thickest end and a lower percentage on its thinnest end. This phenomenon helps to equalize the density on a radiograph by aligning the thinnest part of the filter to the thickest part of the patient. Wedge filters have been used (1) in chest radiography to help increase the density in the bases of the lungs without overexposing the apices, (2) in the feet to help increase the density of the metatarsals without overexposing the toes, and (3) in the lateral view of the pregnant abdomen.

Other types of compensating filters are also available.

The *trough filter,* which is also usually composed of aluminum, has been widely used for radiography of the spine and chest (Figure 12-5). The shape of the trough filter allows the greatest portion of radiation through its central depression. This is very useful in producing a satisfactorily dense spine without overexposing the soft tissues peripherally. In the chest, the trough filter produces a radiograph with an adequately penetrated mediastinum and acceptable density in the lung fields.

With the advent of lead-impregnated Plexiglas, a new group of compensating filters for the chest is being developed. The lead-impregnated Plexiglas has the advantage of using the collimator light to help position the patient, while still providing partial attenuation of the x-ray beam. The ease with which the Plexiglas can be carved allows the production of compensating filters with the proper shape to correct the density differences in a complex body part, such as the chest. These new filters are currently under investigation in a number of sites. Lead-impregnated Plexiglas is also being used to manufacture wedge and trough filters, replacing the more traditional use of aluminum.

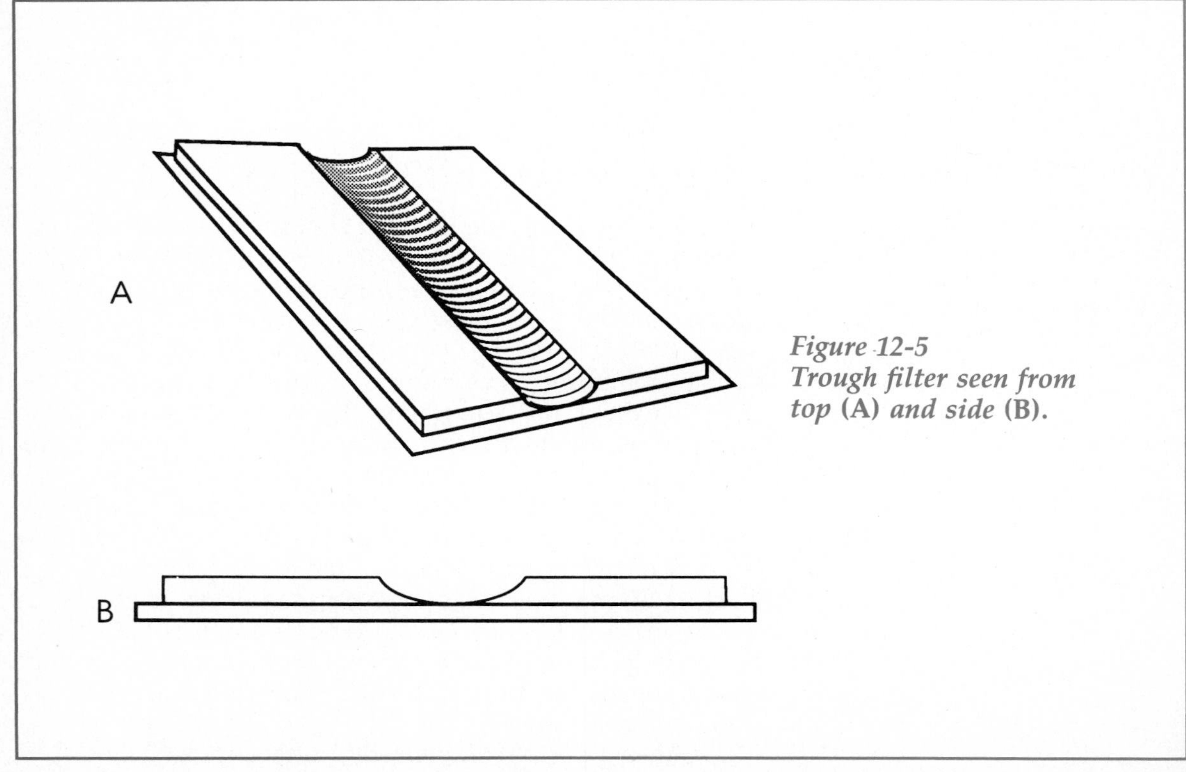

Figure 12-5
Trough filter seen from top (A) *and side* (B).

Technique Considerations with Compensating Filters

Compensating filters require an increase in technique to produce a given density on a radiograph.

Compensating filters require an increase in technique to produce a given density on a radiograph. The amount of increase depends on the filtering material used and the thickness of the material. Compensating filters do not produce a significant increase in patient exposure, despite the increase in technique, because of the absorption by the filter material. The patient exposure will be somewhat higher in the areas exposed by the thinnest parts of the filter; however, the resultant radiograph will have a more satisfactory density in this area. Because of their thickness, compensating filters provide additional filtration and will likely result in a loss of contrast on the radiograph. This effect may not be objectionable and may be outweighed by the benefit of a more uniform radiograph.

Chapter 12—Review Questions

1. What is the primary purpose of filtration?
   a. to increase the average energy of the beam
   b. to improve radiographic contrast
   c. to reduce patient exposure
   d. to harden the x-ray beam
   e. none of the above
2. Which of the following does not contribute to inherent filtration?
   a. an aluminum filter
   b. the mirror used in a collimator to project the light field
   c. the port of the x-ray tube
   d. two of the above
   e. all of the above
3. What factor plays a part in determining total filtration required?
   a. the kVp range being used
   b. the inherent filtration of the collimator
   c. the inherent filtration of the x-ray tube
   d. two of the above
   e. all of the above
4. Which of the following is true as total filtration exceeds 3 mm of aluminum?
   a. Patient dose is dramatically reduced, with small increases of total filtration.
   b. Patient dose increases due to the dramatic increase in the average energy of the beam.
   c. There is a reduction in the x-ray beam intensity, requiring additional exposure.
   d. two of the above
   e. all of the above
5. Which of the following materials is routinely used as a filter during mammographic studies?
   a. aluminum
   b. yttrium
   c. molybdenum
   d. none of the above

6. What effect does filtration have on the density and contrast of the radiographic image?
   a. Increasing filtration increases density and contrast.
   b. Increasing filtration decreases density and contrast.
   c. Increasing filtration increases density and decreases contrast.
   d. Increasing filtration decreases density and increases contrast.
   e. none of the above
7. What is half-value layer?
   a. a convenient measure of attenuation
   b. that thickness of material that will reduce the intensity of an x-ray beam by 50 percent
   c. an indication of the quality of an x-ray beam
   d. two of the above
   e. all of the above
8. What is the half-value layer, given the following factors? (1) An initial exposure with no attenuating material in the beam had an intensity of 1040 mR. (2) A second exposure with 1 mm of aluminum in the beam had an intensity of 820 mR. (3) A third exposure with 2 mm of aluminum had an intensity of 520 mR. (4) A fourth exposure with 3 mm of aluminum had an intensity of 410 mR.
   a. 520 mR
   b. 3 mm of aluminum
   c. 2 mm of aluminum
   d. none of the above
9. Which of the following factors increases the half-value layer?
   a. increased kVp
   b. increased mAs
   c. increased total filtration
   d. two of the above
   e. all of the above
10. Which of the following statements concerning compensating filters is *not* true?
    a. They require an increase in exposure factors, and they increase patient dose.
    b. They result in lower radiographic contrast.
    c. They help to equalize the density on a radiograph.
    d. two of the above
    e. all of the above

13

Geometry of Image Formation

OBJECTIVES

After completing Chapter 13, you should be able to:

1. Define the following terms:
   distortion
   penumbra
   resolution
2. Discuss image geometry, its impact on radiographic detail, and its control.

The goal of radiography is to produce a detailed and accurately represented image of an object. Several geometric phenomena occur during the production of the radiograph that alter the accuracy of the image produced. The technologist must understand these phenomena and minimize their effect on the radiograph.

Penumbra

If we could produce a point source of x-rays and use that point source to radiograph a very thin, square lead sheet, we would produce an image with very sharp and well-defined edges (Figure 13-1). As long as the film and the square lead sheet were kept parallel to each other and the point source was centered to the lead sheet, the image on the film would continue to show sharp, well-defined edges. This would be true regardless of how far the lead sheet is from the film. Moving the lead sheet up from the film would only impact the size of the image. As the sheet moves up from the film, the size of the image would increase because of the diverging nature of the point-source

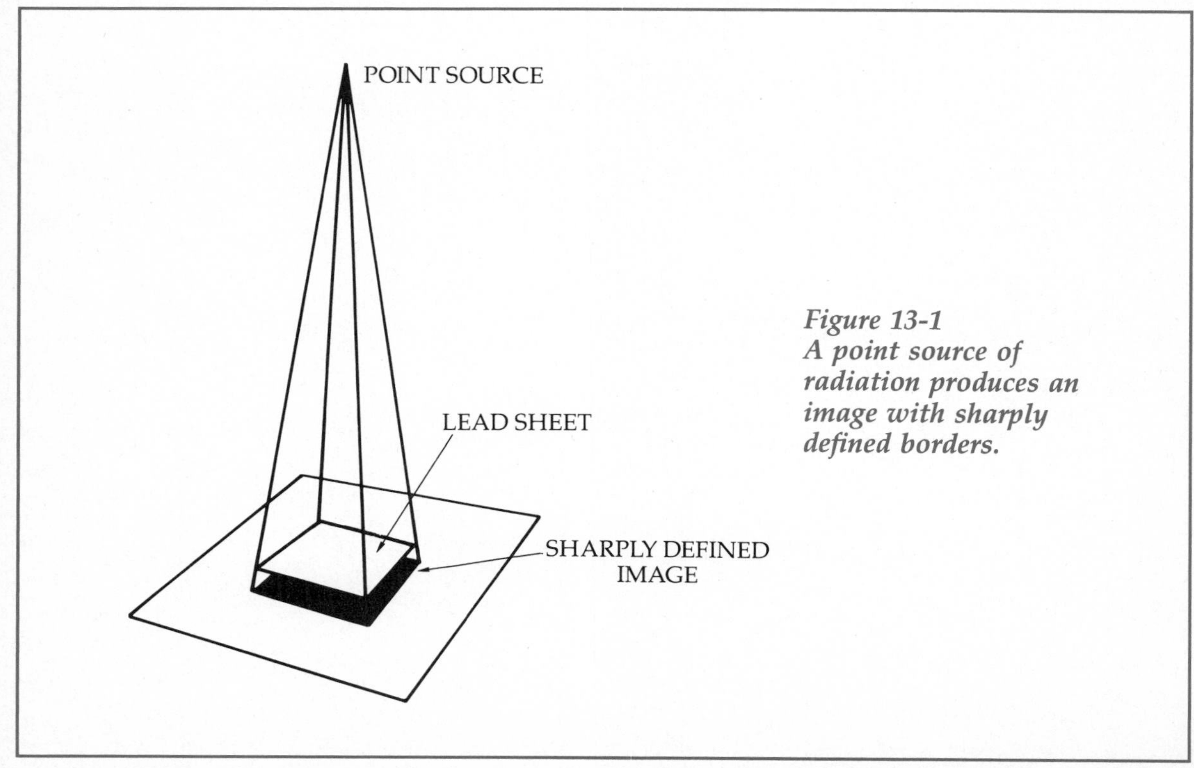

Figure 13-1
A point source of radiation produces an image with sharply defined borders.

Penumbra *is unsharpness of the edges of the image that is the result of the area source of x-rays.*

x-ray beam (Figure 13-2). In addition, if the lead sheet was at a fixed distance from the film, moving the point source of x-rays farther from the film would reduce the size of the image. Moving the point source of x-rays closer to the film would increase the size of the image (Figure 13-3).

A point source of x-rays is helpful in explaining what happens during image formation. Unfortunately, the x-ray tube is not a point source of x-rays, and no such source exists. The x-ray tube is an area source and generates x-rays over the entire focal area of the target. Many x-rays interact with the object to produce the image. If we radiographed our lead sheet with an area source of radiation, we would notice that the edges were not as sharp or well defined as they were with our point source of x-rays. The unsharpness of the edges would be the result of the area source of x-rays (Figure 13-4). This area of unsharpness is termed the *penumbra,* and excessive penumbra is undesirable on a radiograph.

In the radiographic environment, the technologist can control certain conditions to reduce the amount of penumbra in a radiograph. The focal spot size is a controllable fac-

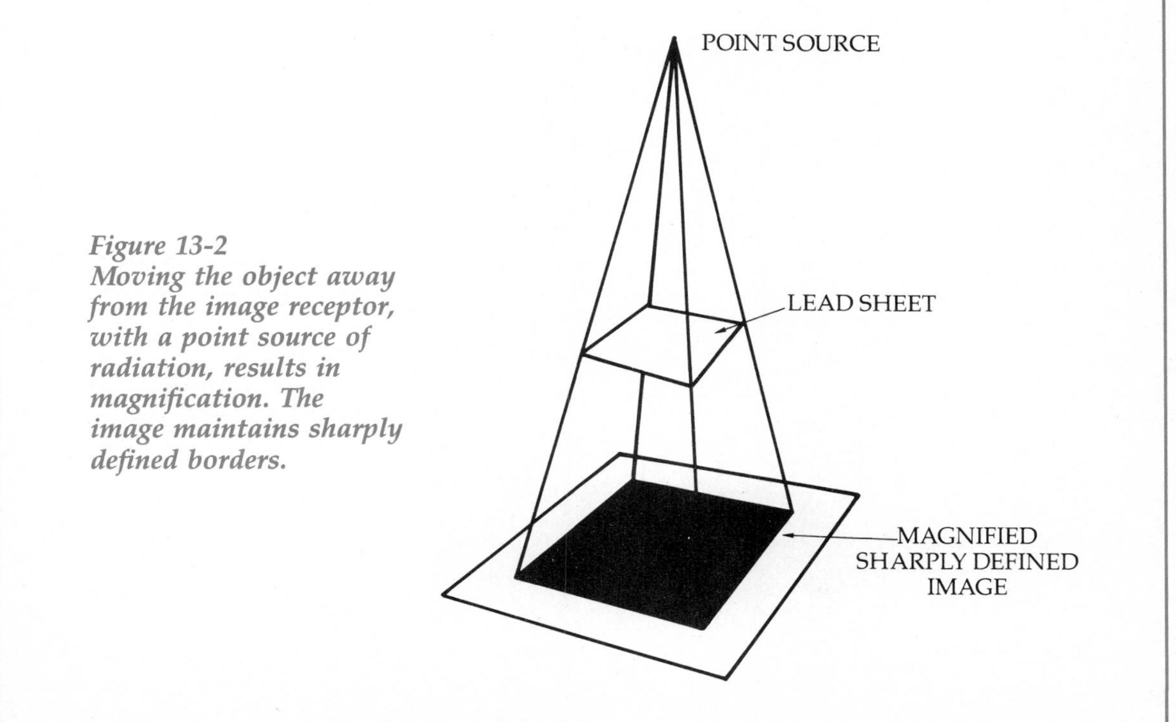

Figure 13-2
Moving the object away from the image receptor, with a point source of radiation, results in magnification. The image maintains sharply defined borders.

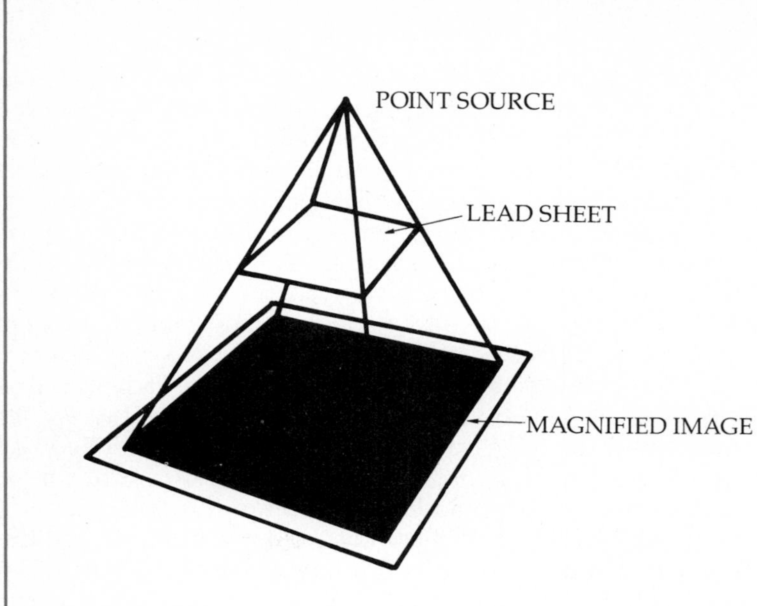

Figure 13-3
Moving the point source of radiation closer to the image receptor also results in magnification. The image still maintains sharply defined borders.

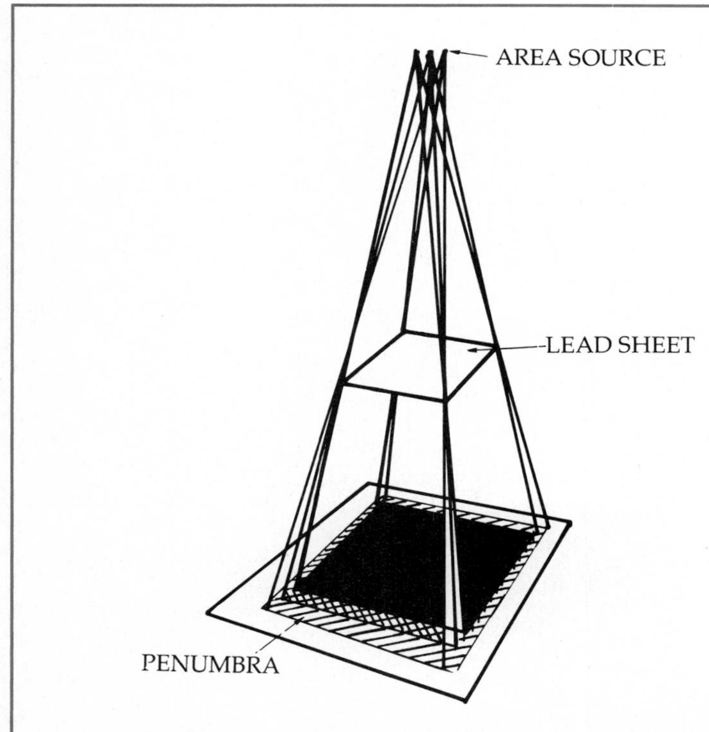

Figure 13-4
An area source of radiation produces an image with unsharp borders. The unsharpness is called penumbra.

Reducing the size of the focal spot, increasing the SID, or decreasing the OFD results in less penumbra on the radiograph.

tor. Reducing the size of the focal spot reduces the area over which x-rays are produced, resulting in less penumbra on the radiograph (Figure 13-5). Additionally, increasing the source-to-image receptor distance (SID) will decrease penumbra for a given focal spot (Figure 13-6). Finally, moving the object radiographed closer to the image receptor, or reducing the object-to-film distance (OFD), will minimize penumbra (Figure 13-7).

The ideal condition for demonstrating detail and minimizing penumbra would be to use a small focal spot, with a long SID and a short OFD. Of course, these conditions are not always possible to achieve. The use of small focal spot size limits the amount of milliamperage (mA) and therefore requires longer exposure time, potentially allowing patient motion. Increasing SID requires increasing technique according to the inverse square law, and not every body part can be placed in proximity to the image receptor. However, the technologist can often use one or more of these factors to increase the detail and decrease the penumbra on a radiograph.

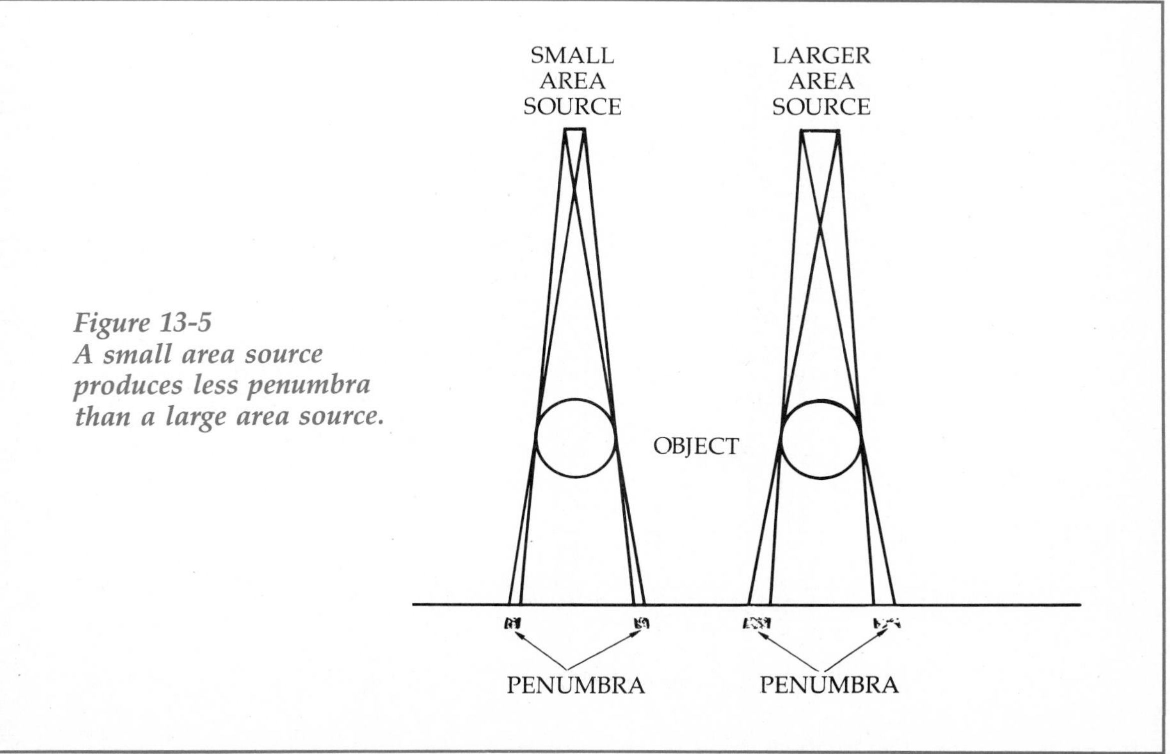

Figure 13-5
A small area source produces less penumbra than a large area source.

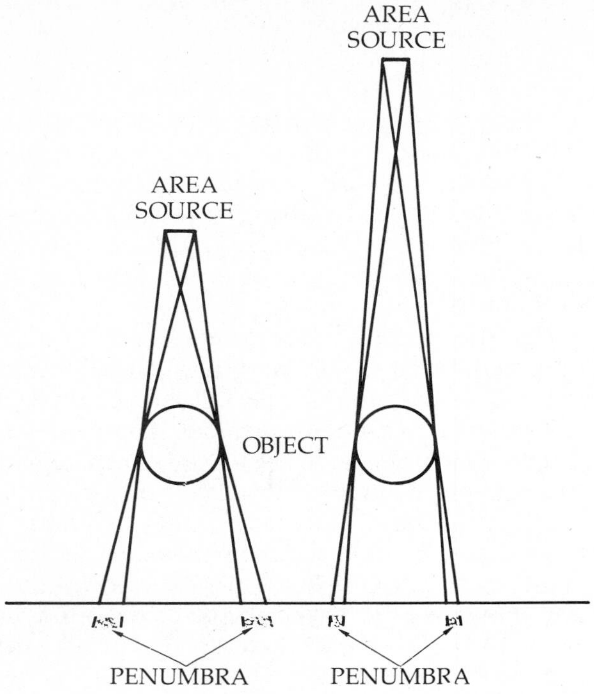

AREA SOURCE

AREA SOURCE

OBJECT

PENUMBRA

PENUMBRA

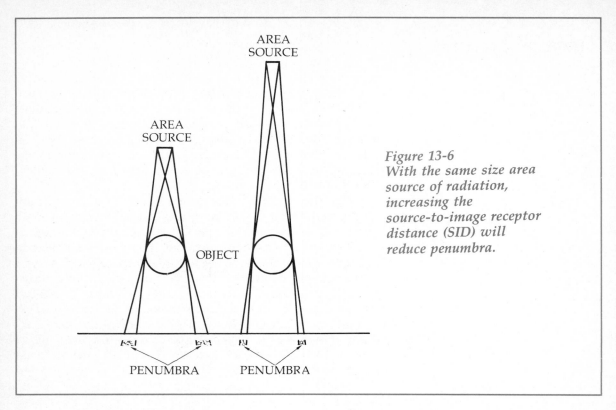

Figure 13-6
With the same size area source of radiation, increasing the source-to-image receptor distance (SID) will reduce penumbra.

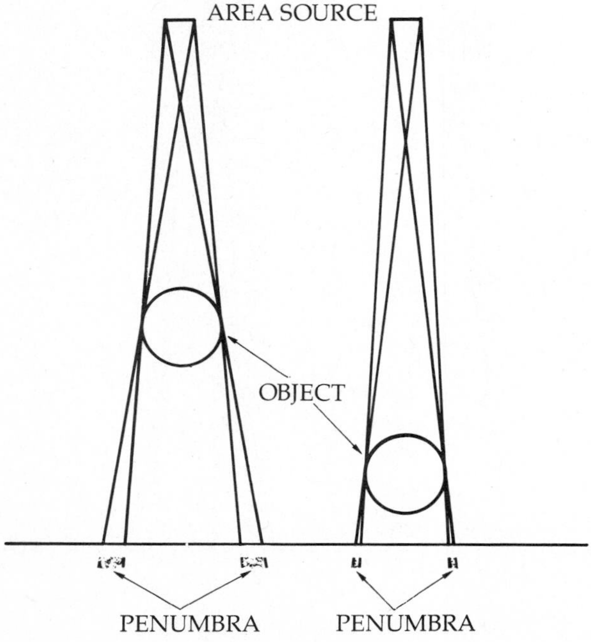

AREA SOURCE

OBJECT

PENUMBRA

PENUMBRA

Figure 13-7
Reducing the object-to-film distance (OFD) will reduce penumbra.

Radiographic detail is the information recorded on the film that constitutes the diagnostic image.

Radiographic Detail

Radiographic detail is the information recorded on the film that constitutes the diagnostic image. *Resolution* or *definition* are terms used to describe the sharpness with which the detail is recorded on the film. Three separate phenomena affect radiographic detail:

1. Geometric unsharpness is influenced by focal spot size, OFD, and SID.
2. Motion unsharpness is the result of either patient or equipment motion.
3. Screen unsharpness is described in Chapter 6.

Motion unsharpness has the greatest negative impact on radiographic detail.

One must recognize that motion unsharpness has the greatest negative impact on radiographic detail. Motion unsharpness can result from voluntary and involuntary patient motion or vibration in the x-ray equipment. Although vibration in the equipment may be difficult for the technologist to correct, she or he can usually control patient motion in several ways:

1. The use of high-mA and short-exposure times helps to "freeze" the image and minimize the effect of motion.
2. Immobilization of the patient helps prevent motion and may negate the need for high-mA, short-time exposures.
3. Explaining the procedure and securing the patient's cooperation may help to reduce motion. If patients understand the need to remain motionless for the examination, they will usually do their best to cooperate.

Screen unsharpness may be the result of defective equipment or simply a result of the screen-film combination selected. As stated in Chapter 6, high-resolution screen-film combinations are available that use a single high-resolution screen and single-emulsion film. These high-resolution screen-film systems should be used when excellent detail is necessary for the examination and when the additional exposure necessary is not a significant consideration.

Magnification

Magnification is a normal occurrence in the production of a diagnostic radiographic image. Since the x-ray beam diverges from the target of the x-ray tube, an object that is not in intimate contact with the film will be magnified. Intimate body part/film contact with a patient is often impossible due to the equipment used or anatomic and positioning considerations. The distance between a radiographic table top and the film is often several inches.

Magnification does not necessarily detract from the quality of a radiograph. The radiograph of the object may have excellent resolution and no distortion of shape. The image is only displayed larger than its actual size. The radiologist is accustomed to viewing normally magnified images. If absolute measurement of size is important, an object of known dimension can be radiographed at the same level as the patient, and the degree of magnification can be calculated.

Magnification does not necessarily detract from the quality of a radiograph.

Magnification can be a useful technique in radiography when it is necessary to display very fine detail. Magnification radiography can overcome the resolution limits of intensifying screens by magnifying the detail to be visualized. When performing magnification radiography, one must use very small focal spots because penumbra, as well as detail, is enlarged. *A 0.3 mm focal spot is required for 2× magnification.* Even smaller focal spots are often used to produce high-resolution magnification studies. Magnification radiography has found widespread use in angiography, extremity radiography, and mammography.

When performing magnification radiography, one must use very small focal spots because penumbra, as well as detail, is enlarged.

The degree of magnification is a function of SID and OFD. Magnification is calculated using the following equation:

$$\text{Magnification} = \frac{\text{SID}}{\text{SID} - \text{OFD}}$$

$$\textit{Magnification} = \frac{\textit{SID}}{\textit{SID} - \textit{OFD}}$$

For example, if the SID is 40 inches and the OFD is 10 inches, magnification can be calculated as follows:

$$x = \frac{40}{40 - 10}$$

$$x = \frac{40}{30} = 1.33$$

The magnification formula is also quoted as SID divided by source-to-object distance (SOD). Of course, SID minus OFD gives the SOD.

The use of long SID and short OFD can reduce magnification during radiography. The primary reason most chest radiography is performed at 72-inch SID is to reduce magnification of the heart. Lateral cervical spine radiographs are performed at 72-inch SID to minimize the magnification caused by the distance between the spine and the film.

Distortion is the misrepresentation of the true shape of an object in the radiographic image. Distortion is the result of unequal magnification of an object.

Distortion

Distortion is the misrepresentation of the true shape of an object in the radiographic image. Distortion is the result of unequal magnification of an object. Magnification does not necessarily distort an object; however, unequal magnification does. If an object is flat, parallel to the film, in intimate contact with the film, and directly beneath the focal spot, its image will be undistorted. Raising the object off the film will magnify but will not distort it. Tilting the object so that it is no longer parallel to the film will cause unequal magnification, distorting the image (Figure 13-8).

Radiographs of three-dimensional objects always possess some distortion. The portions that are farther from the film are more magnified than those closest to the film. For example, if we were to radiograph an upright can, an accurate representation would display a single circle, representing the superimposed top and bottom edges of the can. Actually, we see two concentric circles, the larger one representing the top of the can and the smaller one represent-

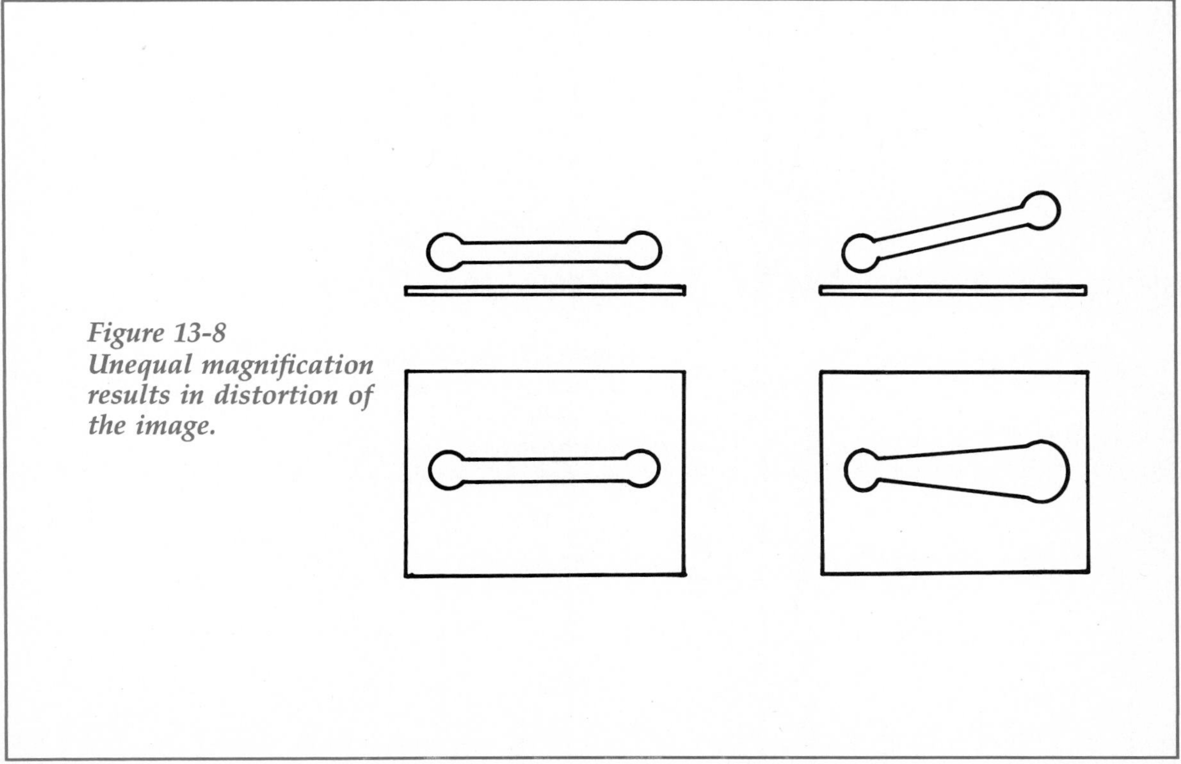

Figure 13-8
Unequal magnification results in distortion of the image.

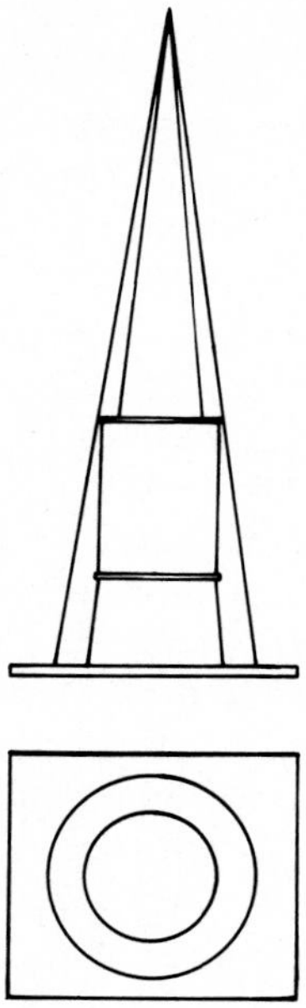

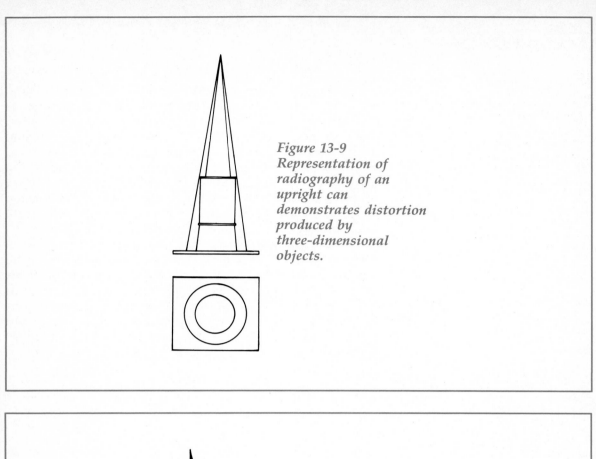

Figure 13-9
Representation of radiography of an upright can demonstrates distortion produced by three-dimensional objects.

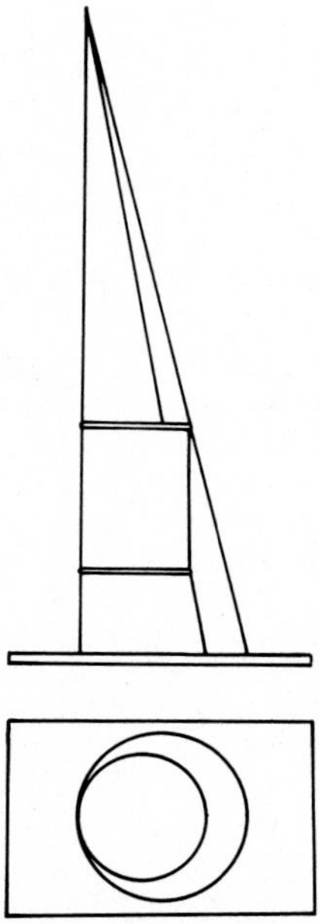

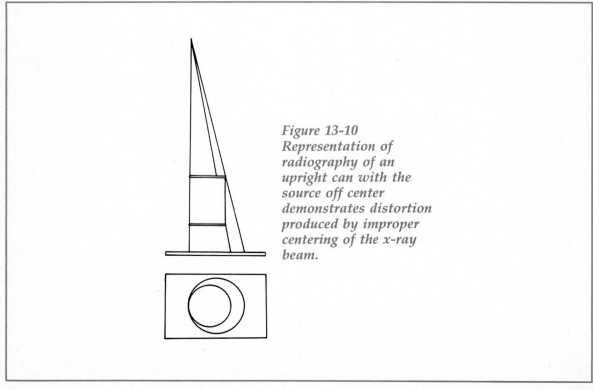

Figure 13-10
Representation of radiography of an upright can with the source off center demonstrates distortion produced by improper centering of the x-ray beam.

ing the bottom of the can (Figure 13-9). If the x-ray tube is moved from the center of the can to one side, additional distortion is introduced. The resultant image now has two circles that are not concentric. Again, the larger outer circle is the top of the can, whereas the smaller circle is the bottom of the can. Shifting the x-ray tube has projected the top of the can in the opposite direction of the tube shift (Figure 13-10).

Distortion can be reduced by centering the x-ray tube directly over the object, keeping the object parallel to the film, and positioning it as close to the film as possible.

Distortion can be reduced by centering the x-ray tube directly over the object, keeping the object parallel to the film, and positioning it as close to the film as possible. Since decreasing magnification can decrease distortion, a long SID also helps minimize distortion. The standard radiographic positions have been developed to achieve these conditions for specific body parts.

Chapter 13—Review Questions

1. What term describes the area of unsharpness at the edge of a structure on a radiograph?
   a. density
   b. distortion
   c. penumbra
   d. detail
   e. magnification
2. Which of the following factors will result in decreased penumbra?
   a. reduced focal spot size
   b. reduced SID
   c. increased focal spot size
   d. increased OFD
   e. none of the above
3. What term describes the information recorded on the film that constitutes the diagnostic image?
   a. density
   b. distortion
   c. penumbra
   d. detail
   e. magnification
4. Which of the following has the greatest negative impact on radiographic detail?
   a. geometric unsharpness
   b. motion unsharpness
   c. screen unsharpness
   d. focal spot size
   e. object-to-film distance
5. Which of the following terms best describes an image of a flat object that is directly beneath and centered to the focal spot, raised above the film, and parallel to the film?
   a. distorted
   b. magnified
   c. both of the above
   d. none of the above

6. Which of the following combinations of SID and OFD minimize magnification during radiography?
   a. long SID and long OFD
   b. long SID and short OFD
   c. short SID and long OFD
   d. short SID and short OFD
   e. none of the above
7. What is the magnification factor of an object being radiographed with an SID of 60 inches and an OFD of 20 inches?
   a. 1.33
   b. 1.50
   c. 2.0
   d. 3.0
8. Which of the following factors have a detrimental effect on radiographic detail?
   a. low mA techniques (without patient motion)
   b. small focal spot
   c. large OFD
   d. large SID
   e. none of the above
9. What term describes the misrepresentation of the true shape of an object?
   a. density
   b. distortion
   c. penumbra
   d. detail
   e. magnification
10. What impact does magnification have on distortion?
    a. Magnification does not influence distortion.
    b. Increased magnification decreases distortion.
    c. Decreased magnification increases distortion.
    d. Decreased magnification decreases distortion.

14

Radiographic Quality and Exposure Control

OBJECTIVES

After completing Chapter 14, you should be able to:

1. Define the following terms:
   diagnostic radiograph
   subject contrast
2. Discuss the impact of subject contrast and attenuation on the production of a diagnostic radiograph.
3. Describe the methodology of the development and use of technique charts.
4. Discuss the function and use of automatic exposure controls.

The Diagnostic Radiograph

The term "diagnostic radiograph" is frequently used but difficult to define. What is diagnostic to one individual may not be diagnostic to another. Most radiologists and technologists, however, agree on several qualities of a diagnostic radiograph.

A diagnostic radiograph has sufficient density, being neither underexposed nor overexposed. The detail of the radiographed object is sharply defined. An appropriate kVp for the radiographed object is used, resulting in the variations in the tissue densities being readily evident. The radiographed object is properly positioned and centered so its image is not distorted. Finally, the radiograph is properly identified and labeled with right or left markers.

Subject Contrast

Understanding subject contrast requires an understanding of anatomy and body composition. Not only do various body parts differ from each other in density, but the same part may differ in density from one individual to another. Subject contrast, as represented on the radiograph, is influenced by three factors:

1. Atomic weight (composition) of the material
2. Thickness of the material
3. Wavelength of the radiation employed

The more dense a material, or the greater its specific gravity, the more radiation it will attenuate. Obviously, lead is a better attenuator than water. One can make certain generalizations about the attenuation properties of the various tissues in the body. Most soft tissues, such as muscle, viscera, skin, cartilage, tendons, and nerves, have about the same attenuation properties as water. Fat is somewhat less dense than water, and air-laden tissues, such as the lungs, are significantly less dense than water and attenuate less radiation than other soft tissues. Calcified structures, such as bone and dentin, are significantly more dense than water and attenuate far more radiation than the soft tissues. The following is a list of body tissues in descending order of their density: dentin, bone, muscle, water and soft tissues, fat, and air-laden tissues.

The more dense a material, or the greater its specific gravity, the more radiation it will attenuate.

Thickness of the body part also plays an important part in attenuation properties. A 40-cm abdomen theoretically requires twice as much milliampere-seconds (mAs) to produce the same density as found with a 20-cm abdomen. The mAs are doubled because twice as much similar mate-

Thickness of the body part also plays an important part in attenuation properties.

rial exists to attenuate approximately twice as much radiation. The knee, however, which is about one-half the thickness of the chest, requires twice the mAs as the chest for a satisfactory density. In this case, even though the knee is one-half the thickness of the chest, it is composed of water-density tissues and bone. These tissues attenuate substantially more radiation than do the air-laden tissues of the chest.

Use and Development of Technique Charts

Although technique charts can serve as a guide in the selection of technical factors, they are not the ultimate answer to radiographic quality.

Technique charts can be valuable tools to a technologist, especially when performing an unusual procedure or working in an unfamiliar environment. Although technique charts can serve as a guide in the selection of technical factors, they are not the ultimate answer to radiographic quality. The success of technique charts depends on many factors, including:

1. Consistent equipment function (mA, time, kVp)
2. Consistent examination performance (SID, screen-film combination, grid ratio, positioning, collimation, estimation or measurement of part size, selection of technical factors)
3. Consistent processing of radiographs (thus the need for sensitometric evaluation of the processor)

Fixed-kVp versus Variable-kVp Charts

Essentially, two types of technique charts exist: fixed kVp and variable kVp. Normally, fixed-kVp technique charts are preferred for the following reasons:

1. Optimum kVp is used, regardless of part thickness.
2. Part measurement is less critical.
3. mAs has a linear relationship to density.
4. Use of fixed kVp typically results in lower patient dose.
5. Use of fixed kVp typically results in fewer heat units per exposure.

A 35 percent change in mAs is required to produce a noticeable change in density.

In many respects, technique charts are developed through trial and error. Typically, average techniques are established first, and techniques for small and large patients are calculated from the average. One must remember that it requires at least a 35 percent change in mAs to produce a noticeable change in density. Therefore, the technique for small and large patients should be established at 50 percent and 200 percent of the average mAs, respectively. In some anatomic sites, such as the chest and abdomen, patient size can vary greatly. In these cases it may be necessary to create several technique classifications.

When using technique charts, technologists must pay particular attention to *pathology*. The presence of many pathologic conditions can greatly alter the density of the tissue being examined, requiring alteration of the technique. Examples of pathology affecting tissue density include ascites (additive), pneumonia (additive), emphysema (subtractive), and severe osteoporosis (subtractive).

The presence of many pathologic conditions can greatly alter the density of the tissue being examined, requiring alteration of the technique.

The kVp selected for each body part may vary from institution to institution. The kVp selection should be based on the following:

1. Thickness, density, and tissue composition of the part
2. Preference of the radiologist
3. Common pathologies encountered in the institution

The following is a list of recommended kVps for various body parts. Remember: these are only recommendations; selection of kVp should consider the factors already mentioned.

Skull and facial bones	80 kVp (grid)
Cervical spine	80 kVp (grid)
Chest (lungs, mediastinum)	120 kvP (grid)
Chest (ribs)	80 kVp (grid)
Thoracic spine (anteroposterior [AP] views)	90 kVp (grid)
(lateral)	80 kVp (grid)
Abdomen	80 kVp (grid)
Lumbar spine (AP)	85 kVp (grid)
(lateral)	100 kVp (grid)
Shoulder (AP)	75 kVp (grid)
Upper arm and elbow	70 kVp (nongrid)
Lower arm and hand	55 kVp (nongrid)
Femur	80 kVp (grid)
Knee	70 kVp (grid)
Tibia and fibula	70 kVp (nongrid)
Ankle (AP, lateral)	65 kVp (nongrid)
Foot	60 kVp (nongrid)

Use of Automatic Exposure Devices

Automatic exposure devices measure the amount of radiation reaching the film.

Another method of technique management is the use of automatic exposure devices. Automatic exposure devices are commonly known as *phototimers, amplimats,* and *ionomats.* All these devices work in the same manner: as an exposure is made, these devices measure the amount of radiation reaching the film. Once the proper amount of radiation to produce a predetermined density strikes the film, the exposure is automatically terminated. These devices typically use ionization chambers or photomultiplier tubes. *Ionization chambers* are usually radiolucent and located between the patient and the film. *Photomultiplier tubes* are usually located behind the x-ray cassette and can only be used with phototiming cassettes. As radiation interacts with these devices, an electric charge is created; when the electric charge reaches a given level, the exposure is terminated electronically by the timer circuit.

The mA must be low enough to meet or exceed the minimum response time of the device.

The technologist selects the kVp and mA; the automatic exposure device terminates the exposure at the proper time. When using automatic exposure control, the technologist must select the proper kVp and mA. The mA must be low enough to meet or exceed the minimum response time of the device (or the shortest exposure that it can control) and high enough to terminate the exposure before reaching the backup time. The *backup time* is a safety feature that limits the maximum exposure possible in the case of operator error or equipment failure.

Positioning of the patient relative to the radiation sensor is an important consideration for the technologist.

Another important consideration for the technologist using automatic exposure devices is positioning of the patient relative to the radiation sensor. Typically, most automatic exposure devices have three sensors located in the upper left-hand portion of the field, the upper right-hand portion of the field, and the center of the field (Figure 14-1). These sensors can be used individually or in combination with one another. When more than one sensor has been selected, the electric charges are averaged, as is the density on the resultant radiograph. Ideally, the technologist should position the patient to locate one or more of the sensors in the area of interest. This will ensure that this area has the proper density. Even slight improper positioning may result in unsatisfactory density on the radiograph.

The importance of proper positioning and sensor selection cannot be emphasized enough. Two common examples of this problem are the posteroanterior (PA) chest and the lateral lumbar spine radiographs. In the chest, if the technologist selects to position the sensor in the left lung, a portion of the sensor will be beneath the heart (Figure 14-2). This will result in decreased exposure to this portion of the detector and overexposure of the film to compensate. In the lateral lumbar spine, positioning of the sensor posterior to the vertebral bodies results in increased exposure to the detector and severe underexposure of the film (Figure 14-3).

In some cases it is necessary to alter the density of the film because of anatomic composition or pathology in the area of interest. To allow density variation, most automatic exposure controls have density selections, −2, −1, N, +1 and +2. These density selections can be adjusted by service personnel, typically as follows:

−2 = 50 percent of normal exposure/density
−1 = 75 percent of normal exposure/density
N = 100 percent of normal exposure/density
+1 = 150 percent of normal exposure/density
+2 = 200 percent of normal exposure/density

The density adjustments do not compensate for patient size.

These adjustments do not compensate for patient

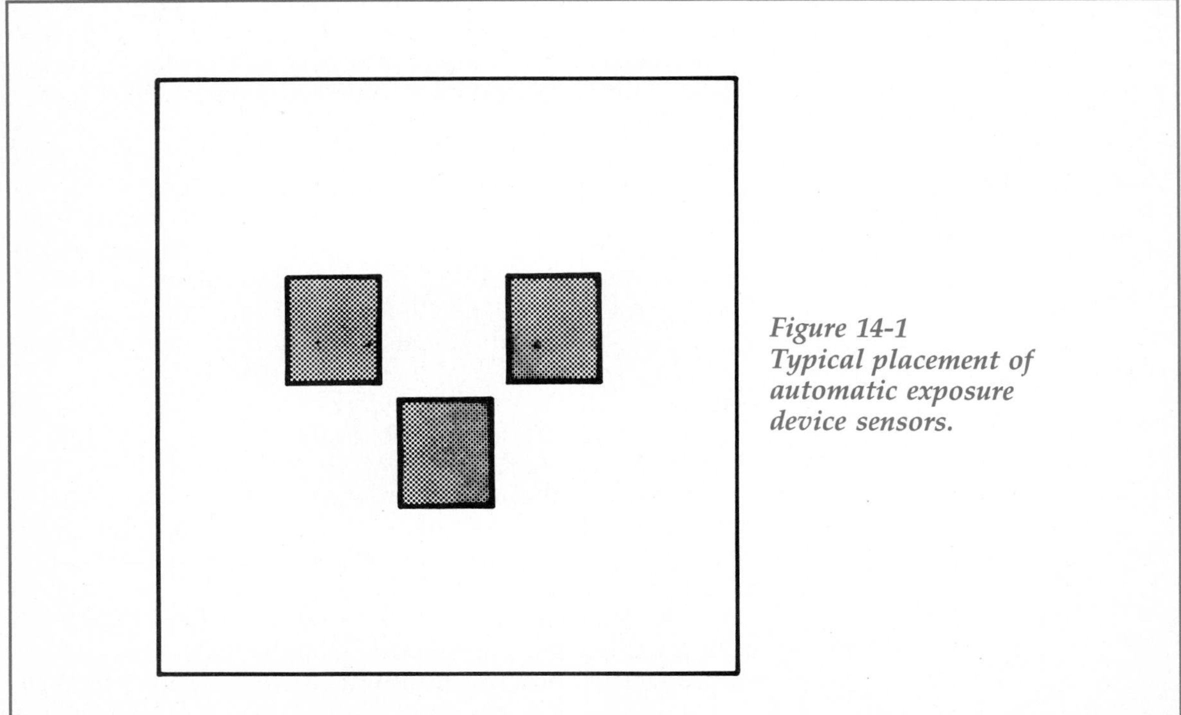

Figure 14-1 Typical placement of automatic exposure device sensors.

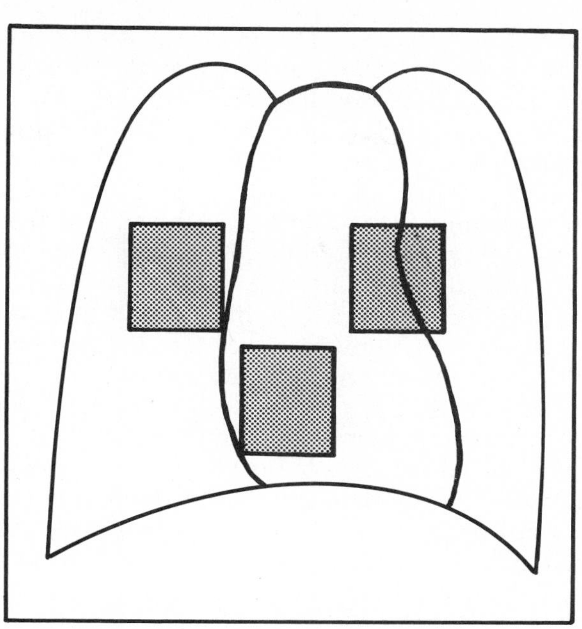

Figure 14-2
During chest radiography, the left-field sensor is partially covered by the mediastinal structures (shaded area of sensor).

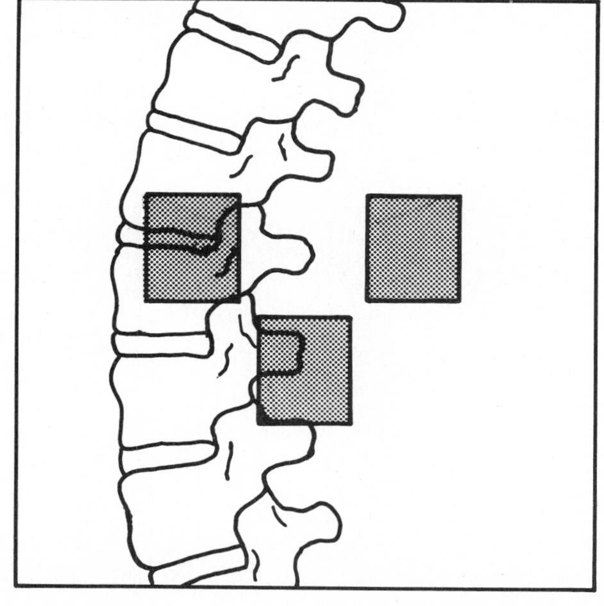

Figure 14-3
During lateral lumbar spine radiography, the portion of the central sensor posterior to the lumbar vertebrae is exposed to unattenuated radiation (shaded area of sensor).

size. The only exception would be an examination with an excessive amount of scatter radiation causing a premature termination of exposure. Common examples of the proper use of density controls include the knee and the ribs. When performing a lateral knee examination, the technologist usually positions the sensor under the superimposed condyles. The condyles are so dense that the proper exposure of the entire film requires the use of −1. With the ribs, the air-filled lungs, which permit most of the radiation to pass through unattenuated, often terminate the exposure too soon to achieve the proper density for a rib examination. In this case, the use of +1 is necessary to obtain adequate density for proper evaluation of the ribs.

Although automatic exposure devices are somewhat complex to use, they can result in the production of superior-quality radiographs and reduced repeat rates once they are mastered. Investment in this device is worthwhile provided technologists are properly trained.

Chapter 14—Review Questions

1. Which of the following factors does *not* influence subject contrast?
   a. the atomic weight of the material
   b. the mAs
   c. the kVp
   d. the thickness of the material
2. Which of the following materials has the highest density?
   a. water
   b. fat
   c. muscle
   d. soft tissue
3. How large a change in mAs is necessary to produce a noticeable change in density?
   a. 25 percent
   b. 35 percent
   c. 45 percent
   d. 55 percent
4. Which of the following pathologies has a subtractive effect on tissue density?
   a. pneumonia
   b. osteoporosis
   c. ascites
   d. two of the above
   e. all of the above
5. What factor plays a role in kVp selection?
   a. the part thickness
   b. the part density
   c. the tissue composition of the part
   d. the radiologist's preference
   e. all of the above
6. What is the primary purpose of the backup timer when using an automatic exposure device?
   a. to determine the minimum exposure time
   b. to prevent equipment malfunction
   c. to limit the maximum exposure possible
   d. none of the above

7. Which of the following factors is most critical when using an automatic exposure device?
   a. accurate measurement of the part thickness
   b. proper selection of exposure time
   c. proper positioning
   d. two of the above
   e. all of the above

8. What is the primary purpose of the density selection adjustment on an automatic exposure device?
   a. to compensate for patient size
   b. to compensate for anatomic composition
   c. to compensate for pathology
   d. two of the above
   e. all of the above

9. What is essential for the successful use of fixed-kVp technique charts, variable-kVp technique charts, and automatic exposure devices?
   a. proper positioning
   b. consistent processing of radiographs
   c. accurate part measurement
   d. two of the above
   e. all of the above

10. Which of the following factors is *not* a quality of a diagnostic radiograph?
    a. sharp definition
    b. appropriate kVp
    c. proper positioning
    d. proper identification
    e. none of the above

15

Radiographic Quality Control

OBJECTIVES

After completing Chapter 15, you should be able to:

1. Discuss the quality control testing of the x-ray tube, the generator, the image intensifier, and radiographic accessories.

Radiographic quality control is a very important aspect of an overall departmental quality control program. Proper function of the radiographic equipment will impact patient dose, the repeat rate, and the diagnostic quality of the radiographs. Subdivisions of radiographic quality control include the x-ray tube, the x-ray generator, the image intensifier, and radiographic accessories.

Quality Control of the X-Ray Tube

When performing quality control testing of the x-ray tube, three parameters should be evaluated: (1) the coincidence of the light field and the radiation field, (2) the nominal size of the focal spot, and (3) the filtration or half-value layer. (Chapter 12 discusses the determination and evaluation of half-value layer.)

Several methods are available to evaluate the coincidence of the light field to the radiation field. The essential elements include delineation of the light field and central ray with radiopaque markers and a method of identifying film placement to aid in any necessary adjustments. To perform the test, collimate the beam at least 1 inch within the edges of the film on all sides. Then mark the edges of the light field with radiopaque markers at the corners. Also, identify the position of the film with respect to the collimator by placing a radiopaque marker. Make an exposure using 1-2 mAs at 60 kVp. Last, open the collimator to cover the edges of the film and make a second exposure. This is necessary to document the location of the radiopaque markers if the radiation field is smaller than, or off center from, the light field. This would result in failure to image some or all the markers (Figure 15-1).

Interpretation of this test is relatively simple. The light-to-radiation field must coincide to a plus or minus 2 percent of the source-to-image receptor distance (SID). Therefore, at a 40-inch SID, the light-to-radiation field must coincide within 0.8 inch.

The light-to-radiation field must coincide to a plus or minus 2 percent of the source-to-image receptor distance (SID).

The nominal focal spot size can be evaluated using numerous commercially available test tools or the pinhole camera method. Both methods require the use of non-screen film. Using the *pinhole camera method* is relatively simple, requiring a lead mask with a small hole in the center. Place the lead mask midway between the focal spot and the film and make an exposure (Figure 15-2). Approximately 50 mAs at 60 kVp is usually satisfactory. The exposure will result in the projection of an image of the focal spot on the film.

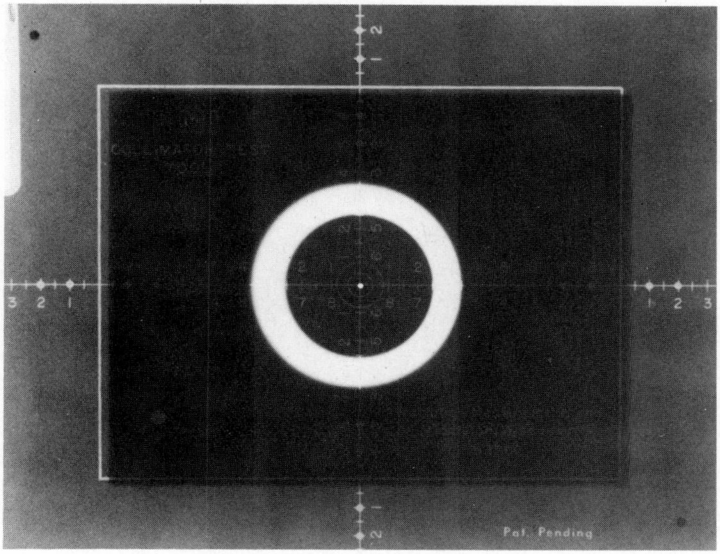

Figure 15-1
Example of a light-to-radiation field coincidence test.

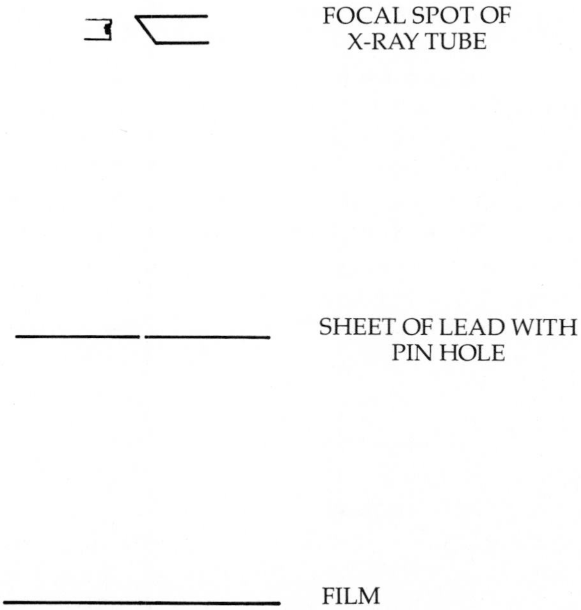

FOCAL SPOT OF
X-RAY TUBE

SHEET OF LEAD WITH
PIN HOLE

FILM

Figure 15-2
Typical setup for a pinhole camera test.

Figure 15-3
Example of a pinhole camera test of focal spot size.

Interpretation of the pinhole test is also simple, requiring the measurement of the image of the focal spot. The image will be the same size as the apparent focal spot (Figure 15-3). The criteria of acceptability will depend on the application of the x-ray tube. The requirements for angiography tubes or tubes used in magnification studies are far more stringent than those for x-ray tubes used in chest radiography.

The criteria of acceptability of the focal spot will depend on the application of the x-ray tube.

Quality Control of the X-Ray Generator

Quality control testing of the x-ray generator requires evaluation of three components: (1) the timer, (2) mA linearity, and (3) the kVp. Evaluation of these parameters requires the use of simple test tools, noninvasive electronic devices, as well as invasive test tools. This discussion centers on the use of simple test tools that the technologist can use independently.

Two basic test tools are available to evaluate the timer circuit. The simplest test tool is the spinning top; however, it can only be used with single-phase generators. The *spinning top* is usually a flat metal disk mounted on an axle that allows it to spin freely (Figure 15-4). Near the outside edge of the disk there is a single slot or hole. This slot or hole passes completely through the thickness of the disk. To use the spinning top, place it on a cassette, centering the x-ray tube directly above. Spin the top by hand and make an exposure. Each pulse of radiation produced by the single-phase equipment produces a dot of density on the film (Figure 15-5). The number of dots produced depends on the length of exposure and the type of rectification used in the generator. Half-wave rectification produces 60 pulses of radiation in 1 second; a 1-second exposure will produce 60 dots on the film. Full-wave rectification produces 120 pulses of radiation in 1 second; a 1-second exposure will produce 120 dots on the film. The proper number of pulses for a given length of exposure can be determined by multiplying the number of pulses per second by the exposure time. For example, for full-wave rectification:

The proper number of pulses for a given length of exposure can be determined by multiplying the number of pulses per second by the exposure time.

120 pulses per second
  × Length of exposure = Number of pulses

120 pulses per second
  × 1/10 second = 12 pulses

Another device used to evaluate the timer is the synchronous timer. The *synchronous timer* is simply a spinning top that is driven by an electric synchronous motor (Figure 15-6). The motor rotates at 1 revolution per second (rps). Use of this device is identical to the spinning top; however, it is used to evaluate the timer on three-phase equipment. Evaluation of three-phase equipment is possible because the disk rotates at a fixed rate of 1 rps. Since the exposure produced by a three-phase generator is essentially continuous, the density produced on the film will be an arc rather than a series of dots (Figure 15-7). Measurement of the arc allows determination of the actual exposure time, which is calculated as follows:

Measurement of the arc allows determination of the actual exposure time when using the synchronous timer.

Time of exposure
  × 360 degrees/second = Degrees of exposure arc

1/10 second
  × 360 degrees/second = 36 degrees

Proper mA linearity will ensure that a given milliampere-seconds (mAs) selected at any mA station will produce the same density on a radiograph.

Milliamperage (mA) linearity is also an important function of the x-ray generator to monitor. Proper mA lin-

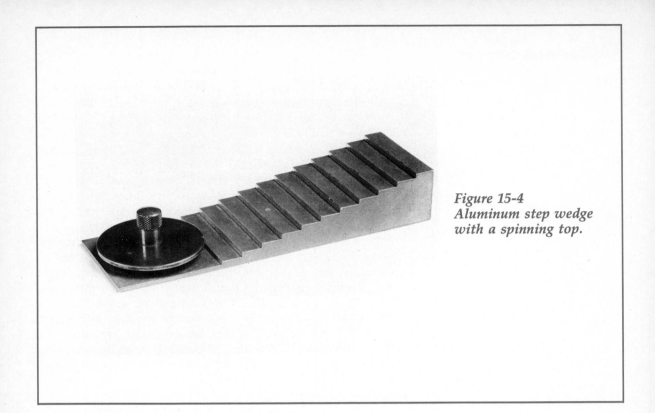

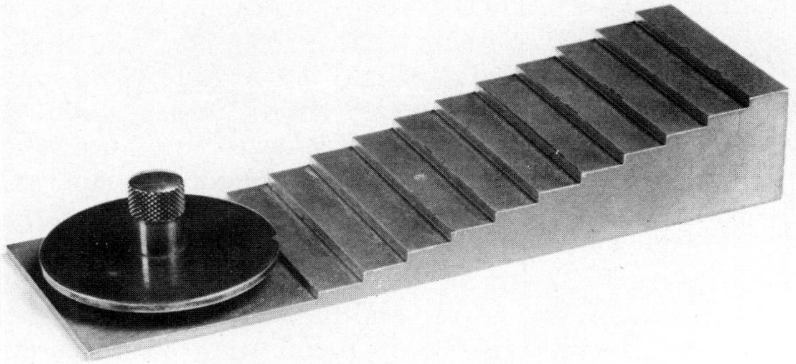

Figure 15-4
Aluminum step wedge with a spinning top.

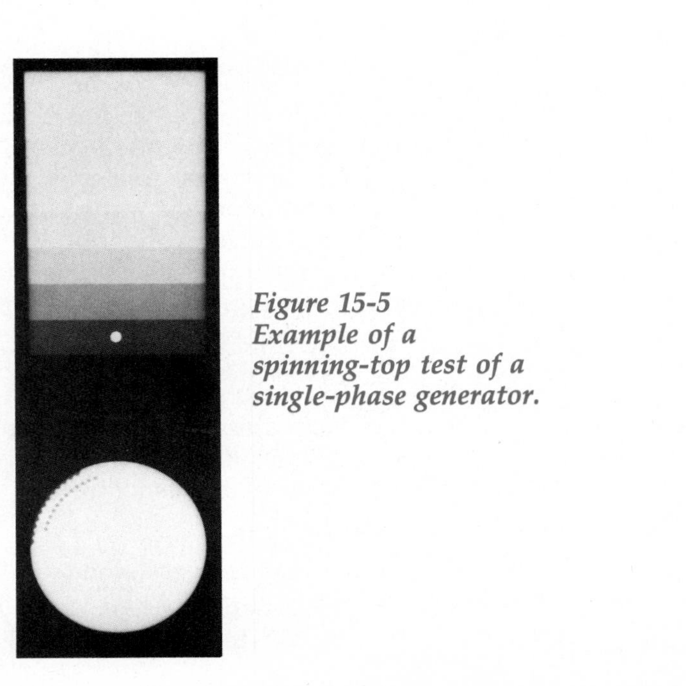

Figure 15-5
Example of a spinning-top test of a single-phase generator.

Figure 15-6
Synchronous timer test tool. Note the dots of density produced by the pulsing radiation. (Courtesy RMI)

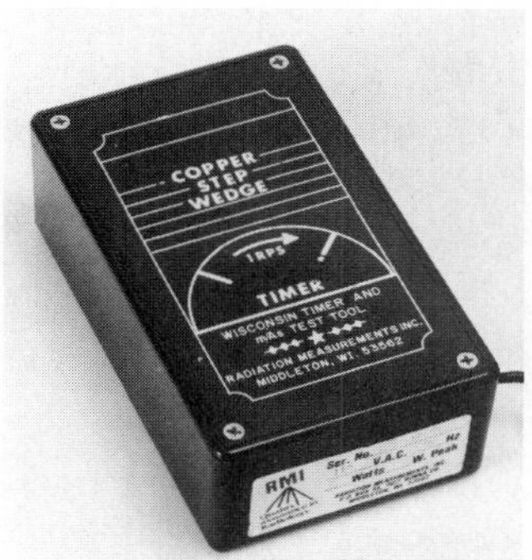

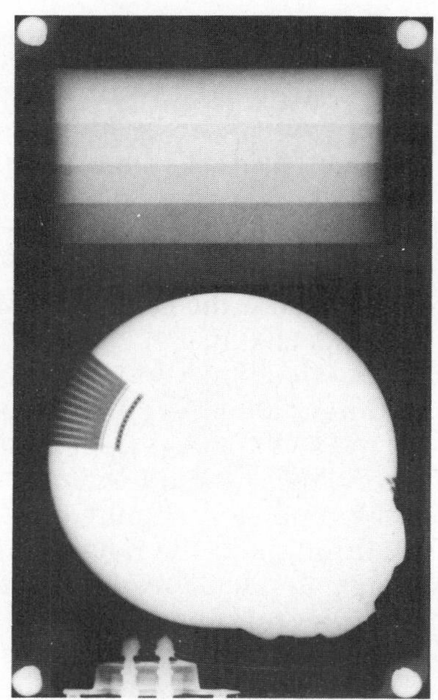

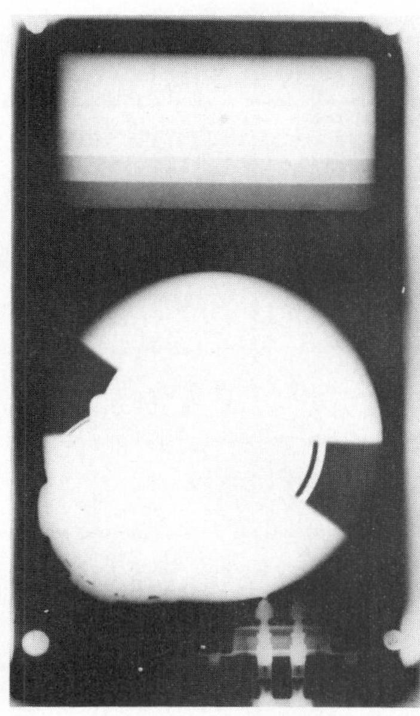

Figure 15-7
Example of a synchronous timer test using three-phase equipment. Note the arc of density produced as opposed to the dots seen with single-phase equipment. (Courtesy RMI)

earity will ensure that a given milliampere-seconds (mAs) selected at any mA station will produce the same density on a radiograph. This is important because the technologist frequently changes the exposure time to reduce motion or overcome generator limitations. A simple step wedge is adequate for mA linearity evaluation. The technologist obtains a radiograph of the step wedge at each mA station using the same mAs and kVp. For example:

10 mAs (100 mA × 1/10 second) at 60 kVp
10 mAs (200 mA × 1/20 second) at 60 kVp
10 mAs (300 mA × 1/30 second) at 60 kVp
10 mAs (400 mA × 1/40 second) at 60 kVp

The technologist should evaluate the film using a densitometer. No one step should vary more than 30 percent in density throughout the range of mA stations. When trying to measure the densities of the steps, it is helpful to identify one or more steps of the step wedge with lead markers to serve as reference points. One often finds step wedges built into timer test tools. This permits the evaluation of both timer accuracy and mA linearity at the same time.

When performing the mA linearity test no one step should vary more than 30 percent in density throughout the range of mA stations.

Evaluation of kVp is possible with the use of a simple test cassette or a digital kVp meter (Figure 15-8). A kVp

A

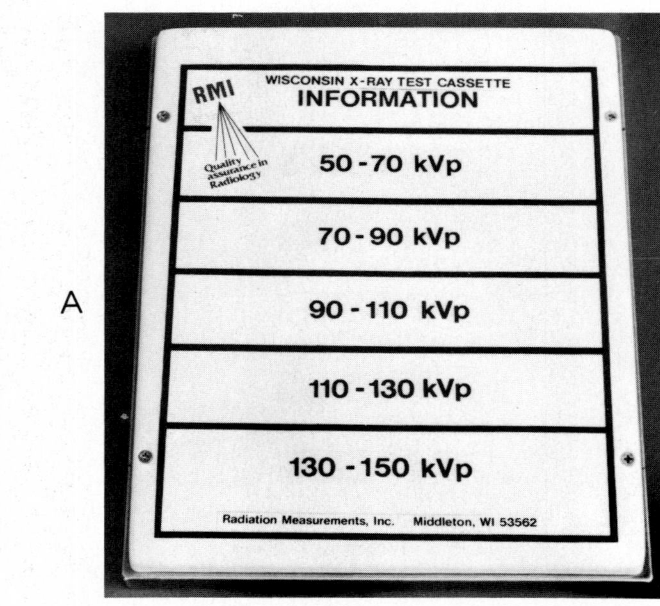

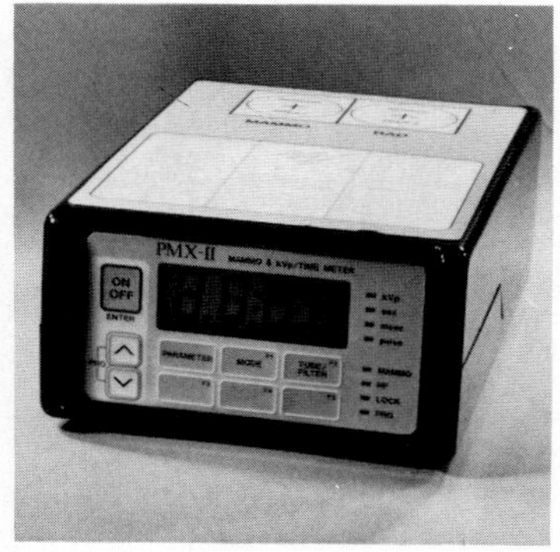

B

Figure 15-8
A, A kVp test cassette (Courtesy RMI) and B, digital kVp meter. (Courtesy RTI Electronics AB)

test cassette uses calibrated step wedges and optical attenuators to permit evaluation of the kVp (Figure 15-9). A digital kVp meter electronically measures and displays the kVp on a numerical readout. Either of these devices is simple to use and accurate. The kVp cassette is less expensive than a digital kVp meter. Half-value layer, another measure of beam quality, should also be a part of the evaluation process (see Chapter 12).

Quality Control of the Image Intensifier

Quality control of the image intensifier is relatively simple to perform. The parameters evaluated include high-contrast resolution, both in the center and at the periphery of the field, and low-contrast resolution. High-contrast resolution evaluation requires the use of a *wire-mesh phantom* (Figures 15-10 and 15-11). The technologist positions the device in contact with the face of the image intensifier to reduce magnification and possible distortion. Fluoroscopy of the device permits evaluation of the image. The smallest

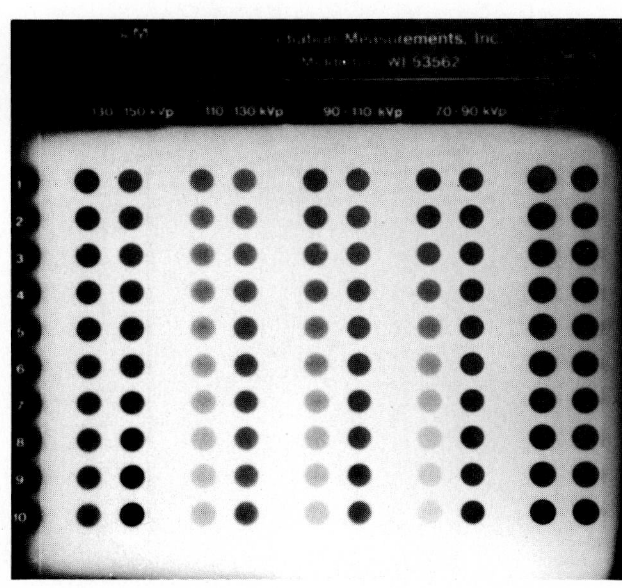

Figure 15-9
A kVp test film.
(Courtesy RMI)

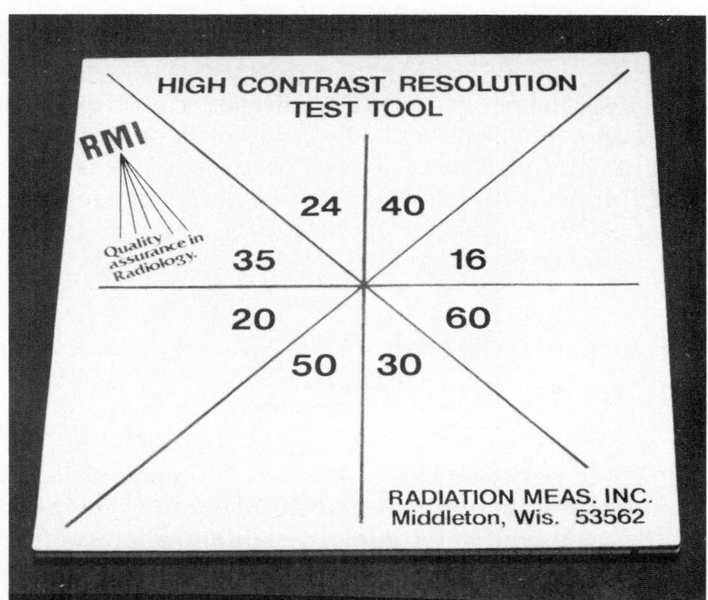

Figure 15-10
Wire-mesh phantom test tool. (Courtesy RMI)

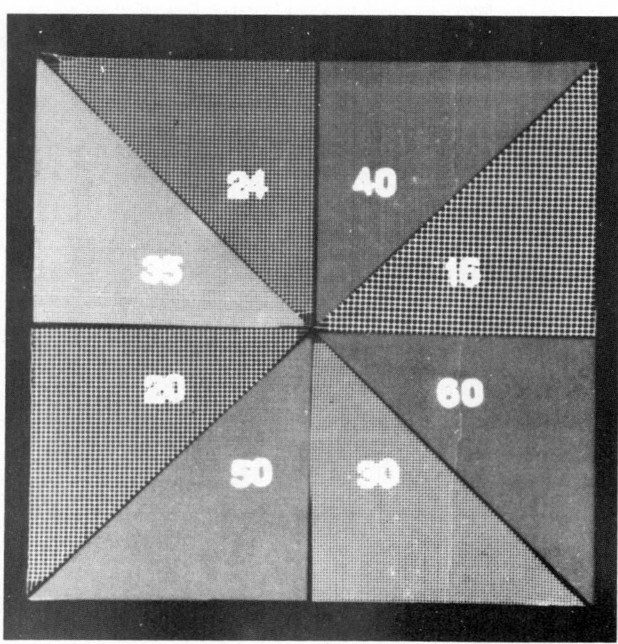

Figure 15-11
Wire-mesh phantom film. (Courtesy RMI)

mesh visible in the center and at the periphery of the image determines image quality. The smaller the mesh visualized, the better is the image quality.

Evaluation of low-contrast resolution of the intensifier takes place at 2 percent and 4 percent contrast levels. A simple tool is available that has a thin aluminum plate with holes of various sizes drilled in it and two thicker aluminum plates (Figure 15-12). Using the thinner plate with holes on one of the thicker aluminum plates, the holes represent 4 percent of the total thickness, and therefore 4 percent contrast. Adding the second thicker plate results in the holes representing 2 percent of the total thickness, and therefore 2 percent contrast. Fluoroscopy of the plate with the holes and one or both of the thick plates permits evaluation of image contrast. The smaller the visualized hole and the lower the contrast (2 percent), the better is the image quality. The results of the contrast evaluation depend on the specifications as well as the age of the machine. Frequently, only higher-quality image intensifiers can easily demonstrate 2 percent contrast. All intensifiers decline in contrast resolution with age.

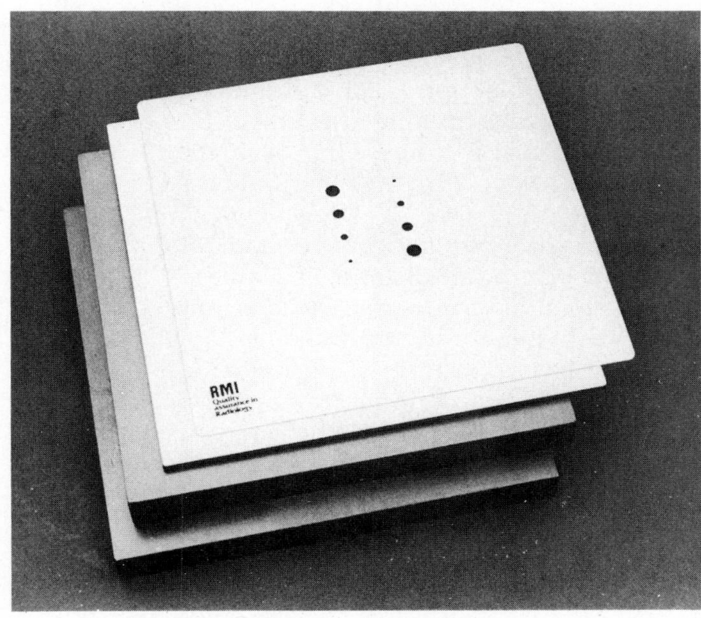

Figure 15-12
Aluminum low-contrast resolution test tool. (Courtesy RMI)

It is very important to evaluate the intensifier when conducting acceptance testing of a new piece of equipment. This will identify the level of detail resolution and contrast resolution with which to compare all future testing. Tolerance of variation from the original standard of detail, resolution, and contrast resolution will depend on the type of procedures performed. A cardiac catheterization suite, for example, will require more critical adherence to the original standard than will a typical fluoroscopic room. Additionally, if any other imaging devices that depend on the fluoroscopic image are present (e.g., cine, spot-film cameras, digital imaging), they must be a part of the total evaluation.

Quality Control of Radiographic Accessories

Many of the radiographic accessories used in the radiology department require evaluation in a quality control program. These items include lead protective devices, grids, cassettes, and intensifying screens. These devices require evaluation on at least an annual basis.

Lead protective devices, including aprons, gloves, gonadal shields, thyroid shields, and fluoroscopic curtains, should undergo annual radiographic or fluoroscopic evaluation. When many protection devices exist and a fluoroscopic unit is available, fluoroscopic examination can result in a substantial savings in film cost. The technologist must identify aprons and document the evaluation appropriately. All damaged devices require immediate replacement.

Lead protective devices, including aprons, gloves, gonadal shields, thyroid shields, and fluoroscopic curtains, should undergo annual radiographic or fluoroscopic evaluation.

Considering the construction of radiographic grids, one can easily appreciate the fragile nature of these devices. Grids are subject to damage and require evaluation annually with radiography. To evaluate a grid, place the grid on a cassette and make an exposure with just enough technique to produce a uniform gray density on the film. Examine the radiograph for density variations across the film or areas of artifact. Evaluation of grids should also be done before initial use to ensure the quality of a new grid.

Grids are subject to damage and require evaluation annually with radiography.

The cassettes and intensifying screens also require regular evaluation. A protocol for screen cleaning and visual inspection is desirable. This will help to keep the screens artifact free. Also, the cassette and intensifying screens require at least annual radiographic evaluation. To evaluate screens and cassettes, place them under the x-ray tube and make an exposure, which will produce a uniformly gray radiograph. Then examine the film for artifacts or density differences. If possible, the problem should be corrected or the cassette or intensifying screens taken out of service. Devices are available that use an ultraviolet light source to help in the visual inspection of the screens. Ultraviolet light often makes defects in the screens readily apparent to the naked eye. However, these devices do not help in the evaluation of the cassette itself.

Other Quality Control

In many respects, quality control of the radiographic environment has no bounds; any part of the imaging process can undergo evaluation. Examples include measurement of the output of radiographic and fluoroscopic units, evaluation of phototimers, and monitoring of the repeat rate. Each of these items, as well as others, plays an important role in quality control.

Measurement of the output of radiographic and fluoroscopic units is accomplished by using an ionization chamber or an *R-meter*. Of these measurements, the most important is the dose rate at the tabletop during fluoroscopic procedures: *this dose rate may not exceed 10 roentgens per minute.*

The fluoroscopic, table-top dose rate may not exceed 10 roentgens per minute.

Evaluation of the phototimer is possible using radiography of a phantom. Making multiple radiographs of the phantom with the phototimer should demonstrate consistency of density (assuming constant kVp). Comparison of the exposures to a previously established standard allows one to detect drifting of the phototimer. Each field of the phototimer requires separate evaluation, including proper density as well as consistency from field to field.

Monitoring of the radiograph repeat rate can be a cost-effective element of quality control. When monitoring the repeat rate, one should keep track of the number of procedures, the number of sheets of film used, the number of repeat radiographs, and the number of wasted films. It is also important to categorize repeats by procedure and the reason for repeat. If possible, collection of information concerning the specific unit and technologist may also prove helpful. Monitoring of the repeat rate may identify specific problems that, when corrected, may reduce repeats and film cost.

Quality control plays a key role in ensuring the quality of radiographic examinations. Remember: the primary goal of a quality control program is to identify problems before they affect the radiograph and detract from the quality of patient care.

The primary goal of a quality control program is to identify problems before they affect the radiograph and detract from the quality of patient care.

Chapter 15—Review Questions

1. Which of the following parameters is evaluated during quality control testing of the x-ray tube?
   a. kVp
   b. half-value layer
   c. mA linearity
   d. two of the above
   e. all of the above
2. If the light-to-radiation field is evaluated at an SID of 72 inches, then the light-to-radiation field must coincide within:
   a. 0.8 inches
   b. 0.72 inches
   c. 1.44 inches
   d. 1.6 inches
3. What is the pinhole camera test used to evaluate?
   a. light-to-radiation field coincidence
   b. focal spot size
   c. half-value layer
   d. none of the above
4. If a spinning-top test is used to evaluate a 500 mA, 150 kVp, three-phase generator, set at 1/20 of a second, how many dots will be present on the film?
   a. 3 dots
   b. 6 dots
   c. 12 dots
   d. 18 dots
   e. none of the above
5. How many dots would appear on the film if a spinning-top test is used to evaluate a self-rectified, single-phase generator, when making an exposure of 1/10 of a second?
   a. 3 dots
   b. 6 dots
   c. 12 dots
   d. 18 dots
   e. none of the above

6. What would the measurement of the arc, in degrees, be for an exposure of 1/20 second?
   a. 18 degrees
   b. 20 degrees
   c. 36 degrees
   d. Not enough information is provided to solve the problem.

7. How often should lead protection devices, grids, and cassettes be evaluated for damage?
   a. monthly
   b. quarterly
   c. semiannually
   d. annually

8. What is the primary purpose of quality control programs?
   a. to meet regulatory guidelines
   b. to identify problems before they detract from the quality of patient care
   c. to provide the basis for a comprehensive quality assurance program
   d. two of the above
   e. all of the above

9. What is the maximum dose rate at tabletop for a fluoroscopic unit?
   a. 5,000 mR
   b. 1.0 R per minute
   c. 10 R per minute
   d. 150 mR per hour at 1 meter
   e. none of the above

10. Which of the following parameters is evaluated during quality control of the image intensifier?
    a. total system gain
    b. high-contrast resolution
    c. low-contrast resolution
    d. two of the above
    e. all of the above

16

Stereoscopic Radiography

OBJECTIVES

After completing Chapter 16, you should be able to:

1. Define the following terms:
   binocular depth perception
   discrepant images
   monocular depth perception
   stereopsis
   stereoscope
2. Discuss the mechanisms of human depth perception.
3. Discuss the principles behind stereo radiography and how to perform a stereoscopic examination.
4. Discuss how proper tube shift is determined for a stereoscopic examination.
5. Identify common clinical applications for stereo radiography.

Depth Perception

The primary mechanism of depth perception in humans is visual. We can determine the relative position of objects that surround us simply by looking at them. Our ability to perceive depth is the result of two separate visual mechanisms.

The first mechanism is monocular depth perception, which depends on four or five visual clues that can be recognized using a single eye. The first visual clue is that objects closest to the viewer may have their borders overlapping the objects behind them. The second visual clue is that objects of similar size appear larger when they are closer to, and smaller when they are farther from, the viewer. Perspective and shading give a sense of depth and are commonly used by artists to give depth to drawings and paintings. Finally, humidity, smog, and dirt in the air result in a graying of objects and a decrease in their sharpness in the far distance.

Monocular depth perception allows us to make relatively accurate estimates about the distances of objects from us. With one eye closed, normal depth perception ability is reduced somewhat, but depth determination is still relatively accurate.

The second mechanism of depth perception is stereopsis. *Stereopsis* is the ability to see two slightly different images, one in each eye, which are converted by the brain into a single picture that has depth. These slightly different images are termed *discrepant images* and are essential for stereopsis (Figure 16-1). The degree of difference between two discrepant images is important to stereopsis. Images that are too discrepant cannot be fused together, while images that are too similar do not produce depth.

Stereopsis *is man's ability to see two slightly different images from each eye that are converted by the brain into a single picture that has depth. These slightly different images are termed* **discrepant images** *and are essential for stereopsis.*

An excellent example of discrepant images producing depth is the children's toy, the View-Master™ (Figure 16-2). This toy is a binocular viewing system in which each eye sees a separate transparency image of objects taken at slightly different angles. Although each transparency is two-dimensional, the fused image appears three-dimensional, giving the perception of depth.

Principles of Stereoscopic Radiography

Monocular depth perception gives minimal information about the relative position of objects on a radiograph. To the individual familiar with radiographic anatomy, the

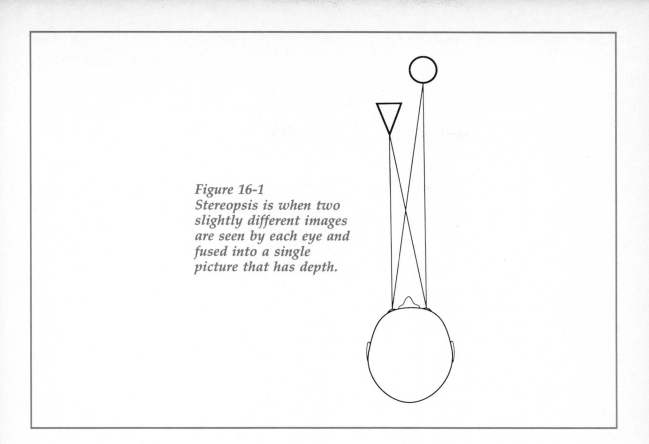

Figure 16-1
Stereopsis is when two slightly different images are seen by each eye and fused into a single picture that has depth.

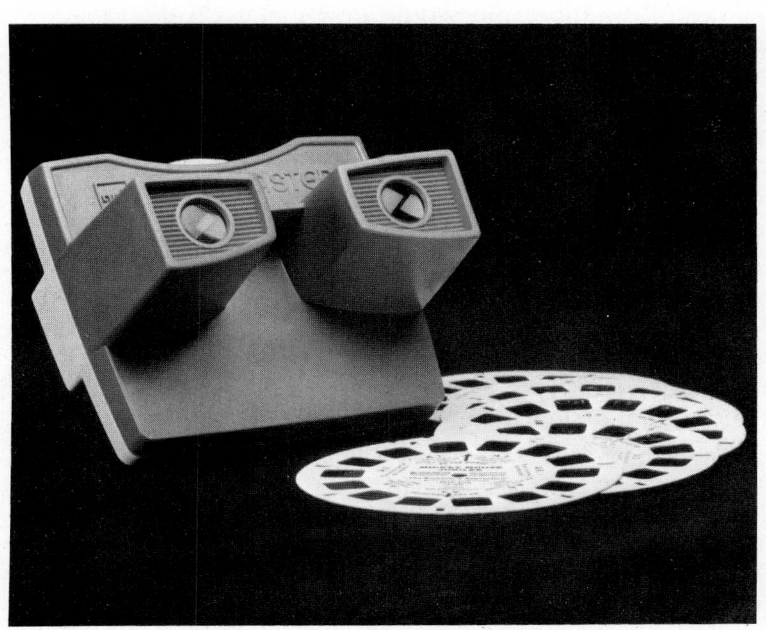

Figure 16-2
The stereoscopic vision toy View-Master™. (The View-Master trademark and picture of viewer are used with permission of View-Master Ideal Group, Inc., a subsidiary of Tyco Toys, Inc., Moorestown, NJ 08057. All Rights Reserved.)

size of the image of an object may indicate that it is closer or farther from the film. Additionally, greater penumbra may indicate that an object is farther from the film than an object with less penumbra. However, these are the only monocular vision clues about the depth of objects on a radiograph.

Stereoscopic radiography, or *stereoscopy,* which was described by J. McKenzie Davidson in 1898, is the technique of taking two slightly discrepant radiographs and viewing them in a manner that fuses them into a single image with depth. The technique is not complicated and can be performed with most equipment on any patient who can cooperate.

Stereoscopic radiography, *or* **stereoscopy,** *is the technique of taking two slightly discrepant radiographs and viewing them in a manner that fuses them into a single image with depth.*

When performing a stereoscopic examination, two films are taken and the tube is shifted, usually a slight distance either side of center, between the exposures. The patient must remain absolutely still between exposures, and the second film must be placed in the same position in the Bucky tray.

The degree of tube shift is important if the resulting stereoscopic examination is to produce the desired effect. Although the amount of the tube shift is not absolutely critical, *10 percent or 1/10th of the focal film distance is the accepted amount of tube shift for stereoscopy.* If the focal film distance for a stereoscopic examination is 40 inches, the total distance of the tube shift would be 4 inches. If the tube is mounted on an arc, such as a head unit, it may be easier to use degrees of tube shift rather than distance. In these cases, at a 40-inch focal film distance a shift of 6 degrees will produce the same effect as a 4-inch tube shift.

10 percent or 1/10th of the focal film distance is the accepted amount of tube shift for stereoscopy.

Tube Shift Techniques

There are three factors of tube shift to consider for stereoscopic examinations. First is the question of how to shift the tube. It is possible to obtain a satisfactory stereoscopic examination by centering the first film as you would for a nonstereoscopic examination and then shifting the tube the total distance and angling back toward the center of the film. To which side the tube is shifted is not important.

A more common technique is to center the patient and the film as you would for a nonstereoscopic examination, and then shift the tube one-half the total tube shift on one side of center, angling back toward the center of the film. The second exposure is shifted one-half the total tube shift from the other side of center and angled back toward

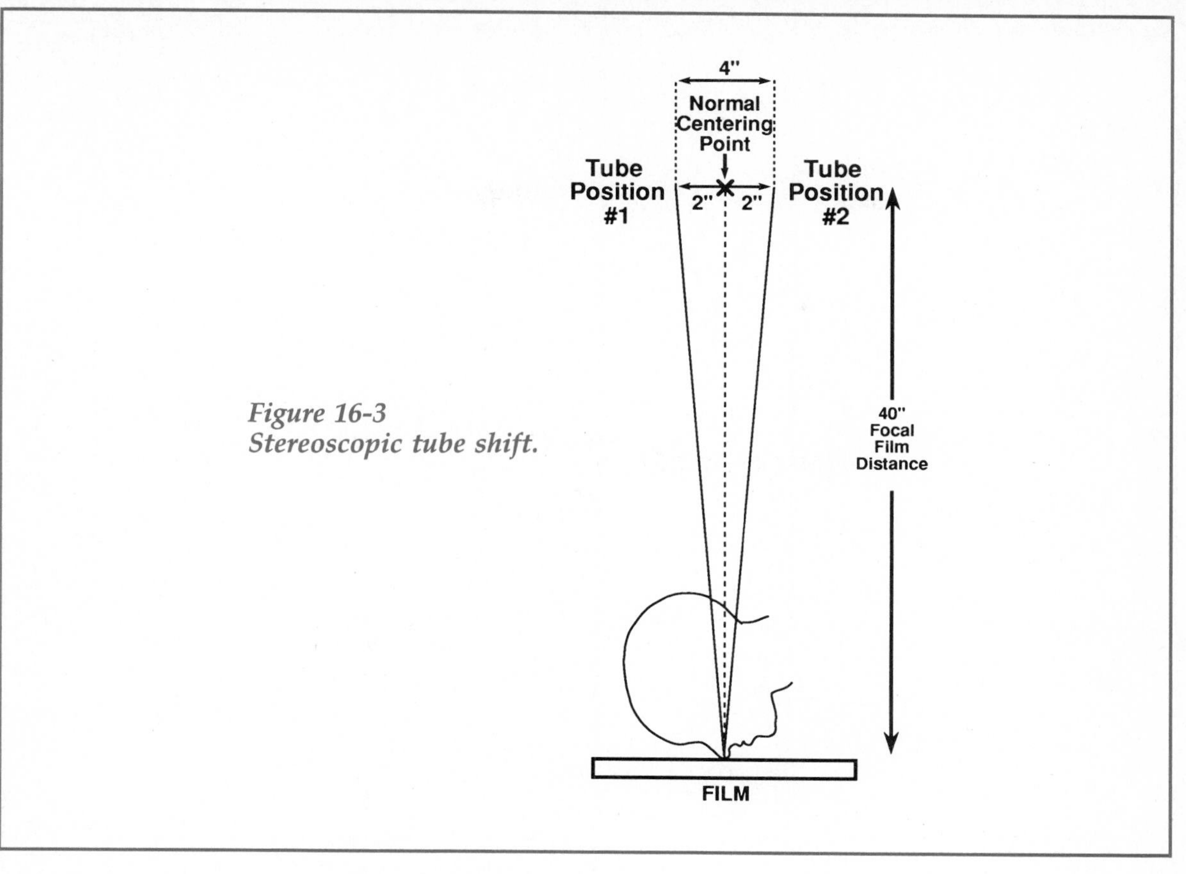

Figure 16-3
Stereoscopic tube shift.

the center of the film. For example, if the focal film distance is 40 inches, the tube would be shifted 2 inches to the left of center and angled back to the center of the film for the first exposure. The second exposure would be made after the tube was shifted 2 inches to the right of center and angled back to the center of the film. Figure 16-3 illustrates this technique of stereoscopic tube shifting.

The second major consideration in tube shift is the direction of tube shift in relation to the body part being radiographed. Since the objective is to produce discrepant images, the tube shift should cross the long axis of the part being examined. For example, if you were performing a stereoscopic examination of a long bone, such as the femur, you would ideally shift across the femur. Shifting along the length of the femur would not produce significantly discrepant images (Figure 16-4). When doing stereoscopic examinations of complex structures, such as the skull, the direction of tube shift is somewhat less critical.

The third important factor of tube shift is the direction of shift and angulation in relation to the grid. As discussed

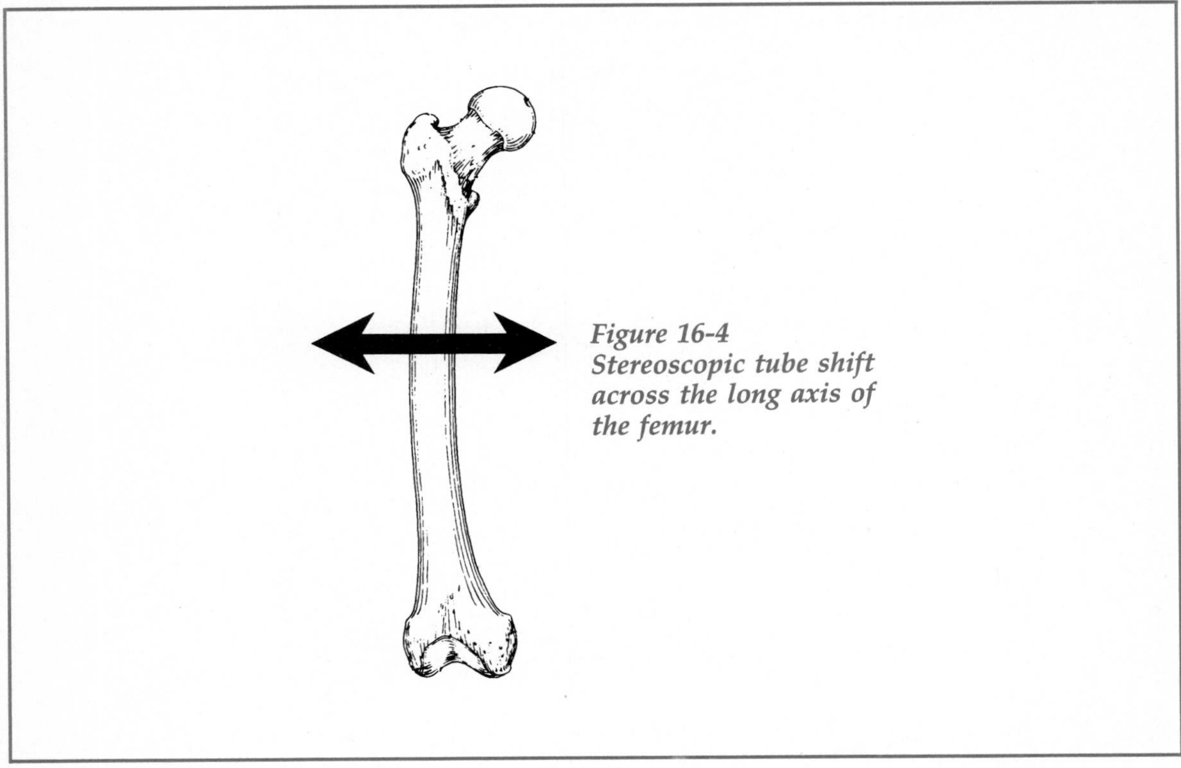

Figure 16-4
Stereoscopic tube shift across the long axis of the femur.

in Chapter 11, shifting or angling parallel to the direction of the lead strips of the grid is acceptable. Shifting or angling across the lead strips of the grid will result in grid cutoff. Therefore, the direction of tube shift must be coordinated with the direction of the grid lines. In a normal stereoscopic examination on a radiographic table, the tube is shifted and angled in line with the long axis of the table. Angling across the long axis would produce grid cutoff. If it becomes absolutely necessary to angle across the long axis of the table, the Bucky grid can be rotated 90 degrees from its normal position to prevent grid cutoff. Sterescopic examinations cannot be performed using a cross-hatch grid.

Considerations for Stereoscopic Viewing

After performing a stereoscopic examination it is necessary to identify three items about the orientation of the

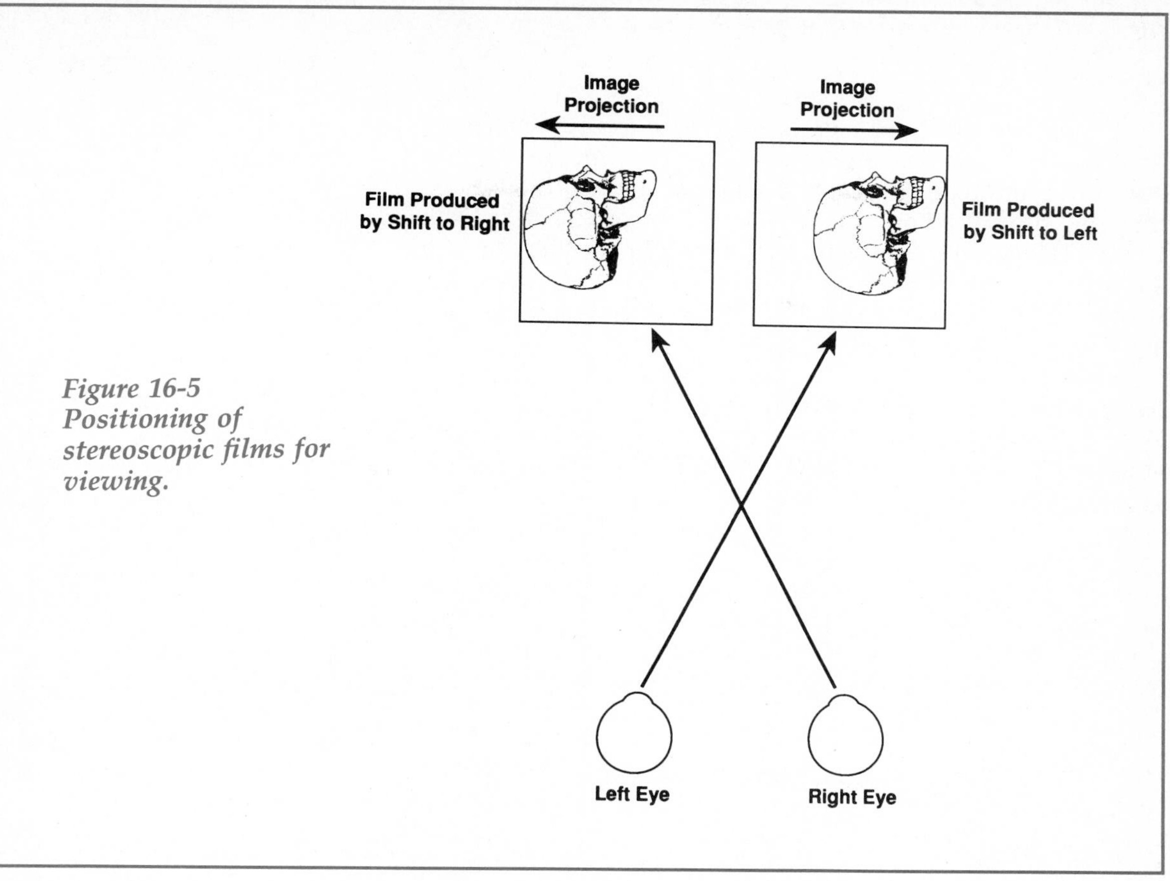

Figure 16-5
Positioning of stereoscopic films for viewing.

films for viewing. If a true stereoscopic effect is to be obtained, the films must be arranged so that the viewer's eyes see the films as the tube projected them.

First, the tube side of the films must face the viewer. Second, the direction of tube shift must be determined and the films hung so that the direction of the shift is horizontal and not vertical. That means that if a set of stereo skull films was obtained by shifting from the top to the bottom of the skull, the films must be hung so a line drawn from the top of the cranium through the foramen magnum would be horizontal to the floor. They could not be hung as they would normally be viewed. The final item to be determined is which film is to be viewed by which eye. The film produced by the shift to the left is viewed by the left eye, and the film produced by the shift to the right is viewed by the right eye. The film produced by the tube shift to the left will have the image projected toward the right side of the film. The film produced by the tube shift to the right will have the image projected toward the left side of the film. Figure 16-5 illustrates how films are positioned for stereoscopic viewing.

Once the films are positioned, there are two methods that can be used to view them. The first method is the cross-eyed method. For this method one hangs the left-eye film on the right and the right-eye film on the left. The viewer crosses his eyes and by looking at the film on the left with the right eye and the film on the right with the left eye, it is possible to converge the images to a single image that possesses depth.

Not everyone can successfully perform cross-eyed stereoscopic viewing. Even for those who can, crossing the eyes and concentrating on a single image can cause eye strain. The major advantage of cross-eyed stereoscopic viewing is that it requires no special equipment.

A variety of viewing devices exists for viewing stereoscopic radiographs. These devices are collectively called *stereoscopes,* and most use mirrors or prisms to enable the viewer to converge the two images into a single image (Figure 16-6). How these devices are used depends on the principles used to deflect the viewer's line of sight. It is im-

A variety of viewing devices exists for viewing stereoscopic radiographs. These devices are collectively called **stereoscopes,** *and most use mirrors or prisms to enable the viewer to converge the two images into a single image.*

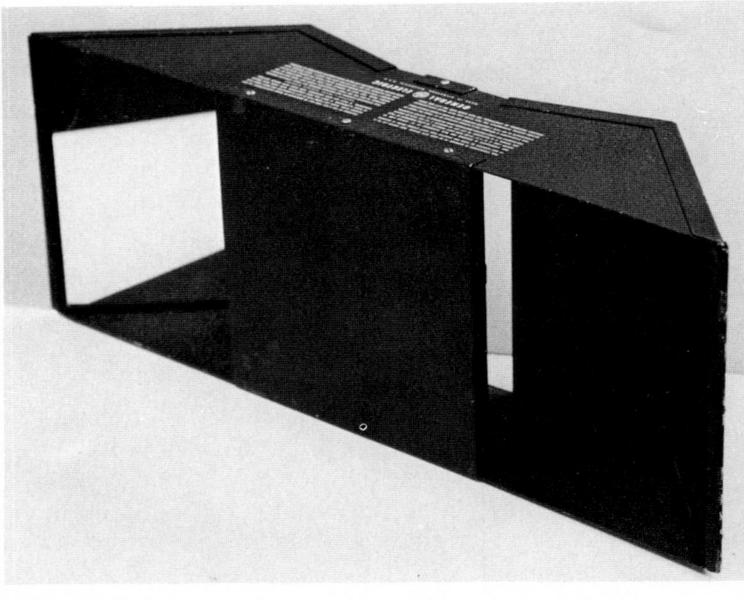

Figure 16-6 ***Hand-held mirror stereoscope.***

portant to read the instructions on how to hang the films for different stereoscopes. While some stereoscopes require positioning films as you would for cross-eyed stereoscopy, others do not. Those devices that use only one set of mirrors probably require viewing the film side opposite the x-ray tube since the single mirrors reverse the image.

The major advantage of stereoscopes is that they are easy to use. When used correctly, they allow those who cannot perform cross-eyed stereoscopy to view stereo radiographs. The major disadvantages of stereoscopes are their cost, their possible unavailability, and that they are easily damaged from mishandling.

Advantages and Disadvantages of Stereoscopy

The major advantage of using stereoscopy is its ability to help sort out confusing structures on the radiograph.

Stereoscopy has been used for a variety of radiographic examinations, but has been abandoned for all but a few. The major advantage of using stereoscopy is its ability to help sort out confusing structures on the radiograph. For example, stereoscopic examinations of the facial bones allow the radiologist to separate the images of the overlapping bones of the sinuses and face. The availability and simplicity of performing stereoscopy also may be considered an advantage, particularly if other more sophisticated technologies are not available.

The primary disadvantage of stereoscopy is the exposure to the patient.

The primary disadvantage of stereoscopy is the exposure to the patient. Two films are required so the patient's exposure is double that of a regular examination. Since the technique is dependent on total patient cooperation, the probability of repeat films is increased, which may further add to the dose. The inability to use stereoscopy on patients who cannot cooperate is another disadvantage. Finally, the declining use of stereoscopy has reduced the technical skills of the technologist and the interpretive skills of the radiologist.

Clinical Applications

As mentioned earlier, stereoscopy is useful for sorting out overlapping images on the film. Stereoscopic examinations have been widely used in the skull to evaluate structures like the facial bones, the sella turcica, and some intracranial calcifications. Additionally, multiple foreign bodies can often be sorted out more effectively with stereoscopy than with other techniques. Radiologists often used stereoscopy to clarify the findings on radiographs in a number of examinations where objects were projected over the structure of interest.

Stereoscopy was used extensively after it was described, but its utility was short-lived. The first decline in its use occurred early in the history of radiology when the harmful effects of ionizing radiation were recognized. The second, and more recent, cause of its decline in use is due to the advent of new technologies such as computed tomography (CT) and magnetic resonance imaging (MRI). These techniques yield a three-dimensional presentation of the structures being examined, and in many instances are a more definitive diagnostic tool than stereoscopy.

For those institutions that do not have access to CT or MRI, stereoscopy continues to be used when appropriate. In certain instances, where the diagnosis depends on simply sorting out the position of structures or objects, stereoscopy is a more cost-effective alternative than CT or MRI. In addition, a properly performed stereoscopic examination will result in less exposure to the patient than computed tomography.

Radiation Protection Considerations

As stated earlier, stereoscopy results in more exposure to the patient than a conventional radiograph of the same body part. There are several things the technologist can do to minimize the exposure to the patient during a stereoscopic examination.

First, the technologist should carefully evaluate the patient's probability of adequately cooperating during the examination. If the patient cannot cooperate, a stereoscopic examination should not be attempted.

The technologist should explain the procedure to the patient and use restraining devices to help maintain the position of the patient. It is important to recognize that the time required to change films and initiate the second exposure is lengthy enough that even cooperative patients may move slightly. The technologist should avoid slamming the Bucky tray closed when changing the film. The noise may startle the patient and cause the patient to move. This is particularly true for lateral skull and facial bone examinations, where the Bucky tray is directly under the patient's ears.

Collimation should be tight, but not so tight that it cuts off part of the anatomy when the tube is shifted from one side to the other. The exposure technique selected should be an optimum kVp technique that produces adequate contrast with minimal exposure. Shielding of surrounding body parts should be appropriately applied.

Chapter 16—Review Questions

1. Which of the following is not a monocular depth perception mechanism?
   a. overlapping borders
   b. discrepant images
   c. perspective
   d. shading
2. If a stereoscopic examination is being performed with a 40 inch SID, what would be the correct amount of tube shift to achieve adequate discrepant images?
   a. 4 inches either side of center
   b. 6 degrees either side of center
   c. 2 inches either side of center
   d. 2 degrees either side of center
3. If a stereoscopic examination is being performed with a 72 inch SID, what would be the total amount of tube shift to achieve adequate discrepant images?
   a. approximately 7 inches
   b. 6 degrees
   c. both a and b
   d. none of the above
4. When performing a stereoscopic examination, which of the following is not an important consideration for the technologist to evaluate?
   a. reduction of technical factors
   b. direction of the tube shift
   c. orientation of the grid
   d. magnitude of the tube shift
5. Which of the following is not a disadvantage of the stereoscope?
   a. cost
   b. potential unavailability
   c. potential for mishandling damage
   d. complexity of operation
6. The primary advantage of stereoscopic radiography is:
   a. reduction of patient exposure
   b. effectiveness on uncooperative patients
   c. ability to help sort out confusing structures
   d. its complementary role in CT and MRI

7. Which of the following would preclude using stereoscopy for a diagnostic examination?
   a. a cross-hatch grid
   b. multiple foreign bodies in the patient
   c. the unavailability of a CT or MRI scanner
   d. all of the above
8. Which of the following would not likely be an appropriate indication for a stereoscopic examination?
   a. evaluation of an orbital fracture
   b. evaluation of a calcified pineal gland
   c. evaluation of a shotgun blast injury
   d. evaluation of fetal development
9. Which of the following are important responsibilities for a technologist about to perform a stereoscopic examination?
   a. evaluation of the patient's ability to cooperate
   b. careful explanation of the procedure to the patient
   c. shielding and collimation
   d. all of the above
10. The primary disadvantage of stereoscopy is:
    a. the need for patient cooperation
    b. patient exposure
    c. the cost of the examination
    d. the need for practice to maintain the technologist's skill

17

Body Section Radiography

OBJECTIVES

After completing Chapter 17, you should be able to:

1. Define the following terms:
   autotomography
   exposure angle or exposure amplitude
   fulcrum
   focal plane
   pantomography
   tomographic angle or tomographic amplitude
   zonography
2. Discuss the principles behind body section radiography.
3. List the synonyms for body section radiography.
4. List the six common tube motions used in body section radiography.
5. Discuss common clinical applications for thick and thin section tomography.
6. Discuss technique considerations as well as radiation protection considerations for body section radiography.

Definition of Body Section Radiography

One of the shortcomings of conventional radiography is the compression of a three-dimensional object into a two-dimensional radiograph. This results in images being superimposed onto each other on the radiograph, which can be quite confusing. Radiologists are proficient at sorting out overlapping images, but in certain complex structures the task may be impossible. In these situations, body section radiography may be required to make an accurate diagnosis.

Body section radiography is a technique utilizing geometric principles to produce an image in which the objects in a selected plane remain well-defined on the radiograph while those above and below that plane are blurred. Body section radiography allows the examination of a subject in one plane at a time, much like looking at a loaf of bread slice by slice. The benefit of body section radiography is that the area, or plane, of interest is imaged in detail while the images of structures above and below the plane are blurred (Figure 17-1). This minimizes the effect of overlapping images and often aids in diagnosis.

Body section radiography *is a technique utilizing geometric principles to produce an image where the objects in a selected plane remain well defined on a radiograph while those above and below that plane are blurred.*

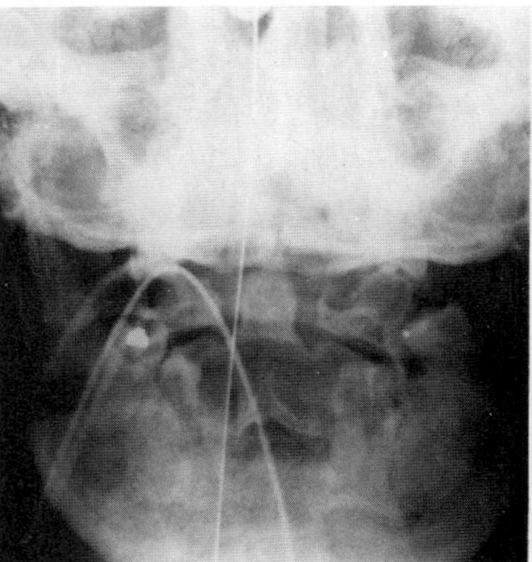

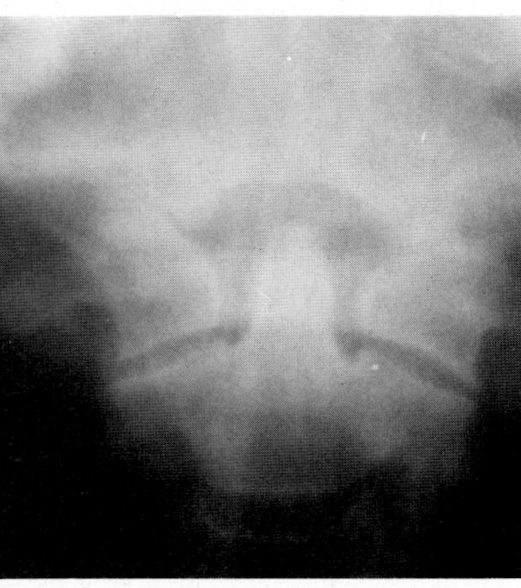

Figure 17-1
A comparison of a conventional radiograph of the odontoid process (left) and a tomogram of the same odontoid (right) showing blurring of the structures outside the plane of focus.

Tomography *is an accepted, widely used synonym for body section radiography.*

Other less frequently used terms for body section radiography include: laminography, stratigraphy, planigraphy, and zonography.

Body section radiography has been known by many names. *Tomography* is an accepted and widely used synonym for body section radiography. Other less frequently used terms include *laminography, stratigraphy, planigraphy,* and *zonography*. Most authors use the term *tomography* interchangeably with *body section radiography*.

Principles of Body Section Radiography

The basic principle behind tomography is that motion is used to blur part of the image. This is most easily explained by examining the simplest type of tomography, which is linear tomography.

The plane in the patient, at the level of the fulcrum, remains in focus while areas above and below the fulcrum are blurred.

In linear tomography, the x-ray tube and the x-ray film holder are attached to a rigid metal rod. The rod is mounted at a point along its length called the *fulcrum,* which acts as an axis or pivot point about which the tube and film move in opposing directions (Figure 17-2). The patient is placed on the table at the level of the fulcrum. Either the patient or the fulcrum is adjusted up or down to select the level of the plane of interest. *The plane in the pa-*

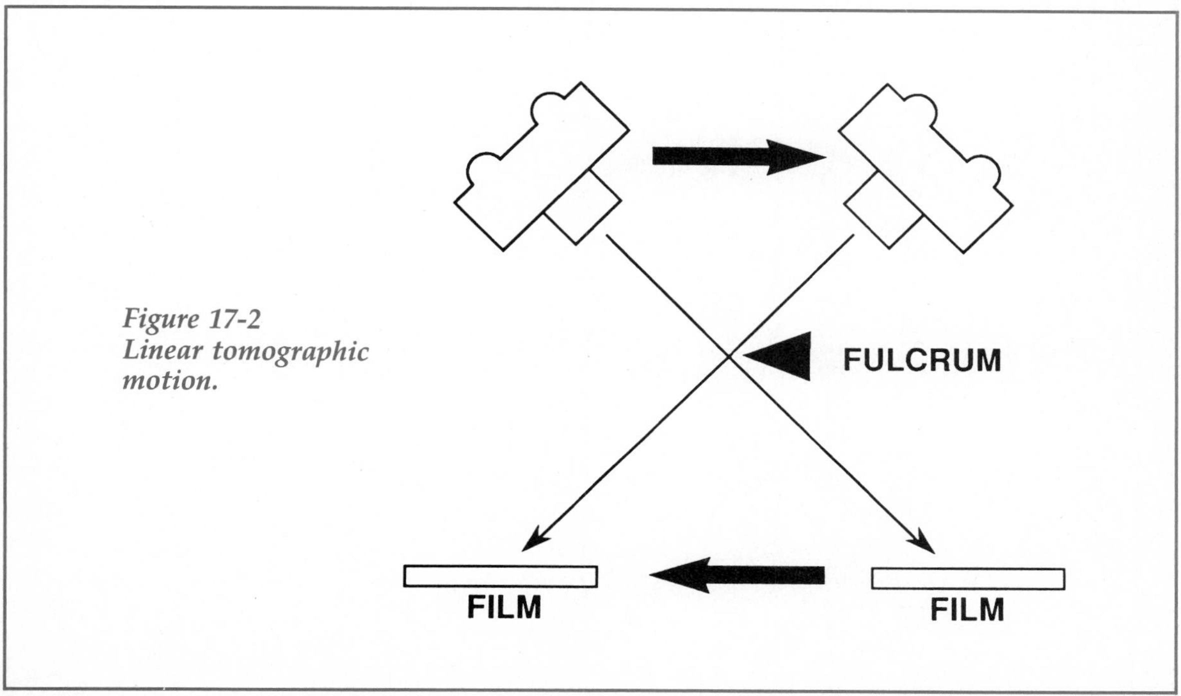

Figure 17-2
Linear tomographic motion.

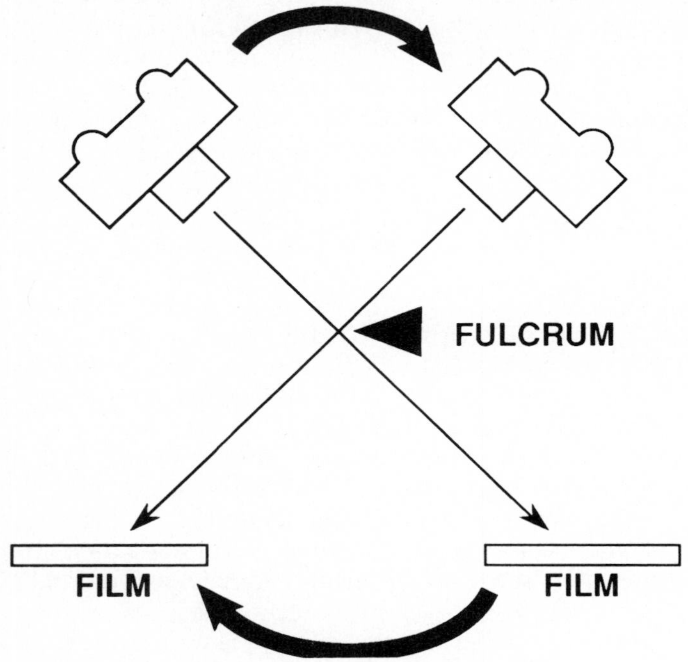

Figure 17-3
Linear tomographic motion with tube and film travel in arcs.

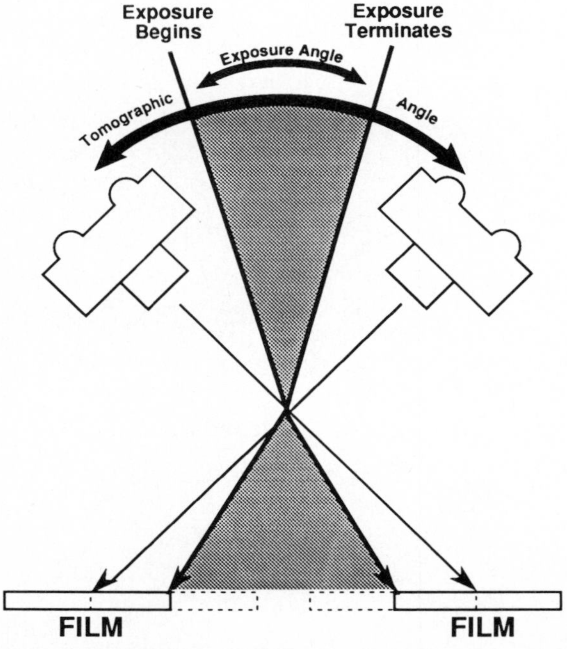

Figure 17-4
Tomographic angle versus exposure angle.

tient, at the level of the fulcrum, remains in focus while areas above and below the fulcrum are blurred.

This method is the one most commonly used on conventional radiographic tables. A variation involves mounting the tube and film on a rigid arm that allows them to move in opposing arcs about the fulcrum (Figure 17-3). This method is more difficult to accomplish on a radiography unit and is normally reserved for dedicated tomography units. Both methods produce similar results.

When performing a tomographic examination, the distance the tube travels is measured in degrees. This measurement is called the **tomographic angle, tomographic arc,** *or* **amplitude of tube travel.**

When performing a tomographic examination, the distance the tube travels is measured in degrees. The actual measurement is derived from the angle that the tube and the rod form with the fulcrum during their travel. This measurement is called the *tomographic angle, tomographic arc,* or *amplitude of tube travel.*

The distance of motion during the exposure is termed the **exposure angle, exposure arc,** *or* **exposure amplitude.**

During tomography, the exposure is usually made for an equal number of degrees either side of center of the tomographic angle. Usually, the exposure is initiated after the tube has begun its travel and moved a small distance. Likewise, the tube normally continues moving a short distance after the exposure is terminated. The distance of motion during the exposure is termed the *exposure angle, exposure arc,* or *exposure amplitude* and is measured in degrees (Figure 17-4). Typically, the tomographic angle is made larger than the exposure angle. This is done to eliminate blurring of the radiograph caused by undesired lateral motion resulting from initiating tube travel.

Tube Motions

Linear tomography *is so named because the tube moves in a straight line if viewed from above.*

Linear tomography is so named because the tube moves in a straight line if viewed from above. There are several other types of tube motions (discussed later in this chapter) that are designed to overcome some of the limitations of linear tomography. Most of the other types of tube motions are circular in nature and require rather complex drive mechanisms. These circular tube motions are generally found only on dedicated tomography units. The most common types of tube motions are linear, elliptical, circular, figure eight, hypocycloidal, and trispiral. These motions are illustrated in Figure 17-5.

The most common types of tube motions are linear, elliptical, circular, figure eight, hypocycloidal, and trispiral.

Exposure Amplitude and Slice Thickness

Tomographic images have thickness. In general, if the blurring of the objects above and below the plane of the

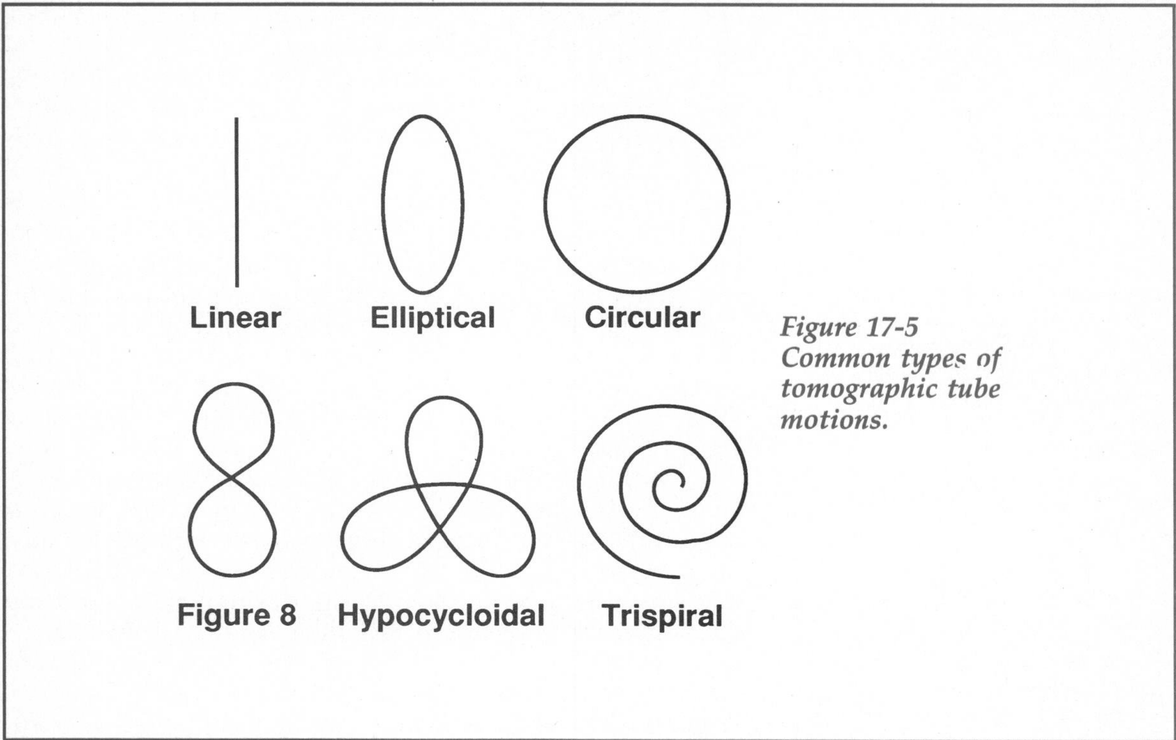

Figure 17-5
Common types of tomographic tube motions.

fulcrum is greater, the tomographic section or "cut" is thinner. Conversely, if the blurring of the objects above and below the plane of the fulcrum is less, the tomographic section or "cut" is thicker.

Several factors affect the blurring during tomography. The greater the tube motion during the exposure, the more objects above and below the plane of the fulcrum will be blurred. *Therefore, the exposure angle, or exposure amplitude, is the primary controller of section thickness.* Many authors use the tomographic angle synonymously with exposure angle. However, it is important to understand that even though the tomographic angle may be 50°, if the exposure angle is 10° a thick section tomogram will result.

The exposure angle, or exposure amplitude, is the primary controller of section thickness.

Tomographic section thickness is inversely proportional to exposure amplitude. The greater the exposure amplitude, the thinner the section thickness. The smaller the exposure amplitude, the greater the section thickness.

Tomographic section thickness is inversely proportional to exposure amplitude.

Blurring

The purpose of body section radiography or tomography is to blur out the images of objects outside the plane of

The purpose of body section radiography, or tomography, is to blur out the images of objects outside the plane of interest.

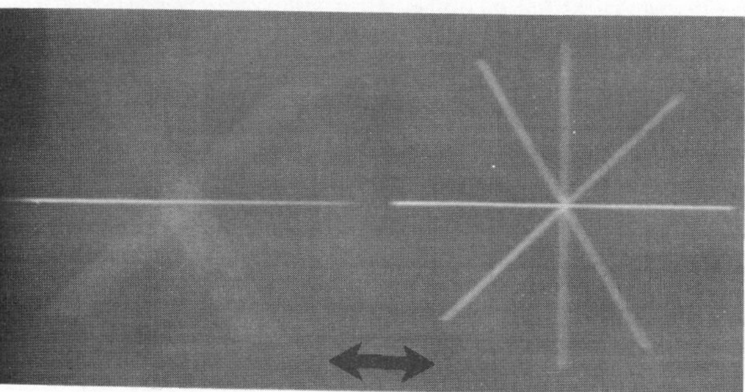

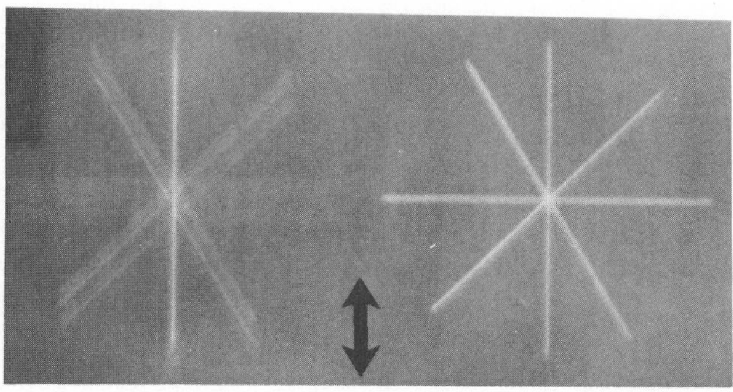

Figure 17-6
Tomography of a tomographic phantom demonstrating how objects aligned with tube travel are not effectively blurred. (Black arrows show tube travel orientation.)

interest. However, the plane of interest is not really a plane at all, and the section or thickness of the "cut" or "slice" that remains in focus is not absolute. There is not a point where objects on one side are in focus and objects on the other are not in focus. Blurring increases as objects become more distant from the plane of the fulcrum. The distance from the fulcrum required to significantly blur an object decreases as exposure amplitude increases and it increases as exposure amplitude decreases.

The orientation of tube travel in relation to the part being tomographed also has a significant effect on blurring. If an object's long axis lies in the same direction as the tube travel, that object will not be effectively blurred unless it is a great distance from the plane of the fulcrum. Objects in line with the tube travel often produce streak-like images or *parasite shadows*. However, if the long axis of an object lies 90° to the direction of the tube travel the blurring will be greater. Figure 17-6 is a tomogram of a tomographic phantom that illustrates this point.

Linear tomography is most effective when the objects to be blurred are perpendicular to the direction of the tube travel.

Linear tomography is most effective when the objects to be blurred are perpendicular to the direction of the tube travel. Since it is not always possible to position patients so that their body parts are perpendicular to the direction of the tube travel, circular tube motions are often used.

The advantage of circular tube motions, including ellipses, figure eights, circles, hypocycloids and trispirals, is their ability to blur objects regardless of their orientation. Circular tube motions can be made in varying exposure angles. The exposure angle or amplitude is measured by the angle formed by the tube and the rod in relation to the fulcrum. The exposure amplitude is never 360 degrees, but usually 50 degrees or less. The amplitude is usually considered equal to the angle formed by the maximum diameter of the circular motion and the fulcrum.

The advantage of circular tube motions, including ellipses, figure eights, circles, hypocycloids, and trispirals, is their ability to blur objects regardless of their orientation.

One disadvantage of circular motion tomography is the cost of the specialized equipment necessary to perform the circular motion. Circular tomography equipment is expensive because of the complexity of the drive mechanism and the need to rotate the grid so it is always aligned with the angle of the tube.

Another disadvantage of circular tomography is the length of the exposure time required to produce the image. While linear tomography can normally be done with 1 second or less of exposure time, circular tomography requires lengthening the exposure to allow the tube to complete its motion. This often requires exposure times of from 3 to 6 seconds. The length of exposure time may preclude its use on patients who are unable to cooperate.

Thin versus Thick Section Tomography

Most tomography units can produce cuts ranging from 1 to 2 millimeters to 30 or 40 millimeters in thickness. It might appear that thin section tomography is always preferable to thick section tomography, but this is not true for several reasons. First, it is often desirable to examine thick structures free of superimposition. An example would be a tomogram of the kidney, where one wishes to remove confusing shadow resulting from bowel gas and fecal material. In this example, a tomogram with a 10-degree exposure amplitude would produce a section thickness of about 6 to 7 millimeters, which would be ideal for examining the kidney while blurring images produced by the bowel.

Thick section tomography of 10-degree exposure amplitude or less is often termed *zonography* because it produces an excellent image of a particular zone. Thick section

Thick-section tomography of 10-degree exposure amplitude or less is often termed **zonography** *because it produces an excellent image of a particular zone.*

tomography has the advantage of producing high contrast, sharply defined tomograms.

Thin section tomography, usually having 30 degrees of exposure amplitude or greater, produces excellent blurring of unwanted structures. It is of great value in examining small parts and complex bony structures. However, thin section tomography results in low contrast images with less definition, even in the plane of focus. In general, the thinner the section or greater the exposure amplitude, the less contrast the tomogram will possess. Conversely, the thicker the section, or smaller the exposure amplitude, the more contrast the tomogram will possess.

In general, the thinner the section or greater the exposure amplitude, the less contrast the tomogram will possess. Conversely, the thicker the section, or smaller the exposure amplitude, the more contrast the tomogram will possess.

Autotomography and Pantomography

Autotomography *is a technique in which the x-ray tube and film remain still, but the patient moves, or is moved, to produce the desired blurring.*

Autotomography and pantomography are special adaptations of the tomographic principle. *Autotomography* is a technique in which the x-ray tube and film remain still, but the patient moves, or is moved, to produce the desired blurring. While several uses of autotomography have been described, only four applications have proven practical.

Autotomography was used to demonstrate the structures of the midbrain during pneumoencephalography, by rotating the patient's head slightly from side to side during a lateral view of the skull. Since new imaging technologies have made pneumoencephalography obsolete, this technique is no longer used.

Another application of autotomography is the Ottonello, or wagging jaw, method of examining the upper cervical spine. In this technique, the patient moves the mandible up and down during a low-mA, long exposure-time film. The motion of the mandible blurs its image, producing a clearer view of the cervical spine structures.

The final autotomographic techniques are breathing films, used to image the thoracic spine, and long exposure films of the sternum, which use heart motion to blur the lung structures.

Pantomography *is a technique which produces a panoramic view of curved structures of the body.*

Pantomography is a technique which produces a panoramic view of curved structures of the body. The most common example of pantomography is the pantomogram of the mandible produced by Panorex dental machines. There is also a specialized pantomographic unit which produces pantomograms of the facial bones, although it is not widely used.

During pantomography, both the tube and film rotate, but the tube is collimated to a slit beam that exposes the film from one side to the other as the film rotates about

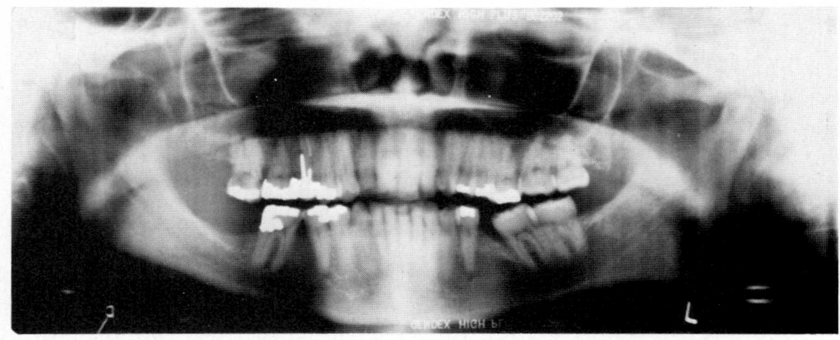

Figure 17-7 Pantomogram of the entire mandible.

a curved surface on the patient. The result is a spread out, flat image of the curved surface. Pantomograms of the mandible demonstrate temporomandibular joints on either side of the film with the teeth and mandible shown in their entirety. Figure 17-7 is an example of a pantomogram of the mandible.

Technique Considerations

Tomography requires several special technique considerations. First, normal radiographic mAs must be adjusted to low-mA, long exposure time to allow adequate time for the x-ray tube to complete its travel. Circular tomography examinations often require the use of 25 mA or less to allow the 3- to 6-second exposure times necessary to complete the motion. In skull and abdominal examinations this is not a problem, but in the chest and extremities, the long exposure times may make it impossible to select a low enough mA without decreasing the normally used kVp.

For thin section tomography, high contrast screen-film combinations are usually indicated to enhance the reduced contrast. Additionally, the technologist may be required to use kVp lower than normal to increase the contrast to produce a diagnostic study. Collimation is also critical, as scatter radiation will reduce the already lowered contrast and negatively impact the quality of the images.

Thin section tomography requires numerous "cuts" or exposures to completely examine the structure in question. Since the exposures are often low-kVp and higher-mAs exposures, heat loading of the x-ray tube may become a problem. Many tomographic units are equipped with x-ray tube anode heat calculators to monitor heat load, but the x-ray tube's housing heat dissipation can also be problematic. The technologist must be aware of the potential to overheat and damage the x-ray tube during multiple tomographic exposures.

Radiation Protection

Three problems make body section radiography a special radiation protection concern. First, the number of exposures required for a thin section examination is high. More than ten exposures are common, and this means that radiation exposure to the area examined will be high. Accurate and tight collimation and proper total filtration are important during tomography.

The second consideration is the low-kVp, higher-mAs techniques often required in tomography. The technologist should use the maximum kVp that will give adequate contrast to the image. Screen-film combination selection should be carefully considered when setting up a tomography unit, as well as when new screen technology becomes available.

The third consideration is the proximity of radiation sensitive organs to the area of interest. Many tomographic studies place the eyes, thyroid, or reproductive organs in or near the x-ray beam. Shielding of areas outside but near the area of interest is important. Tomography does allow certain shielding techniques that could not be used for conventional radiography. Eye shields may be used with circular motions when the eyes must be included in the x-ray beam. Normally the tube motion will blur the eye shields if the structures examined are several centimeters from the eyes.

Another technique to minimize radiation exposure to the eyes or thyroid is to examine the patient in the prone position (posteroanterior projection). This may be less comfortable for the patient, but much of the radiation will be absorbed in the tissues in the back of the neck and head. The radiation reaching the eyes and thyroid will be less than what would occur in the supine position (anteroposterior projection).

Clinical Applications

Conventional tomography reached its height of utilization in the early 1970s. In addition to examinations like nephrotomography, it was widely used to examine the structures of the face, temporal bones, vertebrae, and joints, as well as a wide variety of other skeletal structures. The development of the computed tomography scanner caused a decline in the use of conventional tomography. As the ability of the computed tomography scanner to resolve detail improved, many of the studies done by conventional tomography were lost to computed tomography.

Tomography is still the preferred method to isolate confusing images on a radiograph such as in nephrotomography. Tomography also is still preferred for studies requiring high resolution such as in evaluation of hairline fractures of the carpal bones or vertebrae. Tomography has experienced growth in some areas with large orthopedic practices, where it is used to compliment arthrography in studies referred to as arthrotomography. Although tomography will not likely ever return to the level of use during the early 1970s, it will continue to be a useful diagnostic technique.

Chapter 17—Review Questions

1. The exposure amplitude is determined by measuring:
   a. the angle the tube forms with the floor
   b. the angle the tube is deviated from vertical
   c. the angle the tube forms with the fulcrum during its travel
   d. distance in inches the tube travels during the exposure
2. Which of the following exposure amplitudes would produce the thinnest section tomogram?
   a. 10-degree linear motion
   b. 30-degree circular motion
   c. 40-degree hypocycloid motion
   d. 50-degree linear motion
3. A tomographic image in which structures 5 centimeters above the plane of focus are still relatively well defined would most likely have been done with which of the following motions?
   a. 10-degree linear motion
   b. 30-degree circular motion
   c. 40-degree hypocycloid motion
   d. 50-degree linear motion
4. Which of the following motions cannot be used without considering the orientation of the object in relation to direction of the tube travel?
   a. linear
   b. circular
   c. hypocycloid
   d. trispiral
5. Which of the following motions normally requires the shortest exposure time to complete?
   a. linear
   b. circular
   c. hypocycloid
   d. trispiral
6. Which of the following motions would best demonstrate the kidneys free from superimposed gas and fecal material?
   a. 50-degree linear
   b. 10-degree circular
   c. 48-degree hypocycloid
   d. 50-degree trispiral

7. Which of the following motions would produce the highest contrast tomograph?
   a. 50-degree linear
   b. 10-degree circular
   c. 30-degree circular
   d. 48-degree hypocycloid
8. Which of the following is a possible technique to reduce the exposure to the eyes of a patient undergoing facial bone tomography?
   a. the use of eye shields
   b. the use of high speed screens
   c. examining the patient in the prone position
   d. all of the above
9. Which of the following is not a reason for high heat load on the x-ray tube during tomographic studies?
   a. low mA, low kVp, long exposure time techniques
   b. multiple exposures required
   c. proper filtration of the beam
   d. use of low kVp techniques to enhance contrast
10. Which of the following is a disadvantage of circular tomography?
    a. absence of parasite shadows
    b. complexity of drive mechanism
    c. time required to complete the motion
    d. two of the above

18

Computed Radiography

OBJECTIVES

After completing Chapter 18, you should be able to:

1. Define the following terms:
   latent image
   manifest image
   PACS
   photostimulable phosphor plate
2. Identify the three functions of radiographic film in the production of a radiograph.
3. Discuss the principles behind computed radiography.
4. Discuss the difference between analog and digital information.
5. Identify common clinical applications for computed radiography.
6. Discuss the advantages and disadvantages of computed radiography.

Functions of Radiographic Film

Shortly after the discovery of x-rays, Roentgen produced a radiograph of his wife's hand using photographic plates. Since that time photographic, or radiographic, film has been used as the recording medium for radiography. The refinement of radiographic film has resulted in a recording medium that has served the specialty of radiology well throughout its history.

It is important to recognize that radiographic film serves three functions in the production of a radiograph. The first function of film is to acquire the image. It is the film that stores the invisible electrochemical image, or *latent image,* until processing converts it into a visible or *manifest image.* Radiographic film serves this purpose well and produces an image with high resolution. The only disadvantages of radiographic film are its somewhat nonlinear response to the radiation and its fairly narrow exposure latitude.

It is the film that stores the invisible electrochemical image, or **latent image,** *until processing converts it into a visible or* **manifest image.**

The second function of film is to serve as the display medium for the radiographic image. After processing, the radiologist uses the film to view and interpret the information contained in the manifest image. As a display medium, radiographic film has certain shortcomings. The manifest image is fixed and cannot be altered to suit a particular diagnostic need. The radiologist can only view the film with a standard viewbox or with a "hot light."

The third function of film is to serve as the image storage medium for archival or storage purposes. Film libraries are an integral part of virtually every imaging facility in this country. While film does retain the image very well, the space required to store it and the man hours required to maintain the files are major drawbacks that inevitably lead to lost films.

In the last few decades, the development of digital electronics, high-resolution television systems, and practical, low-cost computers has facilitated the development of alternate methods of acquiring, displaying, and storing radiographic images. The first of these new techniques was computed tomography (CT), followed shortly by digital subtraction angiography (DSA), magnetic resonance imaging (MRI), and others. Each of these techniques acquires images in a digital, rather than an analog, format. Despite the rapid acceptance of these techniques, 60 to 70 percent of the radiology workload is still conventional radiography.

Computed Radiography

Computed radiography (CR), *or* **digital radiography,** *is a relatively recent introduction that allows the direct acquisition of images in a digital format.*

Analog *refers to a continuous presentation of information, while* **digital** *refers to the presentation of information in discrete units.*

Computed radiography (CR), or digital radiography, is a relatively recent introduction that allows the direct acquisition of images in a digital format. The terms analog and digital refer to the way information is represented. *Analog* refers to a continuous presentation of information, while *digital* refers to the presentation of information in discrete units. For example, the standard speedometer in an automobile is a needle that moves across a scale, depending on how fast the car is moving. Its motion up or down is continuous and it can point to an infinite number of locations on the scale. A digital speedometer displays mileage only in discrete units. If the car is moving 10.5 miles per hour, the digital speedometer can only display 10 or 11 miles per hour while an analog speedometer could technically display all the points between 10 and 11 miles per hour. For computers to use information the data must be in discrete units; therefore, computer processing of images is dependent on digital acquisition of the image data.

In **computed radiography,** *a reusable* **photostimulable phosphor plate** *serves as the image receptor and stores the x-ray image until it is generated by the computer in the computed radiography system.*

Computed radiography systems became practical after the introduction of photostimulable luminescent phosphor plates by Fuji Film Company, Ltd. in 1981. In computed radiography, a reusable *photostimulable phosphor plate* serves as the image receptor and stores the x-ray image until it is generated by the computer in the computed radiography system.

Components of the Computed Radiography System

The computed radiography system has four major components: the phosphor plate, identification station, image reader or digitizer system, and monitor. The phosphor plate is contained in a cassette similar to conventional radiography cassettes except the screens and film are replaced by the photostimulable phosphor plate. The similarity of the computed radiography cassette to a conventional radiography cassette allows its use in standard radiographic and fluoroscopic equipment.

The reusable photostimulable phosphor plate is composed of a polyester base on which a support layer is applied. On top of the support layer is a reflective layer which prevents the reflection of the laser light used in the image reader or digitizer. On top of the reflective layer is a layer of very fine crystals of europium-doped barium fluorohalide ($BaFX:Eu^{2+}$), which is the active phosphor material. The phosphor layer is coated with a thin, clear acrylic protective layer. Figure 18-1 shows the construction of the reusable photostimulable phosphor plate in cross-section.

The photostimulable phosphor plate is used in a lightweight aluminum cassette with a carbon fiber front. The cassettes used are similar in size to the cassettes used for conventional film. The cassette and photostimulable plate can be used exactly like a conventional film/screen cassette during a radiographic exam. This is a significant advantage, since the cassette and photostimulable phosphor plate allow the production of digital images using conventional radiographic equipment without modifying it in any way.

The technical factors used with photostimulable phosphor plates do not necessarily need to be changed from standard film techniques. However, the wide latitude of the system may allow the exposure factors to be reduced. Claims of significant dose reduction available with computed radiography must be carefully evaluated. It is possible to produce images with far lower exposure factors than conventional film-screen techniques, but image quality may suffer as a result.

After the plate has been exposed, the patient's identification data is applied to the imaging plate on a device termed the identification station. The information is keyed in manually or read from a barcoded patient identification card on which the data was entered earlier. The information station associates this data with the particular plate in the cassette and stores it to be applied to the film during processing of the image.

Once the identification process is complete, the phosphor plate's image is generated by the image reader or digitizer system (Figure 18-2). The technologist feeds the cassette into the image reader where it is opened and the phosphor plate is removed. The plate is slowly passed in front of a scanning laser beam which causes the emission of light in a quantity proportional to the amount of x-rays that struck the phosphor layer of the plate. This light is carried by high-efficiency light guides to photomultiplier tubes where the light is converted to electrical signals. The phosphor plate is then erased by exposure to bright light, inserted into a cassette, and returned to the technologist for reuse.

The data collected from the imaging plate is then transmitted to the computer portion of the digitizer. Here,

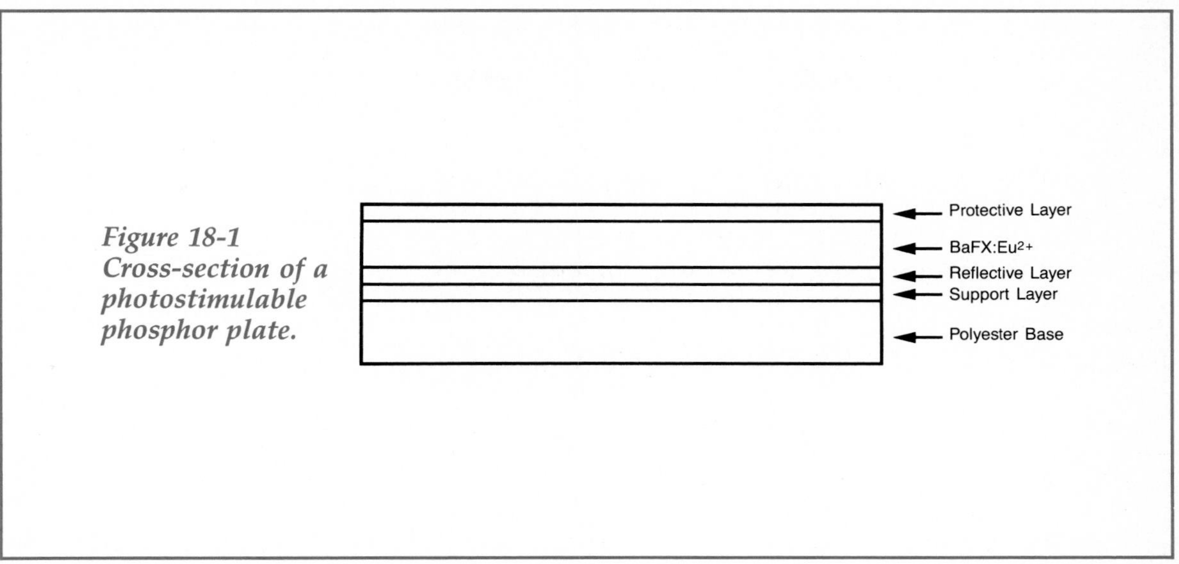

Figure 18-1
Cross-section of a photostimulable phosphor plate.

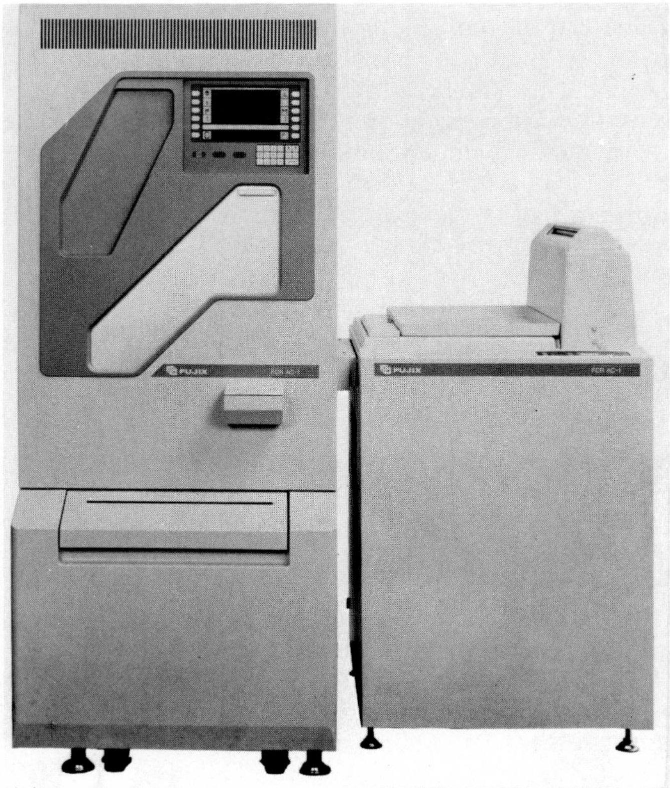

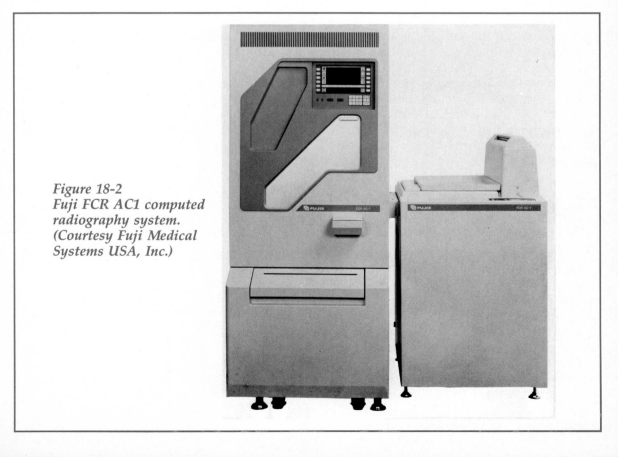

Figure 18-2
Fuji FCR AC1 computed radiography system. (Courtesy Fuji Medical Systems USA, Inc.)

the raw image data can be processed to enhance or suppress features of the image. This is similar to varying window and level settings on a computed tomography scanner to see specific structures. Normally, the digitizer has preprogrammed parameters for various examinations. These settings allow the data to be processed in an optimal fashion for the study that has been performed.

Once the raw image data has been collected and processed, the image can be displayed on a monitor, or the data can be transmitted to an imaging camera or laser imager for printing on film. The raw data can be saved on magnetic disk or optical disk for future use or for archiving in a picture archiving and communication system (PACS).

Clinical Applications for Computed Radiography

Computed radiography is recommended for mobile radiographic exams where inconsistent techniques are frequently a problem. The ability to specify the parameters that govern the display of the image, despite fairly wide variation in technique, is an obvious advantage for the radiologist who must interpret these films.

Computed radiography may also be useful for trauma radiography or for neonatal radiography, where technique errors are fairly common and repeat films may not be easily performed. The wide exposure latitude of the photostimulable phosphor plates will likely result in reduced repeat rates and more consistent film quality.

Advantages and Disadvantages of Computed Radiography

Like many new imaging technologies, computed radiography has both advantages and disadvantages that will determine its acceptance as a diagnostic tool. Computed radiography's major advantage is its high sensitivity and wide exposure latitude. These characteristics permit excellent images of both bone and soft tissue densities from a single exposure (Figure 18-3). The potential to produce diagnostic films with lower exposures and reduce repeat rates because of the wide latitude of the system is another obvious advantage. The ability to interface to a picture archiving and communications system is another potential advantage of computed radiography.

Computed radiography's major advantage is its high sensitivity and wide exposure latitude.

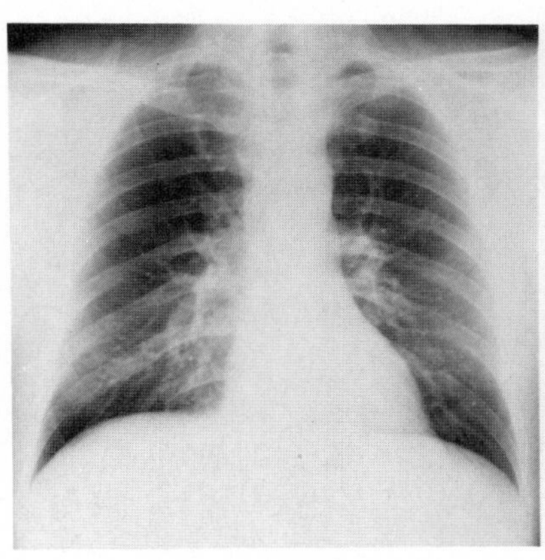

A

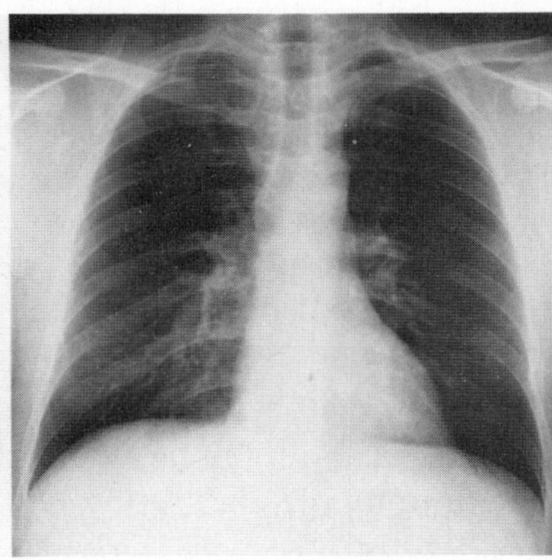

B

Figure 18-3
A comparison of a conventional chest radiograph performed with rare earth screens (A) *to a computed radiograph performed on a Fuji CR imaging plate* (B). *(Courtesy Fuji Medical Systems USA, Inc.)*

The major disadvantage of computed radiography systems is the limited resolution when compared with conventional film.

The major disadvantage of computed radiography systems is the limited resolution when compared to conventional film. This problem may be lessened by the use of ultra-high-resolution display systems; however, this may result in an increase in the cost of computed radiography system hardware.

Summary

Computed radiography systems have the potential to increase the diagnostic accuracy of conventional radiography. Coupled with a picture archiving and communications system, computed radiography will also allow increased efficiency in the operation of the film retrieval and display functions of the department. The consistent image quality and decreases in patient exposure, repeat rates, and lost films have led many imaging facilities to consider computed radiography as a cost-justifiable addition to their operation.

Chapter 18—Review Questions

1. The visible image on a radiographic film is termed the:
   a. latent image
   b. processed image
   c. manifest image
   d. fixed image
2. Which of the following is an advantage of conventional radiographic film?
   a. high resolution
   b. somewhat nonlinear response to radiation
   c. fairly narrow exposure latitude
   d. all of the above
3. Which of the following have allowed the development of computed radiography and other digital imaging techniques?
   a. digital electronics
   b. low-cost, high-efficiency computers
   c. high-resolution television systems
   d. all of the above
4. Which of the following is one of the areas most likely to benefit from the advantages of computed radiography?
   a. mobile radiography
   b. angiography
   c. tomography
   d. arthrography
5. Which of the following is not an advantage of computed radiography?
   a. wide exposure latitude
   b. extremely high resolution
   c. potential reduction of repeat rates
   d. the ability to image both bone and soft tissue on a single exposure

Answers to Review Questions

Answers to Review Questions

Chapter 1	Chapter 2	Chapter 3	Chapter 4	Chapter 5	Chapter 6
1. d	1. b	1. d	1. f	1. b	1. a
2. c	2. a	2. d	2. e	2. b	2. c
3. a	3. e	3. c	3. b	3. c	3. d
4. b	4. d	4. a	4. c	4. d	4. b
5. d	5. f	5. e	5. c	5. b	5. c
6. c	6. h	6. a	6. a	6. d	6. b
7. b	7. c	7. b	7. c	7. c	7. d
8. b	8. e	8. a	8. d	8. e	8. d
9. b	9. d	9. c	9. b	9. e	9. c
10. b	10. c	10. d	10. b	10. e	10. d
11. d	11. d	11. d		11. b	11. c
12. d	12. b	12. d		12. d	12. a
13. c	13. e	13. e		13. e	13. c
14. b	14. c	14. g		14. b	14. c
15. b	15. d	15. d		15. c	15. c
	16. a			16. b	16. b
	17. d			17. b	17. a
	18. e			18. d	18. b
	19. b			19. c	19. c
	20. c			20. e	20. d
	21. d				
	22. c				
	23. b				
	24. d				
	25. d				

Chapter 7

1. b
2. a
3. c
4. e
5. b
6. b
7. a
8. c
9. c
10. b
11. d
12. c
13. b
14. e
15. a
16. b
17. c
18. d
19. c
20. a

Chapter 8

1. a
2. e
3. d
4. c
5. b
6. c
7. b
8. b
9. b
10. a
11. c
12. a
13. b
14. b
15. c

Chapter 9

1. a
2. e
3. h
4. d
5. c
6. b
7. d
8. c
9. c
10. b
11. a
12. f
13. c
14. c
15. c
16. d
17. d
18. a
19. c
20. a

Chapter 10

1. b
2. a
3. b
4. c
5. d
6. c
7. c
8. d
9. b
10. b

Chapter 11

1. c
2. d
3. b
4. b
5. a
6. e
7. d
8. c
9. a
10. c
11. d
12. b
13. c
14. a
15. b

Chapter 12

1. c
2. a
3. a
4. c
5. d
6. b
7. e
8. c
9. d
10. a

Chapter 13	Chapter 14	Chapter 15	Chapter 16	Chapter 17	Chapter 18
1. c	1. b	1. b	1. b	1. c	1. c
2. a	2. c	2. c	2. c	2. d	2. a
3. d	3. b	3. b	3. c	3. a	3. d
4. b	4. b	4. e	4. a	4. a	4. a
5. b	5. e	5. b	5. d	5. a	5. b
6. b	6. c	6. a	6. c	6. b	
7. b	7. c	7. d	7. a	7. b	
8. c	8. d	8. b	8. d	8. d	
9. b	9. b	9. c	9. d	9. c	
10. d	10. e	10. d	10. b	10. d	

Glossary

accelerating anode the positively charged portion of the image intensifier that attracts the photoelectrons toward the output phosphor

added filtration filtering material, usually aluminum, that is inserted in the path of the primary beam to increase the mean energy of the beam; reduces the patient absorbed radiation dose

afterglow the tendency of a phosphor to continue to give off light after the x-ray exposure has stopped; also called phosphorescence

air-gap technique an alternative to the use of a grid accomplished by moving the patient a short distance from the film

ampere (A) a quantitative term of current; indicates the number of electrons passing a given point in a circuit in a period of 1 second

amplimat an automatic exposure device that measures the amount of radiation reaching the film

analog refers to the presentation of information in a continuous format as opposed to the discrete units of digital presentation

angstrom (Å) the unit of measurement for wavelength

anode the positively charged electrode of the x-ray tube; serves to decelerate the electrons as well as store and dissipate heat

antihalation layer the light-absorbing coating on the nonemulsion side of the base of single emulsion film; serves to increase detail by preventing reflection of light transmitted through the film base

aperture diaphragm the simplest type of beam-restricting device

atom the smallest divided part of matter that can enter into combination or chemical reactions with other atoms

atomic number the number of protons or positive charges in the nucleus of an atom

atomic weight the weight of an atom as compared to the weight of a carbon atom

attenuation the total reduction in the number of x-rays remaining in the x-ray beam following penetration through a given thickness of matter

autotomography a tomographic technique in which the x-ray tube and film remain still, but the patient moves, or is moved, to produce the desired blurring

autotransformer a single coil of wire that functions through self-induction; allows selection of the voltage applied across the x-ray tube

average gradient a method used to express film contrast numerically; the slope of a straight line drawn between density levels 0.25 and 2.0 above gross fog on the characteristic curve

backscatter radiation photons that scatter approximately 180 degrees, or in the opposite direction, of the incident photon

backup-time a safety feature that limits the maximum exposure possible when using automatic exposure devices

base the material that provides structural support for the functional layers (photographic emulsion, fluorescent layer or phosphor layer) of film, intensifying screens, or photo-stimulable phosphor plate

beam-restricting device a device that controls the size and shape of the primary beam

becquerel (Bq) the SI equivalent to the curie; quantifies that amount of radioactive material in which one atom disintegrates every second

body section radiography a technique utilizing geometric principles to produce an image where the objects in a selected plane remain well-defined on the radiograph while those above and below that plane are blurred

bremsstrahlung radiation x-radiation produced when a high-speed electron passes near the nucleus of an atom and is deflected and decelerated

brightness gain the increase of image brightness produced by an image intensifier; the product of flux gain and minification gain

Bucky factor also referred to as grid factor; the increase in exposure necessary to compensate for the loss of primary and secondary radiation reaching the film as a result of the use of a grid

cathode the negatively charged electrode in the x-ray tube that serves as the source of electrons

characteristic curve the plotting of the relationship between measurements of exposure and density on radiographic film

characteristic radiation radiation of a characteristic energy that occurs when an incident electron ejects an orbital electron from an inner shell of an atom in the bombarded material

cinefluorography the recording of a fluoroscopic image with a motion picture or cine camera

classical scattering also referred to as unmodified, coherent, Rayleigh, or Thompson scattering; the interaction of an incident photon with an entire atom where the photon's energy is momentarily given to the atom, which then releases the energy as a photon of the same energy in an altered direction

collimator a device to control the size and shape of the primary beam; usually constructed of adjustable lead vanes, it can produce rectangular or square fields of adjustable size

compensating filter a filter that is used to compensate for radiographic density differences caused by differing body thickness or density

Compton effect also referred to as Compton scattering; the interaction of an incident photon with an outer-shell electron which is ejected from orbit resulting in ionization of the atom; the incident photon continues on with lowered energy in an altered direction

computed radiography (CR) also referred to as digital radiography; a relatively recent introduction that allows the direct acquisition of images in a digital format

contrast improvement factor (K) the measurement of a grid's ability to improve contrast

copy film also referred to as duplicating film; film made for the duplication of radiographs

coulomb the unit of electric charge

coulomb per kilogram (C/kg) the SI equivalent to the roentgen; the electric charge per unit mass of air

crosshatch grid also referred to as crossed grid; two linear grids with their grid lines perpendicular to each other

cumulative MPD (maximum permissible dose) the maximum cumulative radiation exposure for an occupational worker based on age and whole-body exposure; prior to 1987 $5(N - 18) = MPD_c$, after 1987 $1 \times N = MPD_c$

curie (Ci) a unit of radioactivity; quantifies the amount of radioactive material and not the radiation emitted

current electricity the flow of electrons along a conductor

cylinder cone an aperture diaphragm with a cylindrical extension that restricts the beam at the distal end

definition also referred to as resolution; describes the sharpness with which detail is recorded on the film

densitometer an instrument that reads density numerically by comparing the incident light to the transmitted light

density the black metallic silver deposit on film; the ratio of the logarithm of the incident light striking the radiograph to the logarithm of the light transmitted through the film

developing the step in photographic processing during which the reduction of exposed silver halide crystals to metallic silver occurs

diagnostic radiograph a radiograph with sufficient density, sharply defined detail, appropriate contrast levels, proper positioning and centering, and appropriate identification and labeling

differential absorption the difference between those photons absorbed photoelectrically and those not absorbed at all

digital refers to the presentation of information in discrete units as opposed to the continuous analog format

digital radiography see computed radiography

direct exposure film film intended for exposure with x-rays and not light from intensifying screens

distortion the misrepresentation of the true shape of an object in the radiographic image

double-emulsion film film with emulsion on both sides of the base

drying the step in film processing which removes water from the emulsion

duplicating film also referred to as copy film; film made for the duplication of radiographs

dynabrake a device that slows the rotating anode after exposure

electromagnetic radiation the movement of electric and magnetic fields through space at the speed of light

electromagnetic spectrum the ranking of electromagnetic radiation in order of wavelength, frequency, and energy

electron a negatively charged particle that revolves around the nucleus of an atom in well-defined orbits

electrostatic focusing lenses a series of metal rings plated around the inside walls of an image intensifier that serve to focus the photoelectrons on the output phosphor

emulsion the light-sensitive layer of photographic film that is made of gelatin and contains the silver halide crystals

energy the capacity for performing work

exposure a term used in radiography to denote the radiation used to expose the film; also the amount of radiation absorbed by the patient during a radiographic examination

exposure amplitude the measure in degrees of the angle the x-ray tube and supporting rod form with the fulcrum, during the time of x-ray exposure, when performing a tomogram

exposure angle the measure in degrees of the angle the x-ray tube and supporting rod form with the fulcrum, during the time of x-ray exposure, when performing a tomogram

exposure arc the measure in degrees of the angle the x-ray tube and supporting rod form with the fulcrum, during the time of x-ray exposure, when performing a tomogram

exposure latitude the range between the minimum and maximum exposure that will produce an acceptable density on the radiograph

film badges radiation exposure monitoring devices which utilize a photographic film strip to measure personnel radiation dose

film speed the sensitivity of film to exposure

filtration the absorption of low energy photons by materials in the path of the x-ray beam

fixing the step in photographic processing that removes undeveloped silver halide from the film emulsion

flare cone an aperture diaphragm with a conical extension that appears to match the divergence of the beam

fluorescent intensifying screen a screen that produces light when exposed to radiation, which in turn exposes radiographic film

fluoroscopy a dynamic imaging technique in which motion is evident

flux gain the acceleration of the electrons from the input to the output phosphor of an image intensifier which results in approximately a 50-fold increase in light output

focal distance also referred to as grid radius or grid focus; the distance from the target of an x-ray tube to the grid

focal range the range of distance through which a focused grid can be used without objectionable grid cutoff

focusing cup a metal cup that surrounds and houses the filament and is negatively charged; its purpose is to condense or focus the electrons produced by thermionic emission

fog the density on film that is not a result of radiation carrying the desired image

fulcrum (tomographic fulcrum) the device which is the point upon which the rigid metal rod supporting the film and x-ray tube rotates; it is also the level of the plane of focus of a tomographic unit

full-wave rectification the conversion of alternating current to pulsed direct current through the use of valve tubes or rectifiers

gelatin a component of film emulsion

general radiation x-radiation produced when a high speed electron passes near the nucleus of an atom and is deflected and decelerated

glass envelope the glass enclosure of an x-ray tube that provides structural support for the components and maintains the vacuum necessary for operation

Gray (Gy) the SI equivalent to the rad

grid cutoff the undesirable attenuation of the primary beam caused by improper alignment of a radiographic grid

grid factor also referred to as Bucky factor; the increase in exposure necessary to compensate for the loss of primary and secondary radiation reaching the film

grid frequency the number of lead strips per inch or per centimeter

grid lines the image of the lead strips projected on a radiograph

grid radius also referred to as focal distance or focal range; the distance at which a focused grid can be used without producing grid cutoff

grid ratio the ratio of the height of the lead strips to the distance between the lead strips

grid selectivity (Σ) the ratio of the amount of primary radiation transmitted through a grid to the amount of scatter radiation transmitted through a grid

half-value layer (HVL) the amount of absorber placed in a beam of radiation that will reduce its intensity by one half

half-wave rectification the conversion of alternating current to pulsed direct current by elimination of the negative portion of the electrical cycle

heat unit the unit of measure of the heat produced in an x-ray tube during the production of x-rays; kVp × mAs × time for single-phase and kVp × mAs × time × 1.35 for three-phase equipment

heel effect the uneven distribution of x-rays produced from the anode to cathode end of the tube; a decrease in x-ray intensity at the anode end of the x-ray tube

high contrast also short scale contrast; a small range of widely different densities; a product of low-kVp techniques

image intensifier an electronic device that receives an x-ray image, converts it to a light image, and substantially increases the light intensity of the image as compared to conventional fluoroscopic screens

image orthicon a type of television tube used in recording image-intensified fluoroscopy

inertia the resistance a body offers to any change in position

inherent filtration the removal of low energy photons from the primary beam by materials used in the construction of the x-ray tube and collimator

input phosphor a fluorescent screen composed of zinc cadmium sulfide or cesium iodide that converts the x-ray image to a light image in the image intensifier

intensification factor the ratio of the exposure needed to produce a density on a film using screens compared to the exposure required to produce the density without screens

intensifying screens a fluorescent screen used to convert x-rays to light and reduce the amount of radiation necessary to expose the radiographic film

intrinsic efficiency the ability of a given phosphor to convert x-ray photons into light photons

inverse square law a physical principle that states the number of x-ray photons per unit area is inversely proportional to the square of the distance from the source

ionization the addition or subtraction of an electron from an atom caused by bombarding matter with x-radiation or electrons

ionization chamber also referred to as an R-meter; a device used to measure the output of radiographic and fluoroscopic units

ionomat an automatic exposure device that measures the amount of radiation reaching the film

isotope an atom of an element that has the same atomic number but more or fewer neutrons

kilovolt (kV) 1000 volts

kilovoltage a technical factor controlling the quality of radiation produced by a radiographic or fluoroscopic unit

kilowatt (kW) 1,000 watts

kinetic energy energy which is the result of a body being in motion

latent image the invisible deposition of metallic silver on photographic film

linear energy transfer (LET) the rate at which energy is deposited in the tissue

linear tomography the simplest motion in tomography, so named because the tube moves in a straight line if viewed from above

line voltage compensator a device that senses changes in incoming voltage and allows for either automatic or manual adjustment for the changes

long scale contrast also referred to as low contrast; a product of high-kVp techniques; a long range of densities with many grays

magnet a substance with the power to attract ferromagnetic substances

magnetic flux the composite of the magnetic lines of force around a magnet

manifest image the visible image on radiographic film produced by processing

matter anything that has mass and occupies space; possesses the property of inertia

maximum permissible dose (MPD) the maximum radiation exposure allowable for an occupational worker for a given body part per unit of time

milliampere (mA) 1/1,000 of an ampere

milliampere-second (mAs) the product of milliamperage and time; a technical unit to determine the quantity of radiation produced during a radiographic exposure

minification gain the increase in brightness produced by an image intensifier resulting from the reduction in image size from the input phosphor to the output phosphor producing more light photons per unit area

mirror optics a series of lenses and mirrors that magnify and reflect the image from the output phosphor of an image intensifier to the viewer

molecule the smallest part of a substance that retains all the characteristics of the original substance

moving grid also referred to as a Bucky device or a Potter-Bucky diaphragm; an electromechanical device that moves the grid during exposure, blurring grid lines from the radiographic image

neutron a particle contained within the nucleus of an atom having no charge

nonphototiming cassettes cassettes with lead-lined steel backs that prevent backscatter radiation from affecting the film

nucleus the central body of an atom, containing protons and neutrons

off-focus radiation also referred to as stem radiation; radiation produced in the x-ray tube when electrons interact with matter other than the target

ohm (Ω) the amount of resistance that permits 1 ampere of current to flow under the pressure of 1 volt in a circuit

output-phosphor the exit end of an image intensifier; a small fluorescent screen composed of a thin layer of very small particles of zinc cadmium sulfide which convert electrons to light

PACS an acronym for picture archiving and communication system

pair production the interaction of a high-energy (1.02 keV minimum) photon with the nucleus of an atom. The photon disappears, and its energy undergoes conversion into matter, resulting in two particles: an electron and a positron

pantomography a tomographic technique which produces a panoramic view of curved structures of the body

parallax the phenomenon resulting from light entering the film emulsion on an angle, passing through the base, and affecting the emulsion on the opposite side of the film in a slightly different area; parallax results in loss of resolution

parasite shadows streak-like, artifactual images produced during linear tomography by incomplete blurring of objects in line with the tube travel

penumbra geometric unsharpness at the edges of the image of an object

phosphor layer the functional layer of an intensifying screen; composed of a plastic substance that contains the phosphor crystals

phosphorescence also referred to as afterglow; the tendency of a phosphor to continue to give off light after the x-ray exposure has stopped

photocathode a component of the image intensifier composed of compounds of cesium and antimony, which convert the light produced by the input phosphor to electrons

photodisintegration a high-energy photon interaction, involving the nucleus of an atom, ejecting part of the nucleus

photoelectric effect the interaction of an incident electron with an inner shell electron of an atom ejecting it from orbit; an outer shell electron moves in to fill in the void and produces a photon of characteristic radiation

photoemissive layer the photocathode of the image intensifier

photographic effect a concept that states the quantity and quality of radiation have a predictable effect on film

photomultiplier tube electronic device that measures light and is sometimes used in automatic exposure devices

photopic vision vision at higher-light levels; the vision where detail resolution is most acute

photostimulable phosphor plate the reusable image receptor plate that stores the x-ray image in a computed radiography system

phototimer automatic exposure device that measures the amount of radiation reaching the film and terminates the exposure

phototiming cassette a cassette that allows radiation to pass through its back to strike the phototimer; a cassette for use with automatic exposure devices

picture archiving and communication system (PACS) a computerized system that stores images and patient information for display and archiving

plumbicon a type of television tube used in recording image-intensified fluoroscopy, with the advantage of better contrast and less image lag

pocket ionization chambers also termed small pocket dosimeters, are radiation exposure monitoring devices which utilize an ionization chamber to measure personnel radiation dose

positive beam limitation (PBL) a motorized collimation system that automatically collimates to the size of the image receptor

positron a positively charged particle with the same mass as an electron

potential energy the energy inherent in a body at rest

protective layer the outermost layer of an intensifying screen that protects the fluorescent layer from damage

proton a particle contained within the nucleus of an atom, having a positive electric charge

rad the unit of radiation absorbed dose received by human beings or animals

radiographic contrast the comparison of two or more radiographic densities on a x-ray film

radiographic density the black metallic silver deposited in the emulsion of x-ray film after exposure to light and processing

radiographic grid a device that reduces the amount of secondary or scatter radiation reaching the film

radiographic rating chart a chart that shows the maximum safe single exposure that can be used for a particular x-ray tube

rare earth phosphor a phosphor that converts x-rays to light approximately four times more efficiently than calcium tungstate

rectification a process that prevents the flow of electrons from the anode to the cathode

rectifier a diode that permits the flow of electrons only in one direction

reflective layer a layer in many intensifying screens composed of a white reflective substance that reflects light, generated away from the film, back toward the film

relative biological effect (RBE) the ability of radiation to produce a biological effect

relative speed a comparison of the speed of one screen-film combination to the speed of another screen-film combination

relative unit the measurement in which one exposure is the basis for comparison of all others

rem the radiation equivalent man; quantifies radiation dose for humans

resistance the hindrance to the flow of electricity encountered in a conductor; measured in ohms (Ω)

resolution also referred to as definition; term used to describe the sharpness with which detail is recorded on the film

R-meter a device used to measure the output of radiographic and fluoroscopic units

roentgen (R) the unit of radiation exposure or intensity; quantifies radiation output or exposure

scotopic vision vision at low-light level; the vision with poorest detail acuity

screen efficiency the ability of light emitted by the phosphor of an intensifying screen to escape the screen and interact with the film

self-rectification the property of the x-ray tube which prevents the flow of electrons from the anode to the cathode and can be used to rectify alternating current to pulsed direct current

sensitivity speck silver sulfide that forms on the surface of a silver halide crystal in film emulsion providing the location for the development of the latent image

sensitometer a device that uses light to make a measured exposure on film

sensitometry the study of the response of film to changes in exposure and processing

short scale contrast also referred to as high contrast; a small range of widely different densities; a product of low-kVp techniques

shoulder that part of a sensitometric curve that represents the area where the film is reaching its maximum exposure

sievert (Sv) the SI equivalent to the rem

silver halide the component of x-ray film emulsion that is sensitive to light or radiation; breaks down into metallic silver on development

single emulsion film film with emulsion on only one side of the base

single phase power an electrical current with 60 cycles per second, and each cycle consists of a positive and negative pulse

space charge liberated electrons that form an electron "cloud" surrounding the filament of an x-ray tube

spinning top a simple test tool that can be used to evaluate the accuracy of the timer of a single phase x-ray unit

static electricity a quantity of electricity in which the electric charge is at rest

stem radiation also referred to as off-focus radiation; radiation produced in the x-ray tube when electrons interact with matter other than the target

step-down transformer a transformer used to decrease voltage

step-up transformer a transformer used to increase voltage

stereopsis man's ability to see two slightly different images, one with each eye, that are converted by the brain into a single picture that has depth

stereoscope a collective term used for a variety of devices used to view stereoscopic radiographs

stereoscopic radiography the technique of taking two slightly discrepant radiographs and viewing them in a manner that fuses them into a single image with depth

stereoscopy a synonym for stereoscopic radiography

straight-line portion that part of the sensitometric curve that represents the area of film response where increases in exposure produce corresponding increases in density on the film

subject contrast the difference in density between two parts of an object or patient

subtraction mask film film used to produce the exact reverse of the scout film when producing subtractions of angiographic films

subtraction print film film used to produce the final print of the angiographic contrast film and superimposed mask film when producing subtractions of angiographic films

synchronous timer a slotted disc that rotates at a fixed rate (often 1 revolution per second) and is used for evaluation of the accuracy of either single-phase or three-phase timers of radiographic units

tabular-grain film film with tabular or flat silver halide crystals

thermionic emission the process by which the electrons are liberated or "boiled off" the filament of an x-ray tube

thermoluminescent dosimeters radiation exposure monitoring devices which use an energy storing crystal, lithium fluoride, to measure personnel radiation dose

three-phase power a type of electric current consisting of three single-phase waveforms that are superimposed 120 degrees out of phase from one another

toe that part of the sensitometric curve that represents the area of exposure that is below the film's ability to respond

tomographic amplitude the measure in degrees of the angle the x-ray tube and supporting rod form with the fulcrum during tomography

tomographic angle the measure in degrees of the angle the x-ray tube and supporting rod form with the fulcrum during tomography

tomographic arc the measure in degrees of the angle the x-ray tube and supporting rod form with the fulcrum during tomography

tomography an accepted widely used term synonym for body section radiography

total filtration the sum of inherent and added filtration

transformer two coils of wire, insulated from one another and wrapped around a single iron core whose purpose is to change voltage from one level to another

trough filter a compensating filter with a depression or trough in its center; often used for radiography of the spine and chest

valve tube a diode that permits the flow of electrons in only one direction

vidicon the least expensive and most widely used television camera for recording image-intensified fluoroscopy

vignetting a "fall off" in brightness at the periphery of the image intensified image usually seen with mirror optic systems

volt (V) the electrical pressure or force that causes electrons to move

washing the step in film processing where the fixer is washed from the emulsion of the film by a water rinse

watt (W) a unit of power required to cause 1 ampere of current to flow

wavelength the penetrating power of any form of radiant energy; the distance between two successive crests or troughs in the waveform

wedge filter a compensating filter that is used to compensate for differences in part thickness

whole body MPD (maximum permissible dose) the maximum allowable radiation exposure for an occupationally exposed individual (5 rem annually)

wire-mesh phantom a simple test tool used to evaluate high-contrast resolution on an image intensifier

work the force applied multiplied by the distance through which the force acts

zonography thick section tomography of 10-degree exposure amplitude or less which produces an excellent image of a particular zone

Index

f indicates figure

F

G

H

I

K

L

M

Z